AF412408

SPECIALTY IMAGING™

GENITOURINARY ONCOLOGY

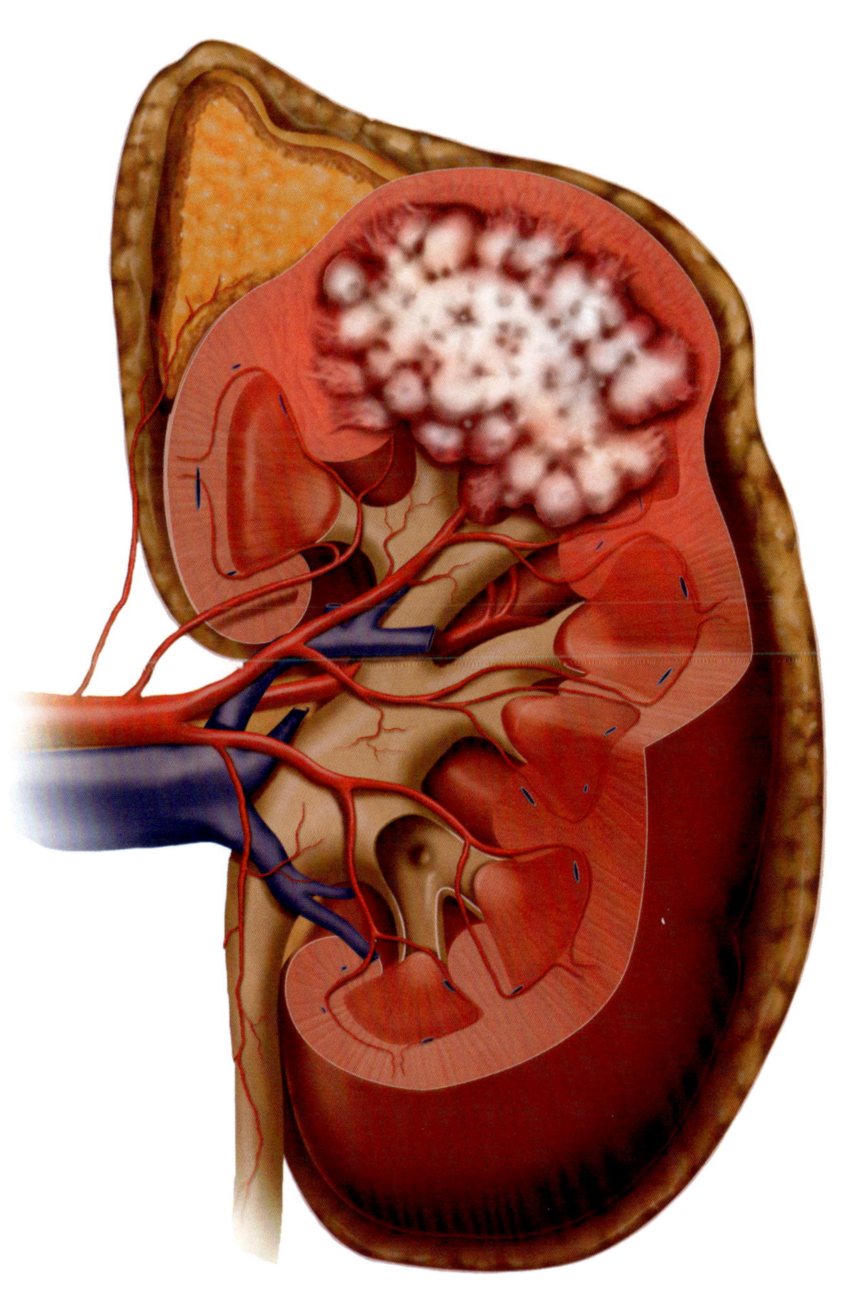

i

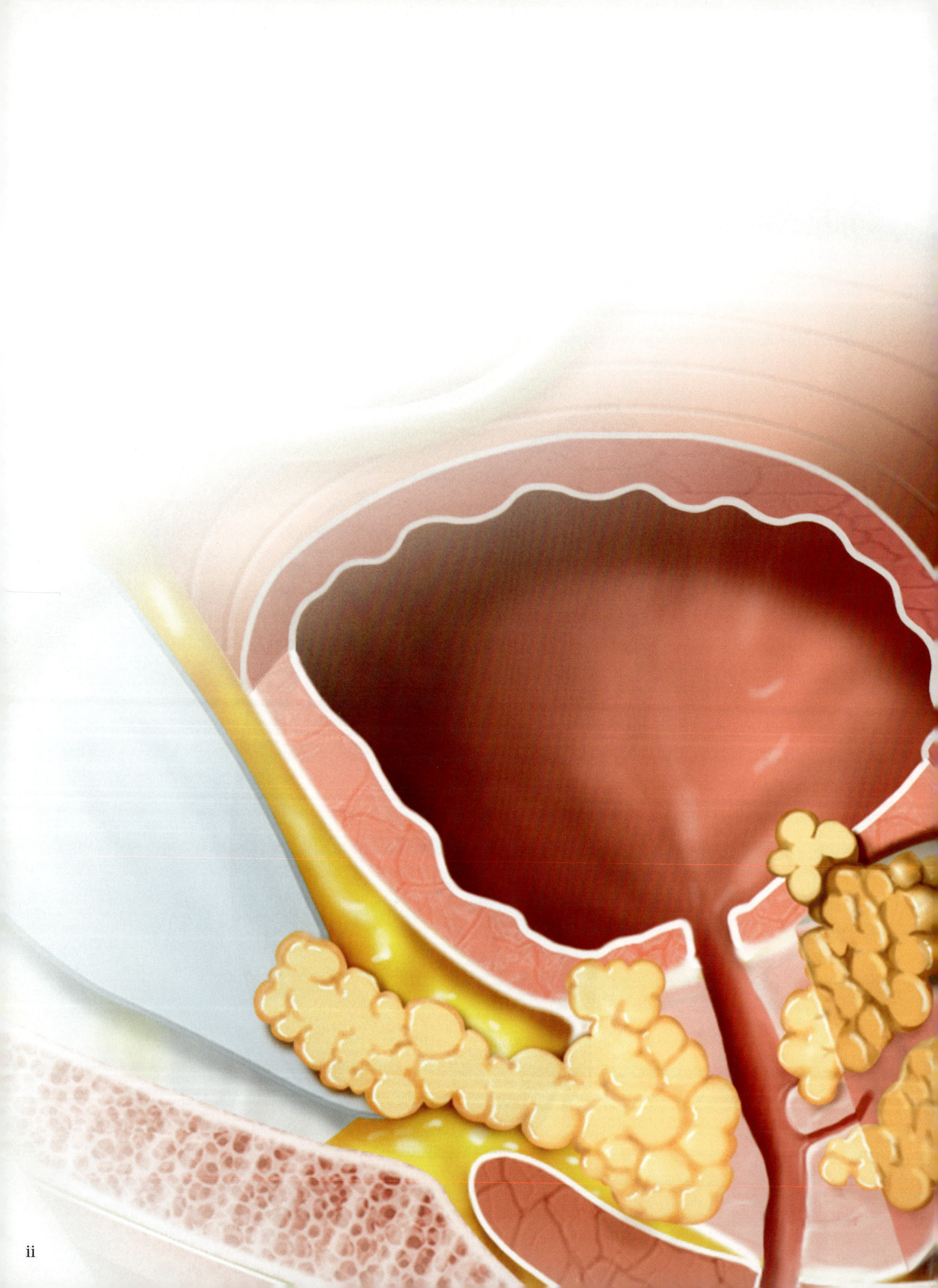

SPECIALTY IMAGING™
GENITOURINARY ONCOLOGY

Akram M. Shaaban, MBBCh

Associate Professor of Radiology
University of Utah School of Medicine
Salt Lake City, UT

Marta E. Heilbrun, MD, MS

Assistant Professor of Radiology
University of Utah School of Medicine
Salt Lake City, UT

Todd M. Blodgett, MD

Adjunct Assistant Professor
University of Pittsburgh Medical Center
President, FRG Molecular Imaging
Foundation Radiology Group
Pittsburgh, PA

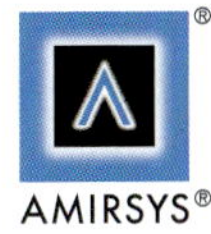

AMIRSYS®

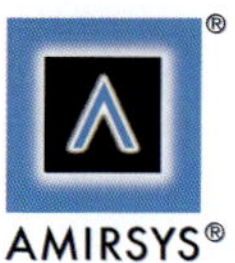

AMIRSYS®

Names you know. Content you trust.®

Notice and Disclaimer

The information in this product ("Product") is provided as a reference for use by licensed medical professionals and no others. It does not and should not be construed as any form of medical diagnosis or professional medical advice on any matter. Receipt or use of this Product, in whole or in part, does not constitute or create a doctor-patient, therapist-patient, or other healthcare professional relationship between the copyright holders and any recipient. This Product may not reflect the most current medical developments, and the copyright holders (individually and jointly), make no claims, promises, or guarantees about accuracy, completeness, or adequacy of the information contained in or linked to the Product. The Product is not a substitute for or replacement of professional medical judgment. The copyright holders, and their affiliates, authors, contributors, partners, and sponsors, individually and jointly, disclaim all liability or responsibility for any injury and/or damage to persons or property in respect to actions taken or not taken based on any and all Product information.

In the cases where drugs or other chemicals are prescribed, readers are advised to check the Product information currently provided by the manufacturer of each drug to be administered to verify the recommended dose, the method and duration of administration, and contraindications. It is the responsibility of the treating physician relying on experience and knowledge of the patient to determine dosages and the best treatment for the patient.

To the maximum extent permitted by applicable law, the copyright holders provide the Product AS IS AND WITH ALL FAULTS, AND HEREBY DISCLAIMS ALL WARRANTIES AND CONDITIONS, WHETHER EXPRESS, IMPLIED OR STATUTORY, INCLUDING BUT NOT LIMITED TO, ANY (IF ANY) IMPLIED WARRANTIES OR CONDITIONS OF MERCHANTABILITY, OF FITNESS FOR A PARTICULAR PURPOSE, OF LACK OF VIRUSES, OR ACCURACY OR COMPLETENESS OF RESPONSES, OR RESULTS, AND OF LACK OF NEGLIGENCE OR LACK OF WORKMANLIKE EFFORT. ALSO, THERE IS NO WARRANTY OR CONDITION OF TITLE, QUIET ENJOYMENT, QUIET POSSESSION, CORRESPONDENCE TO DESCRIPTION OR NON-INFRINGEMENT, WITH REGARD TO THE PRODUCT. THE ENTIRE RISK AS TO THE QUALITY OF OR ARISING OUT OF USE OR PERFORMANCE OF THE PRODUCT REMAINS WITH THE READER.

The respective copyright holders, individually and jointly, disclaim all warranties of any kind if the Product was customized, repackaged or altered in any way by any third party.

Library of Congress Cataloging-in-Publication Data

Specialty imaging. Genitourinary oncology / Akram M. Shaaban ... [et al.]. -- 1st ed.
   p. ; cm.
  Other title: Genitourinary oncology
  Includes bibliographical references and index.
  ISBN 978-1-931884-24-2 (alk. paper)
  1. Genitourinary organs--Cancer--Imaging--Handbooks, manuals, etc. I. Shaaban, Akram M. II. Title: Genitourinary oncology.
  [DNLM: 1. Urogenital Neoplasms--diagnosis. 2. Diagnostic Imaging. WJ 160 S741 2010]

RC280.G4S64 2010
616.99'46--dc22

          2010021619

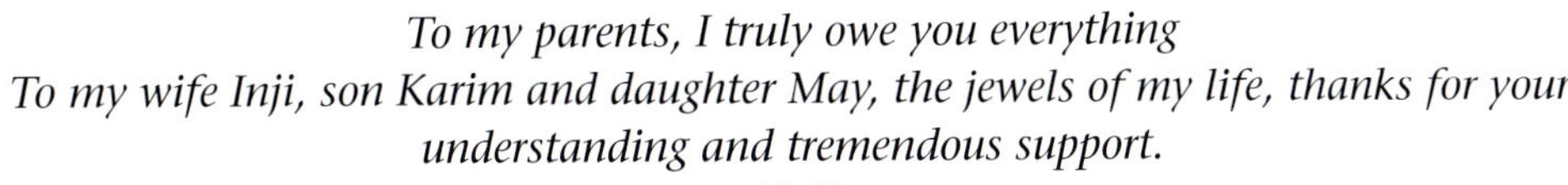

*To my parents, I truly owe you everything
To my wife Inji, son Karim and daughter May, the jewels of my life, thanks for your
understanding and tremendous support.
AMS*

*To my father, M. Peter Heilbrun, MD, an inspiration and the greatest role model for how
to be a physician, a mentor, a parent, and a spouse. Thank you for all you have shared
with me.
MEH*

*To Mary Lou Magee, a great friend, confidant, and mother,
who developed a malignant brain tumor during the creation of this book.
I love you!
TMB*

PREFACE

In *Specialty Imaging: Genitourinary Oncology*, Amirsys proudly presents the most up-to-date staging and imaging for genitourinary cancers—less than one year after the introduction of the 7th edition of the AJCC Cancer Staging Manual. This includes the brand new TNM and prognostic stage grouping for adrenal carcinoma, as well as the inclusion of Gleason score and preoperative prostate-specific antigen levels in the determination of prostate cancer staging. You'll also find the redefined TNM and prognostic stage grouping for cancers of the penis, kidney, urinary bladder, and urethra, along with thorough discussion of cancers of the testes and renal pelvis and ureter.

Each lavishly illustrated chapter offers multiple ways to make sense of a particular genitourinary cancer. Quick reference tables provide the definitions for TNM and AJCC prognostic groups. Rich drawings illuminate these stages. High-quality images of practically every stage of every tumor demonstrate clinical appearances. All of these vivid images—more than 450 in the volume—are fully annotated to maximize their illustrative potential. Bulleted text distills the pertinent information to the essentials. Whether you are looking for routes of spread, imaging techniques for local staging, or treatment options, you will find it quickly in this easy-to-use yet comprehensive reference.

Like other Amirsys books, *Specialty Imaging: Genitourinary Oncology* was designed with you, the reader, in mind. We think you'll find this new volume a handy and wonderfully rich resource that will significantly enhance your practice—and find a welcome place on your bookshelf.

Paula J. Woodward, MD
David G. Bragg, MD and Marcia R. Bragg Presidential Endowed
Chair in Oncologic Imaging
Professor of Radiology
University of Utah School of Medicine
Salt Lake City, UT

ACKNOWLEDGEMENTS

Contributing Author

David Bauer, MD
Radiology Resident
University of Utah School of Medicine
Salt Lake City, UT

Text Editing

Arthur G. Gelsinger, MA
Katherine Riser, MA
Dave L. Chance, MA

Image Editing

Jeffrey J. Marmorstone
Danny C. La

Medical Editing

Jonathan Shakespear, MD

Illustrations

Lane R. Bennion, MS
Richard Coombs, MS
Laura C. Sesto, MA

Art Direction and Design

Laura C. Sesto, MA

Associate Editor

Ashley R. Renlund, MA

Production Lead

Kellie J. Heap

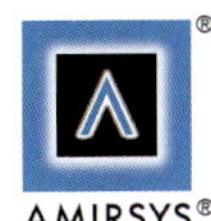

TABLE OF CONTENTS

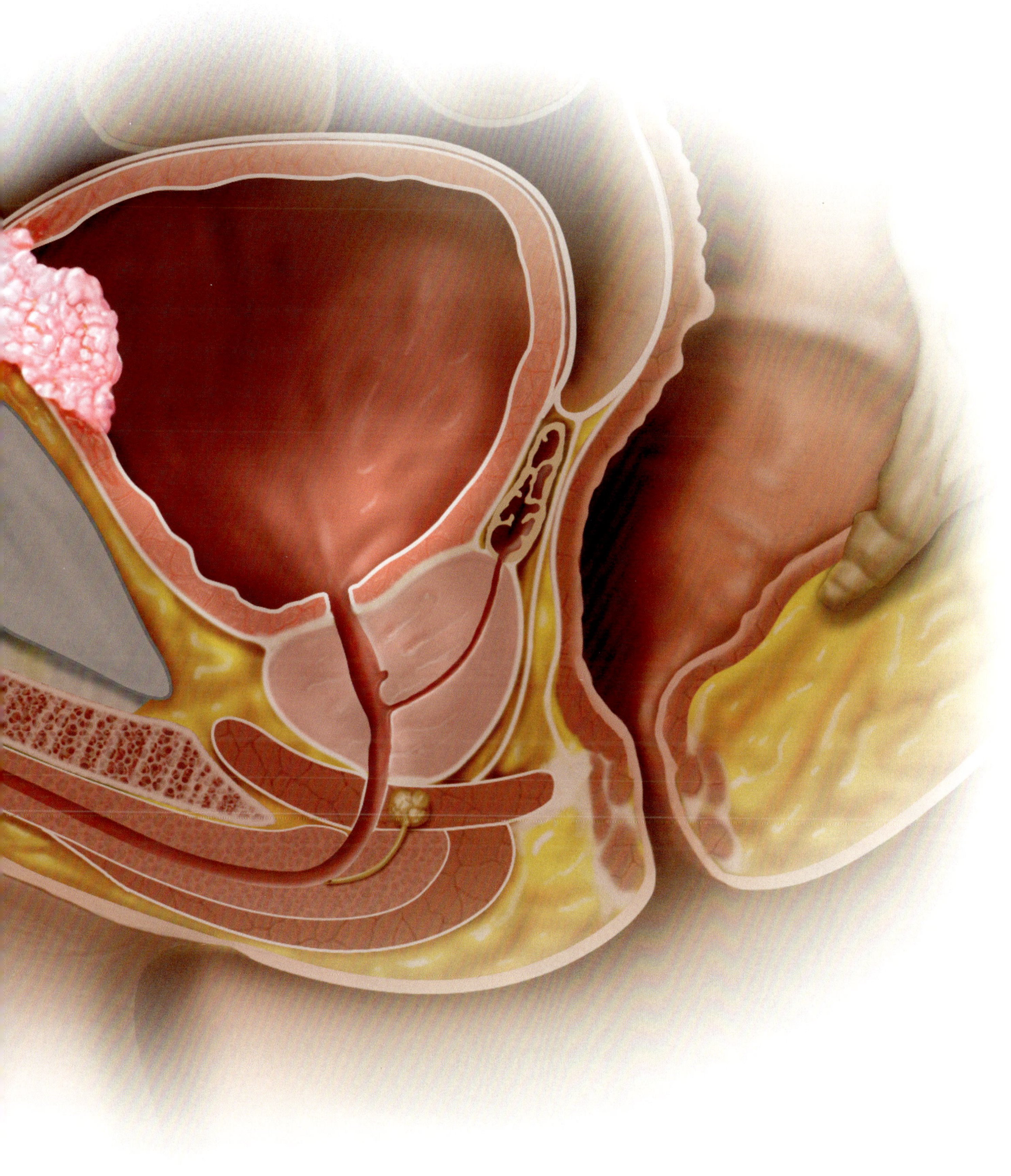

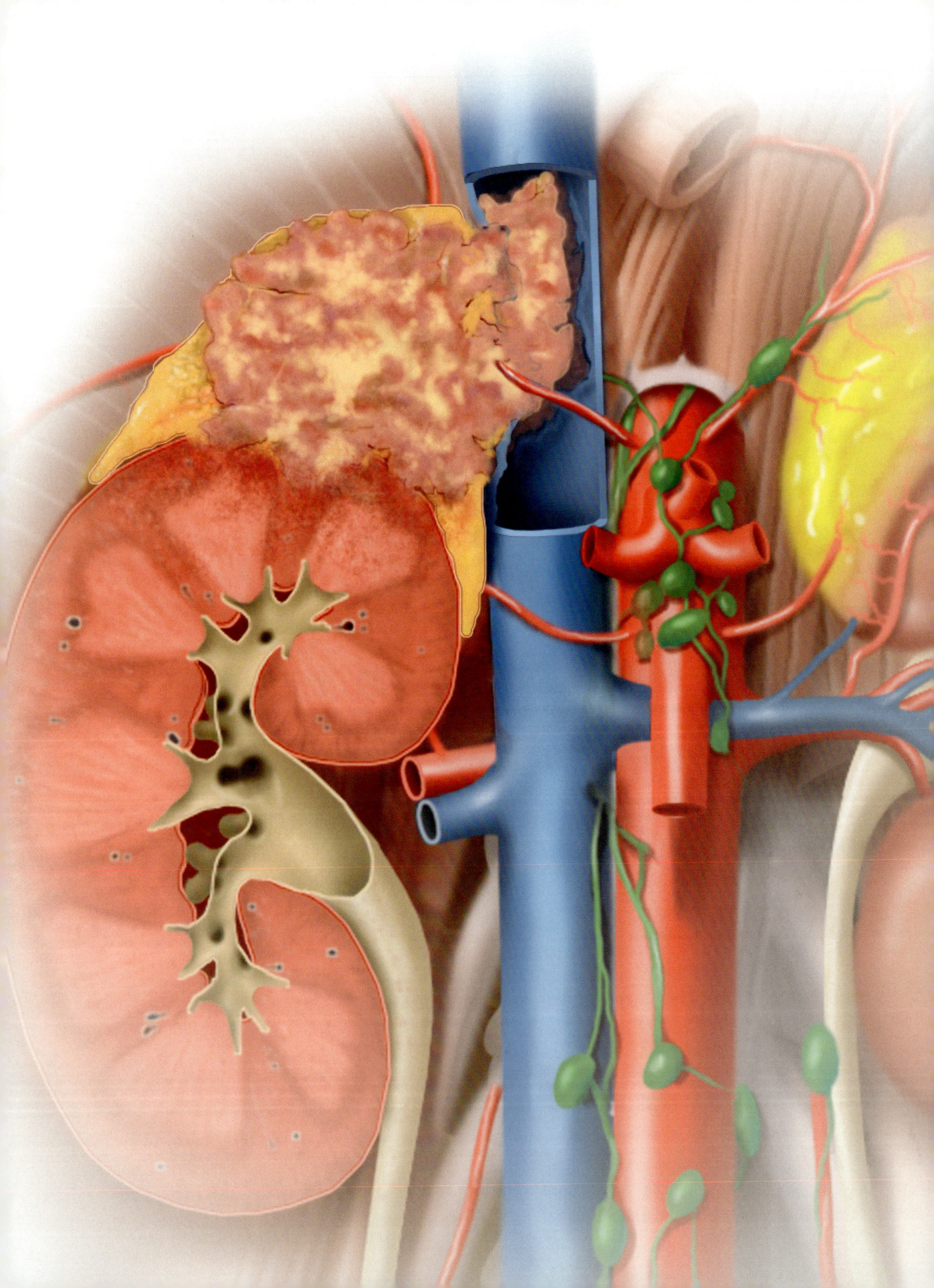

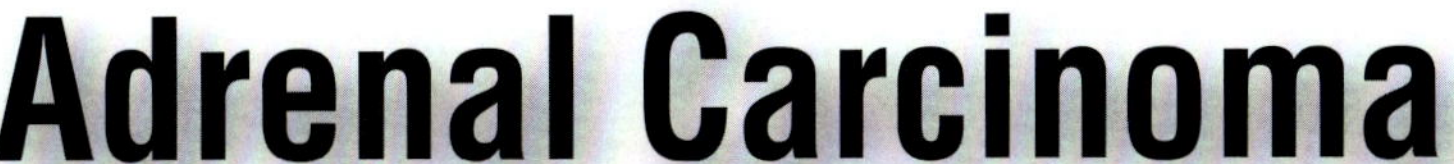

Adrenal Carcinoma

ADRENAL CARCINOMA

(T) Primary Tumor

Adapted from 7th edition AJCC Staging Forms.

TNM	Definitions
TX	Primary tumor cannot be assessed
T0	No evidence of primary tumor
T1	Tumor ≤ 5 cm in greatest dimension, no extraadrenal invasion
T2	Tumor > 5 cm, no extraadrenal invasion
T3	Tumor of any size with local invasion but not invading adjacent organs*
T4	Tumor of any size with invasion of adjacent organs*

(N) Regional Lymph Nodes

NX	Regional lymph nodes cannot be assessed
N0	No regional lymph node metastasis
N1	Metastasis in regional lymph node(s)

(M) Distant Metastasis

M0	No distant metastasis
M1	Distant metastasis

Adjacent organs include kidney, diaphragm, great vessels, pancreas, spleen, and liver.

AJCC Stages/Prognostic Groups

Adapted from 7th edition AJCC Staging Forms.

Stage	T	N	M
I	T1	N0	M0
II	T2	N0	M0
III	T1	N1	M0
	T2	N1	M0
	T3	N0	M0
IV	T3	N1	M0
	T4	N0	M0
	T4	N1	M0
	Any T	Any N	M1

ADRENAL CARCINOMA

T1

Low-power magnification of an H&E section shows sheets of adrenal cortical neoplastic cells ▷ that are limited to the adrenal gland (T1). Adipose tissue ▷ surrounding the adrenal gland is negative for tumor. (Original magnification 40x.)

T2

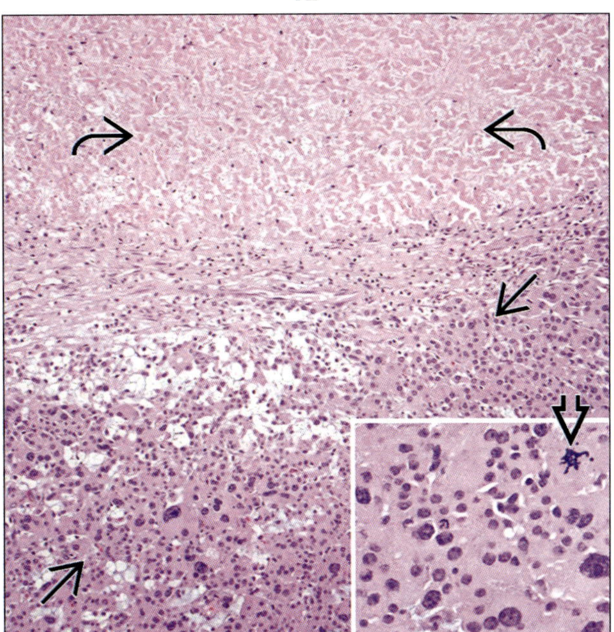

Photomicrograph shows an H&E section from adrenal cortical carcinoma ▷ with large areas of necrosis in the upper aspect of the slide ▷. The inset shows the particularly striking nuclear pleomorphism (large vs. small nuclei) as well as a mitotic figure ▷. (Original magnification 400x.)

T3

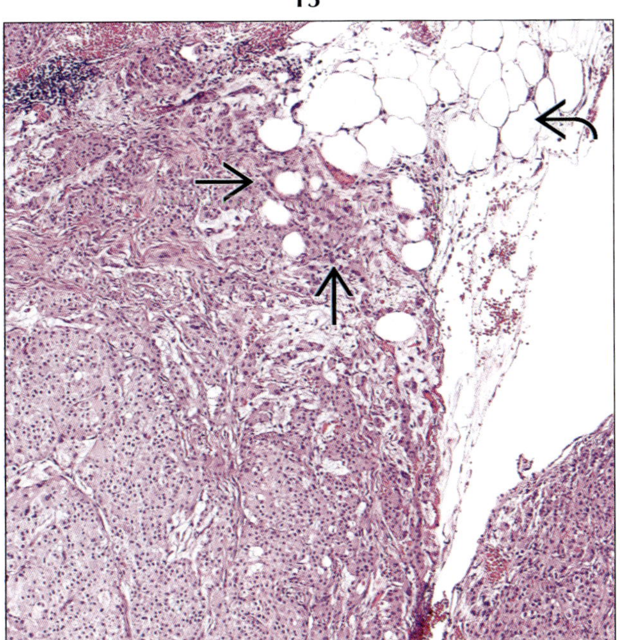

H&E stain shows tumor with local invasion but no extension into adjacent organs, consistent with T3 disease. The adrenal cortical carcinoma invades ▷ locally into the surrounding adrenal fat ▷. (Original magnification 100x.)

T4

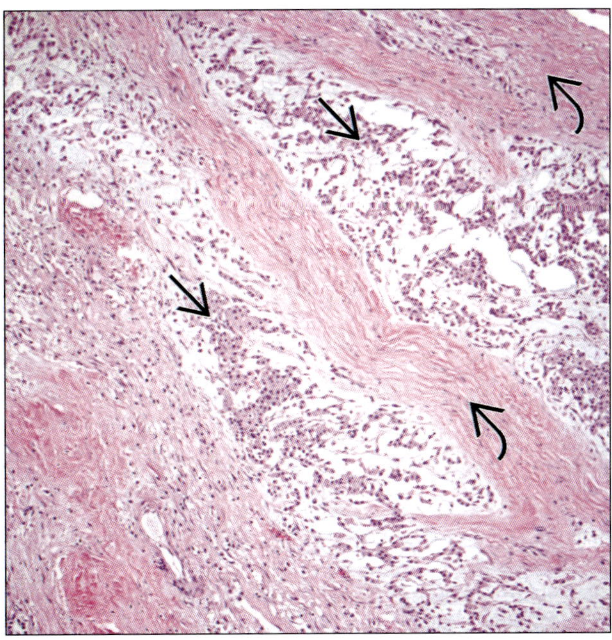

In T4 disease, tumor invades into adjacent organs. This tumor extends to involve the diaphragm. This photomicrograph shows the neoplastic tumor cells ▷ extending into surrounding fibrotic connective tissue ▷. (Original magnification 400x.)

ADRENAL CARCINOMA

T1

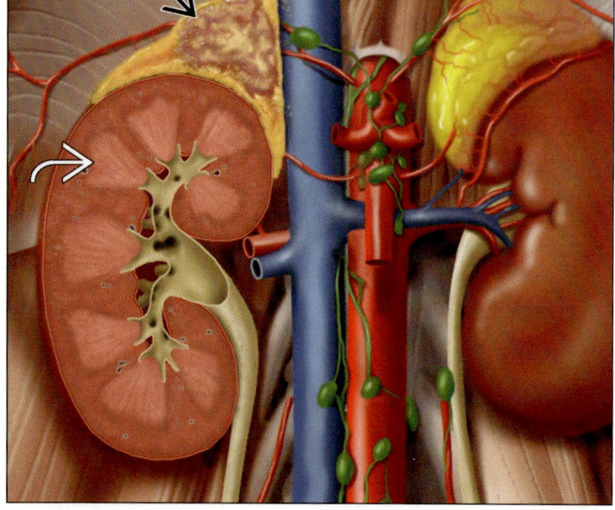

Coronal graphic demonstrates T1 disease. The primary tumor ⊡ is ≤ 5 cm in greatest dimension, without invasion of adjacent organs, including kidney ⊡ or inferior vena cava ⊡.

T2

Coronal graphic demonstrates T2 disease. The primary tumor ⊡ is > 5 cm in greatest dimension, without invasion of adjacent organs, including kidney ⊡ or inferior vena cava ⊡.

T3

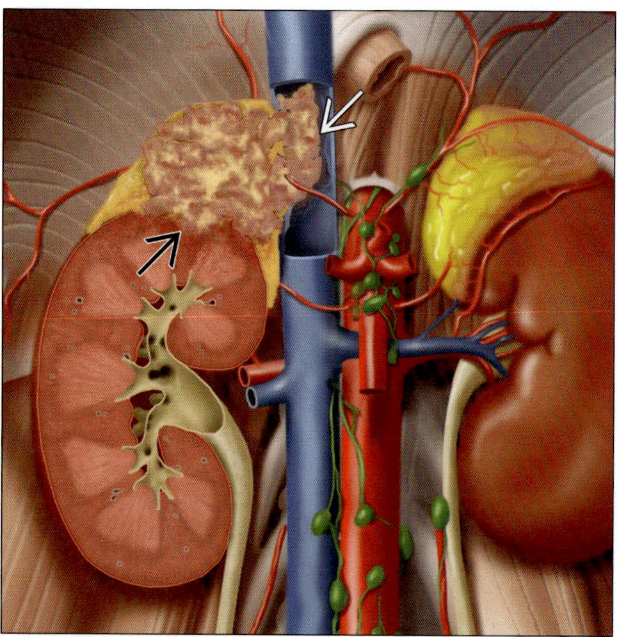

Coronal graphic demonstrates T3 disease. The primary tumor may be any size, with local invasion beyond the confines of the adrenal capsule, shown in the superolateral margin ⊡, but no involvement of adjacent organs such as the kidney ⊡.

T4

Coronal graphic demonstrates T4 disease. The primary tumor can be any size, with local invasion beyond the confines of the adrenal capsule and into adjacent organs, including the kidney ⊡. Direct extension into the inferior vena cava is illustrated ⊡.

T4

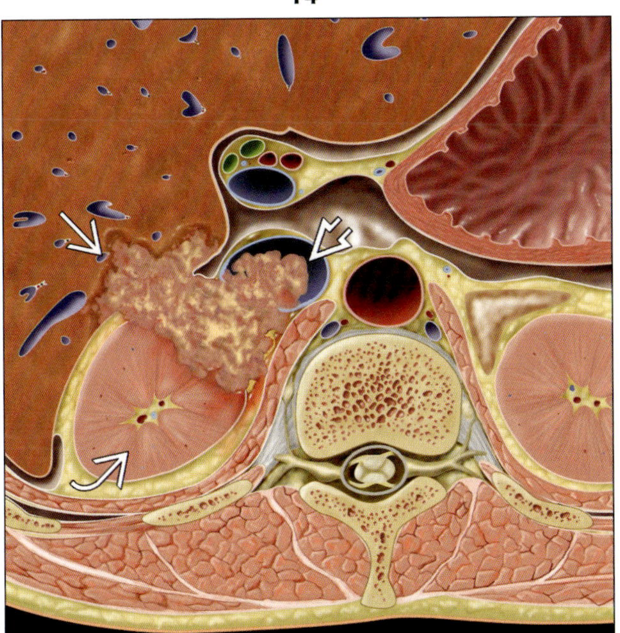

Axial graphic demonstrates right-sided adrenal cortical carcinoma, invading adjacent organs, including the right kidney ➔, the liver ➔, and the inferior vena cava ➔.

N1 and M1

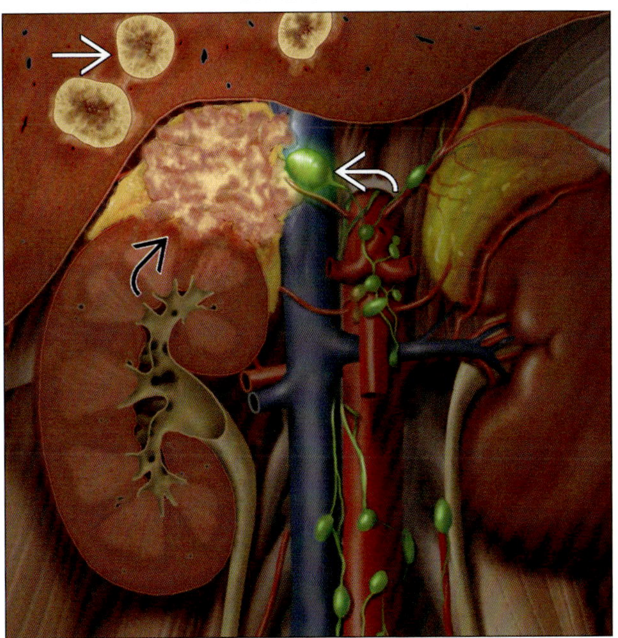

Coronal graphic shows primary adrenal cortical carcinoma with invasion into adjacent kidney ➔. N1 and M1 disease with an enlarged paraaortic lymph node ➔ and multifocal hepatic metastases ➔ are also illustrated.

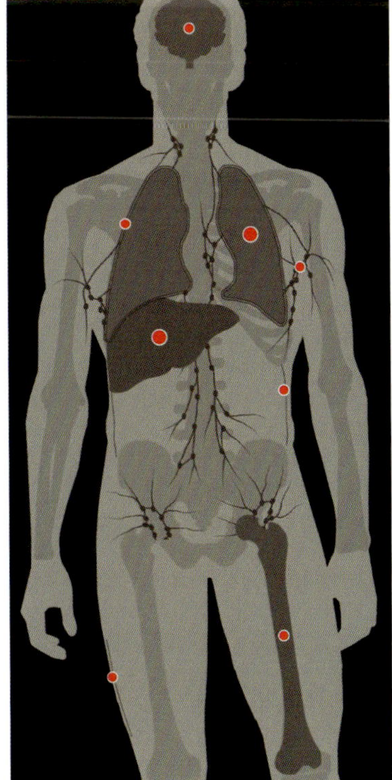

METASTASES, ORGAN FREQUENCY

Liver	11%
Lung	9%
Bone	3%
Distant lymph nodes	2%
Peritoneum	1%
CNS	< 1%
Pleura	< 1%
Skin	< 1%

Data from Bilimoria KY et al: Adrenocortical carcinoma in the United States: treatment utilization and prognostic factors. Cancer. 113(11):3130-6, 2008.

ADRENAL CARCINOMA

OVERVIEW

General Comments
- AJCC staging system applies only to adrenal cortical carcinoma (ACC)
  - Adrenal medullary tumors such as pheochromocytoma and neuroblastoma are not included in this staging system

Classification
- Histological classification
  - Differentiated are usually functioning tumors
  - Anaplastic are rarely hormone producing
- Hormonal: ~ 60% hormone producing
  - Clinical syndromes with functioning tumors
    - Hypercortisolism: Cushing syndrome (30-40%, most common)
    - Adrenogenital syndrome
    - Virilization in females
    - Feminization in males
    - Precocious puberty
    - Hyperaldosteronism
    - Primary hyperaldosteronism: Conn syndrome

PATHOLOGY

Routes of Spread
- Local invasion
  - Only 30% confined to adrenal gland at presentation
    - Almost 20% present with IVC involvement
  - Common to spread via extracapsular infiltration locally into adjacent organs, including
    - Kidney
    - Diaphragm
    - Great vessels
      - Commonly extends into IVC
      - May occlude adjacent vessels
    - Pancreas
    - Spleen
    - Liver
    - Bone
- Lymphatic metastases
  - Regional lymph nodes are
    - Paraaortic and periaortic nodes
    - Other retroperitoneal nodes
- Hematogenous metastases
  - > 30% present with metastases, commonly to
    - Liver
    - Lung

General Features
- Comments
  - Large, solid, unilateral suprarenal mass
    - < 10% present bilaterally
      - Metastases may be bilateral in up to 50%
  - Poorly defined or invasive margins
  - Very heterogeneous lesions
    - Usually contain hemorrhagic, cystic, and calcific areas
  - Functioning tumors
    - Usually ≤ 5 cm at presentation
  - Nonfunctioning tumors
    - May be ≥ 10 cm at presentation

- Benign lesions and metastases much more common than primary adrenal cortical carcinoma
- Genetics
  - ↑ incidence of tumor in genetic syndromes
    - Beckwith-Wiedemann syndrome
      - ↑ secretion of insulin-like growth factor 2 (IGF-2) → hemihypertrophy, diabetes mellitus, and adrenocortical tumors in children
    - Li-Fraumeni syndrome
      - Rare neoplasia syndrome caused by mutations of tumor suppressor gene *p53* that predispose patients to tumors of several organs (brain, breast, adrenal, etc.)
    - Carney complex
    - Multiple endocrine neoplasia 1 (MEN1) syndrome
      - ACC occurs in 25-40% of patients
- Etiology
  - Unknown for sporadic adrenal carcinoma
- Epidemiology & cancer incidence
  - Rare tumor
    - Affects 1-2 persons/1,000,000 population
  - Responsible for only 0.2% of annual cancer deaths in USA
  - M:F ratio approximately 1:1
  - Median age at diagnosis: 44 years; range: 30-70 years
    - Bimodal occurrence
      - 1st peak in 1st decade of life
      - 2nd peak in 4th-5th decades of life
- Associated diseases, abnormalities
  - Clinical presentation related to hyperfunctioning tumors

Gross Pathology & Surgical Features
- Usually large & predominately yellow on cut surface
- Necrotic, hemorrhagic, calcific, lipoid, & cystic areas

Microscopic Pathology
- H&E
  - No absolute histologic criteria for malignancy
    - Documented distant metastases &/or local invasion required for definitive diagnosis
  - Weiss histopathologic system is most commonly used; ≥ 3 of the 9 criteria predict malignant clinical behavior
    - Nuclear grade III or IV, based on Fuhrman criteria
    - Mitotic rate > 5 per 50 high-power fields (HPF)
    - Atypical mitotic figures
    - ≥ 25% clear cells
    - > 1/3 diffuse architecture
    - Necrosis
    - Venous invasion
    - Sinusoid invasion
    - Invasion of tumor capsule
- Special stains
  - MIB-1: Cell cycle-associated marker
  - Ki-67 LI > 5%

IMAGING FINDINGS

Detection
- CT
  - Study of choice to differentiate benign from malignant adrenal mass
  - Solid > 5 cm adrenal mass

- If < 5 cm, ACC is usually functioning
- < 3 cm lesions are probably benign, if no history of primary malignancy
  - Irregular margins
  - ± necrosis and calcification
    - Calcification seen in up to 30%
    - Variable enhancement due to necrosis & hemorrhage
  - Usually unilateral, may be bilateral
  - On NECT mean attenuation of adrenal carcinoma tends to be > mean attenuation of adenoma
    - Some overlap in attenuation between carcinoma and adenoma on NECT and 60-sec CECT
  - 10 minute delayed CECT
    - Significantly less washout of adrenal carcinomas than that seen in adenomas
      - Typically < 40% washout in carcinomas compared to > 50% washout for adenomas
- **MR**
  - T1WI: Hypointense adrenal mass compared to liver
    - T1 (in phase and out of phase [OOP]): No significant loss of signal on OOP imaging to suggest adrenal adenoma
      - Pitfall: ACC may contain foci of intracytoplasmic lipid
      - Loss of signal may be seen in small portions of mass
    - Hemorrhagic byproducts may produce ↑ T1 SI
  - T2WI: Hyperintense heterogeneous adrenal mass compared to liver
    - Necrosis may contribute to ↑ T2 SI
  - T1 C+: Heterogeneous enhancement due to variable necrosis
    - Multiplanar imaging shows vascular invasion into renal vein, IVC, and adjacent solid organs such as kidney
    - Coronal imaging very good for showing IVC invasion
- **Ultrasound**
  - Best imaging tool for initial screening
  - Grayscale ultrasound
    - Small tumors: Echopattern similar to renal cortex
    - Large tumors: Mixed heterogeneous echopattern with hypoechoic/anechoic areas (due to necrosis & hemorrhage)
    - "Scar" sign: Complex, predominately echogenic pattern with radiating linear echoes
      - When seen in large adrenal mass, suggestive of adrenal carcinoma
    - Enlarged regional and periaortic lymph nodes are reliable sign of malignancy
    - Large tumor may cause compression/mass effect on upper pole and anterior surface of adjacent kidney
    - US cannot reliably differentiate between adrenal carcinoma, adrenal adenoma, & neuroblastoma
  - Color Doppler
    - Invasion or occlusion of adrenal vein, renal vein, and IVC
    - Visualization of intraluminal tumor thrombus ± vascularity
- **Nuclear medicine**
  - FDG PET
    - Increased FDG uptake in adrenal carcinoma
    - Adenoma demonstrates limited FDG uptake
    - Not useful to differentiate ACC from mets, lymphoma, or pheochromocytoma
- **Angiography**
  - Historically used to assess renal vein and IVC involvement
  - Replaced by noninvasive imaging including Doppler US, MR and CT angiography
- **Radiography**
  - May see mass effect from tumor
  - Calcifications infrequently identified

Staging

- CT
  - T stage
    - Cross-sectional diameter
    - Extracapsular tumor invasion
    - Patency of adjacent vessels
    - IVC extension
  - N stage
    - Assess local nodal size
  - M stage
    - Liver, bone, and lung lesions
  - Important to perform venous phase imaging through base of heart
    - Evaluate for renal vein and IVC invasion
- MR
  - Best contrast resolution to determine local extension to adjacent organs and vascular involvement
  - Adds specificity to CT characterization

Restaging

- Consider 2 years of surveillance imaging after removal of adrenal nodules
  - Every 3 months for 1st year
  - Every 6 months for 2nd year
- CT
  - Local recurrence, liver and lung metastases
  - Because liver and lung are most common sites for metastases, may be able to image chest and abdomen only with CECT
- Contrast-enhanced ultrasound
  - Microbubble enhancement may add sensitivity for detection of hepatic mets < 1 cm
    - Early enhancement compared to normal liver parenchyma
  - Hypoechoic and sharply marginated lesions
- MR
  - May have increased sensitivity for small hepatic mets
- FDG PET/CT
  - May be very useful for detection of local recurrence and distant metastases

CLINICAL ISSUES

Presentation

- Non-hormonally active
  - Abdominal pain, fullness and palpable mass
  - Incidentally discovered mass on imaging study
  - Presence of metastases
  - More common in males
- Hormonally active

ADRENAL CARCINOMA

- ○ ~ 60% of patients present with symptoms of excessive hormone secretion
- ○ Hormonally active tumors are more common in females
- ○ Cushing syndrome due to ↑ cortisol
  - Most common presentation in symptomatic patients
    - Moon facies
    - Truncal obesity
    - Purple skin striae
    - Buffalo hump
- ○ Female virilization or male feminization due to ↑ androgens
  - Most common presentation in children
  - Virilization present in 95% of functioning childhood tumors
- ○ Conn syndrome (primary hyperaldosteronism)
  - Hypertension & weakness
- ○ Other clinical syndromes
  - Hypoglycemia, polycythemia, & non-glucocorticoid-related insulin resistance

Cancer Natural History & Prognosis
- Radical surgical excision only method by which long-term disease-free survival achieved
  - ○ Recurrence in 70-80% after resection
  - ○ Overall 5-year survival for tumors resected with curative intent ~ 40%
- Stage IV survival usually < 9 months
- Poor prognostic factors
  - ○ Age > 55 at presentation
  - ○ Positive resection margins
  - ○ Lymph node positive disease
  - ○ Invasion of contiguous organ requiring resection
  - ○ Poorly differentiated primary tumor
  - ○ Distant metastases at presentation

Treatment Options
- Major treatment alternatives
  - ○ Radical surgical excision for early stage disease with curative intent
  - ○ If metastatic and functioning, removal of primary tumor and metastatic disease for palliation of symptoms
- Major treatment roadblocks
  - ○ 30% metastatic at presentation
- Treatment options by stage
  - ○ Stage I & II: Radical surgical excision
    - Adjuvant radiation or chemotherapy not demonstrated to improve survival
  - ○ Stage III: Radical surgical excision ± lymph node dissection
    - Clinical trial enrollment recommended for patients with regional lymphadenopathy
    - Possible role for radiation therapy in localized but unresectable disease
    - Mitotane may be indicated if radiographically measurable metastases identified
  - ○ Stage IV: All therapy considered palliative rather than curative
    - Mitotane
    - Systemic chemotherapy
    - Radiation therapy (local control)
    - Surgical resection of functioning localized metastases
    - Clinical trials using cisplatin and other agents

REPORTING CHECKLIST

T Staging
- Important to note if size of tumor is < or > 5 cm
  - ○ > 5 cm considered very high risk for carcinoma
- Presence or absence of extraadrenal invasion
  - ○ Precise definition of cephalad extension of tumor thrombus essential for surgical planning
- Sparing or invasion of adjacent organs
  - ○ Essential to document tumor/kidney fat plane and tumor/liver fat plane if on right

N Staging
- Presence or absence of nodal metastases

M Staging
- Is tumor in adjacent organs due to direct extension or mets?

Rule Out Other Adrenal Tumors
- Most common adrenal mass is benign adrenal adenoma

Vascular Involvement
- Not discrete component of staging
- Recommended for comment; may have therapeutic and prognostic significance

SELECTED REFERENCES

1. American Joint Committee on Cancer: AJCC Cancer Staging Manual. 7th ed. New York: Springer, 2010
2. Bauditz J et al: Improved detection of hepatic metastases of adrenocortical cancer by contrast-enhanced ultrasound. Oncol Rep. 19(5):1135-9, 2008
3. Bilimoria KY et al: Adrenocortical carcinoma in the United States: treatment utilization and prognostic factors. Cancer. 113(11):3130-6, 2008
4. Fareau GG et al: Diagnostic challenges in adrenocortical carcinoma: recommendations for surveillance after surgical resection of selected adrenal nodules. Endocr Pract. 13(6):636-41, 2007
5. Leboulleux S et al: Diagnostic and prognostic value of 18-fluorodeoxyglucose positron emission tomography in adrenocortical carcinoma: a prospective comparison with computed tomography. J Clin Endocrinol Metab. 91(3):920-5, 2006
6. Mackie GC et al: Use of [18F]fluorodeoxyglucose positron emission tomography in evaluating locally recurrent and metastatic adrenocortical carcinoma. J Clin Endocrinol Metab. 91(7):2665-71, 2006
7. Szolar DH et al: Adrenocortical carcinomas and adrenal pheochromocytomas: mass and enhancement loss evaluation at delayed contrast-enhanced CT. Radiology. 234(2):479-85, 2005
8. Elsayes KM et al: Adrenal masses: mr imaging features with pathologic correlation. Radiographics. 24 Suppl 1:S73-86, 2004
9. Aubert S et al: Weiss system revisited: a clinicopathologic and immunohistochemical study of 49 adrenocortical tumors. Am J Surg Pathol. 26(12):1612-9, 2002
10. Lockhart ME et al: Imaging of adrenal masses. Eur J Radiol. 41(2):95-112, 2002

ADRENAL CARCINOMA

Stage I (T1 N0 M0)

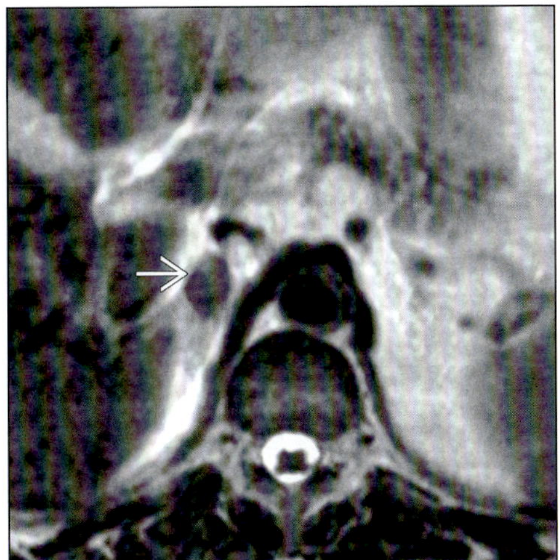

Stage I (T1 N0 M0)

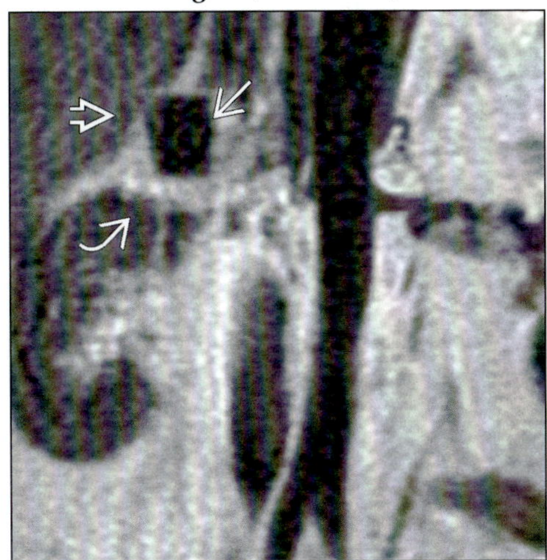

(Left) Axial T2WI MR demonstrates a well-circumscribed T2 dark adrenal nodule ➡, measuring < 3 cm. *(Right)* Coronal T1WI MR shows a T1 dark, well-circumscribed right adrenal nodule ➡. There is a clear fat plane between the nodule and the adjacent kidney ⮕ and liver ⮕.

Stage I (T1 N0 M0)

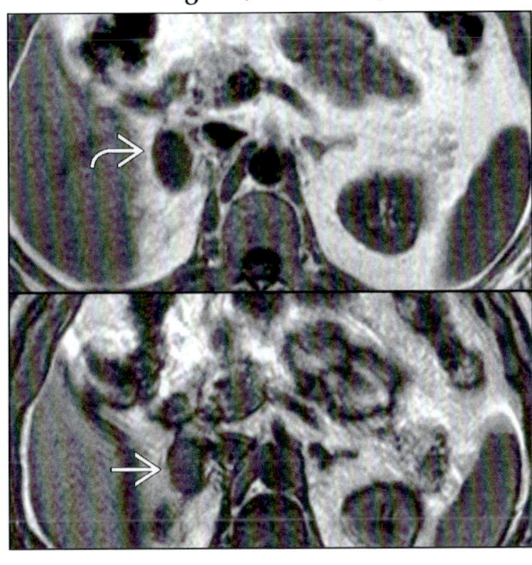

Stage I (T1 N0 M0)

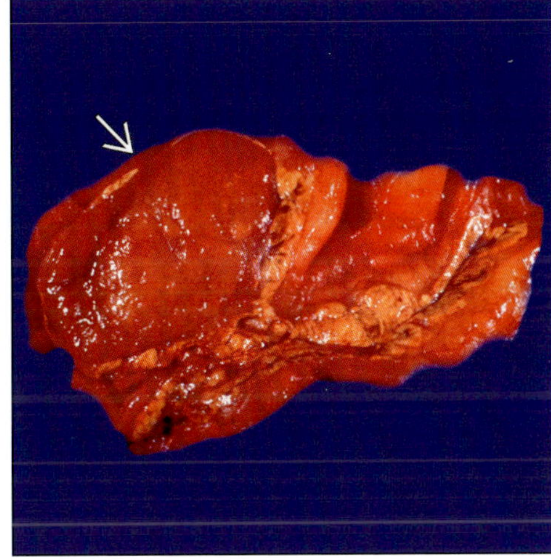

(Left) Axial T1WI MR in the same patient demonstrates that the nodule gains signal intensity ➡ on the out-of-phase imaging (bottom) compared to the in-phase ➡ imaging (top). A benign adrenal nodule would lose signal on the out-of-phase imaging. *(Right)* Gross image shows the well-circumscribed rubbery adrenal mass ➡ corresponding to the lesion seen in the preceding MR images.

Stage I (T1 N0 M0)

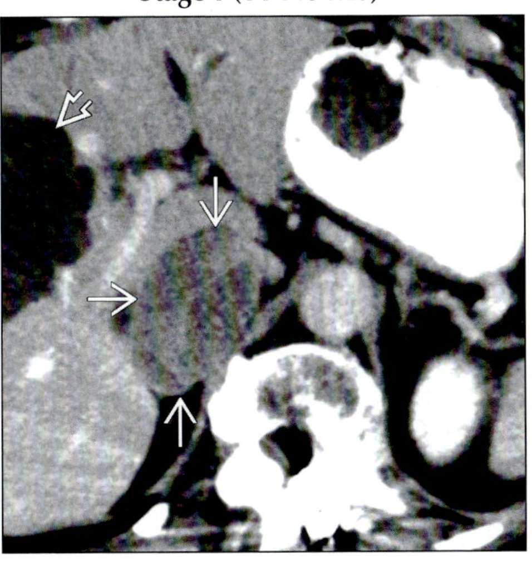

Stage I (T1 N0 M0)

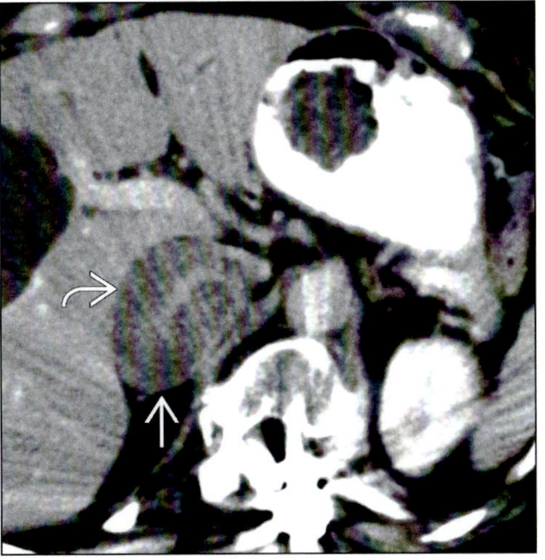

(Left) Axial CECT shows a 4.5 cm, moderate-sized, heterogeneous right adrenal tumor ➡. This typical appearance of an adrenal cortical carcinoma overlaps with the appearance of metastases and pheochromocytoma on CT. An incidental hepatic cyst is seen ⮕. *(Right)* A more inferior image in the same patient at the level of the portal vein shows that the tumor is confined within the adrenal capsule ⮕ and that an intact plane exists between the mass and the liver ⮕.

ADRENAL CARCINOMA

Stage II (T2 N0 M0)

Stage II (T2 N0 M0)

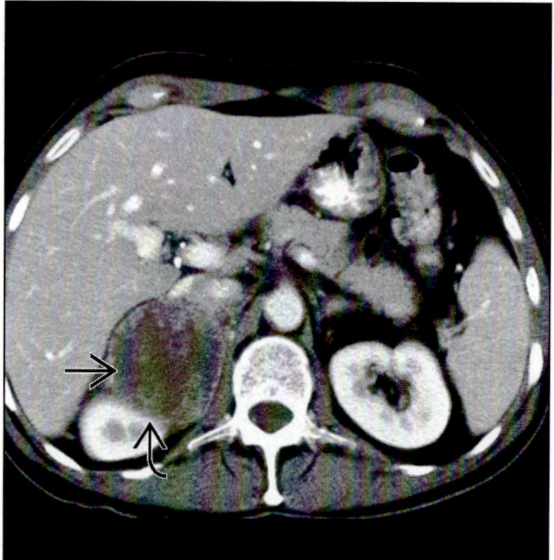

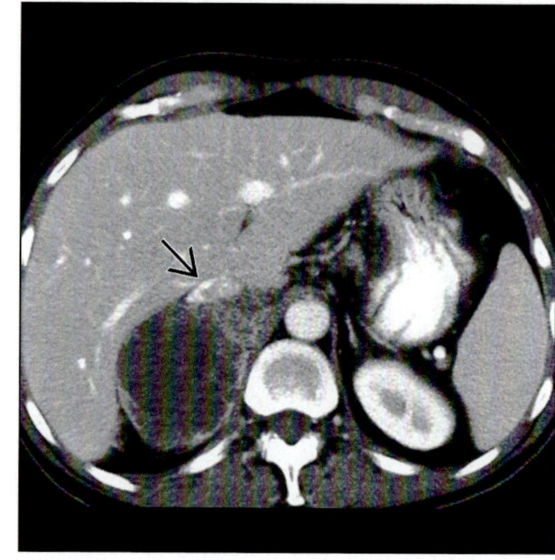

(Left) Axial CECT shows a large heterogeneous right adrenal mass with areas of low density ➡. Note preservation of distinct margin of right kidney ➡, denoting that the mass neither arises from nor invades the kidney. The mass size > 5 cm makes the lesion T2. *(Right)* Axial CECT in the same patient more cranially shows intact planes between the mass and adjacent organs, including liver. The inferior vena cava is compressed ➡ but uninvolved.

Stage II (T2 N0 M0)

Stage II (T2 N0 M0)

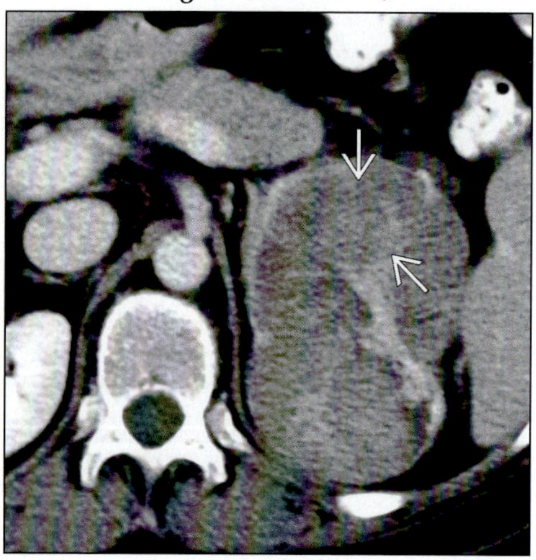

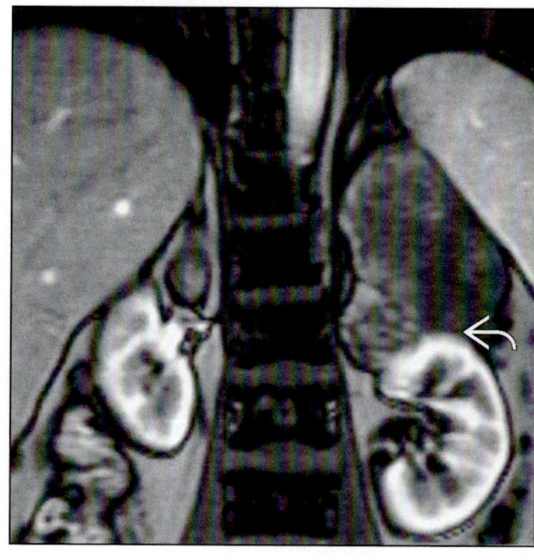

(Left) Multimodality imaging can be very helpful for characterizing tumor margins for preoperative staging. This CECT demonstrates a large (> 5 cm), heterogeneous left adrenal mass ➡ that appears very well circumscribed in a 30-year-old woman presenting with Cushing syndrome. *(Right)* Coronal T1WI C+ MR in the same patient suggests that an intact plane is present between the mass and the adjacent kidney ➡. This was confirmed on resection.

Stage III (T3 N0 M0)

Stage III (T3 N0 M0)

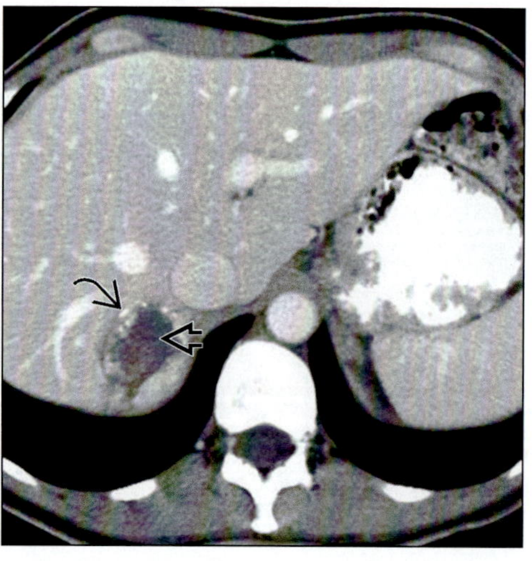

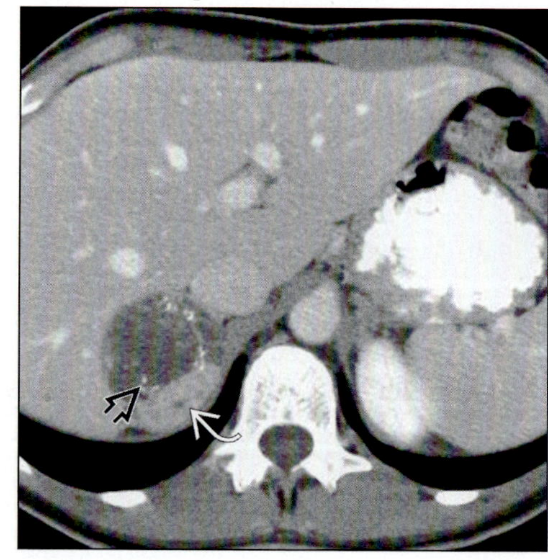

(Left) Axial CECT demonstrates a right adrenal mass with areas of calcification ➡ as well as necrosis ➡. *(Right)* A more caudal image in the same patient again shows the mass demonstrating extensive necrosis with calcification ➡ and areas of heterogeneous enhancement ➡. On this image, an intact tissue plane is suggested between the mass, liver, diaphragm, and inferior vena cava.

ADRENAL CARCINOMA

Stage III (T3 N0 M0)

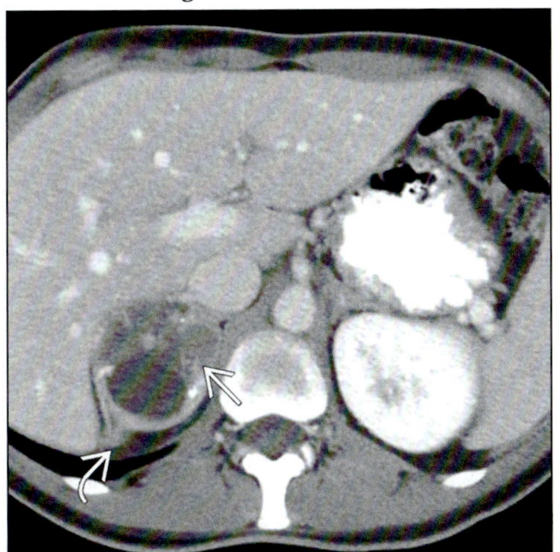

Stage III (T3 N0 M0)

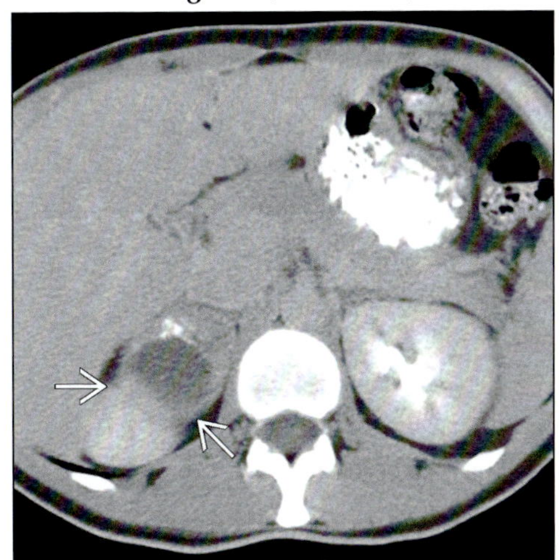

(Left) Axial CECT in the same patient shows a suggestion of soft tissue nodularity and infiltration in the adjacent fat, which would indicate T3 disease. An intact plane is difficult to appreciate, but it is present between the mass ➡ and the liver ➡. *(Right)* Delayed CECT in the same patient illustrates the difficulty of documenting an intact plane between the mass and the kidney ➡, especially on delayed CECT.

Stage IV (T4 N0 M0)

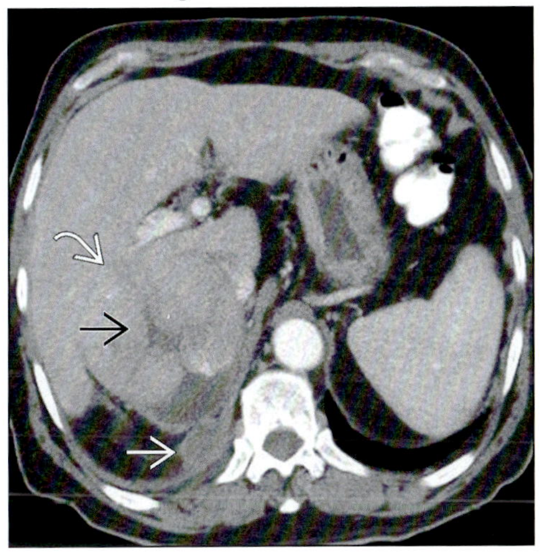

Stage IV (T4 N0 M0)

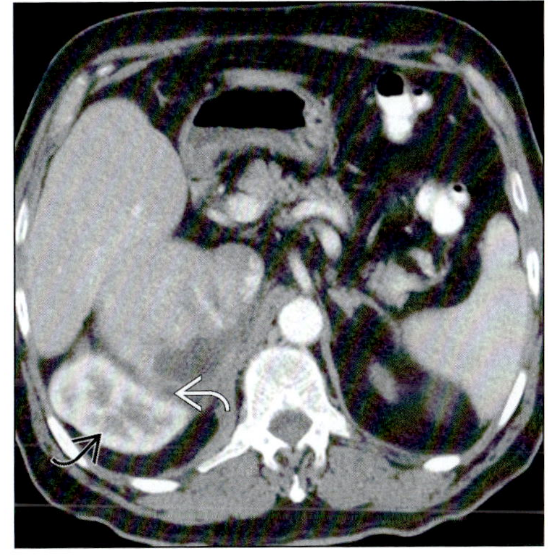

(Left) Axial CECT shows a very large, partially necrotic, heterogeneous adrenal mass ➡ with infiltration beyond the adrenal capsule into adjacent perinephric space. The infiltration into the right diaphragm ➡ makes this T4 disease. No distinct plane is seen between the mass and adjacent liver ➡. *(Right)* Axial CECT in the same patient shows the infiltrated fat ➡ between the mass and the kidney. There is no frank invasion into the adjacent kidney ➡.

Stage IV (T4 N0 M0)

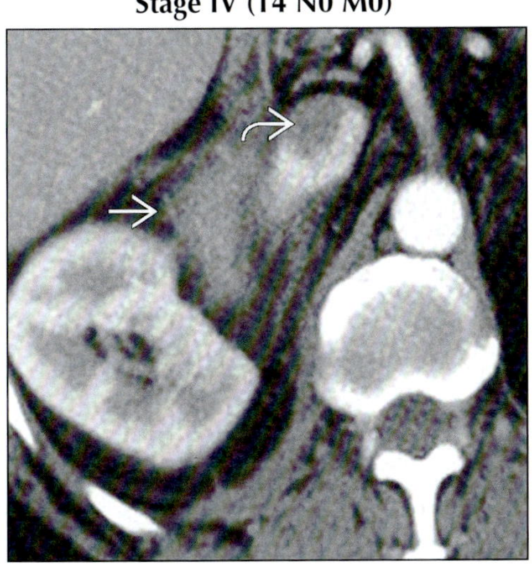

Stage IV (T4 N0 M0)

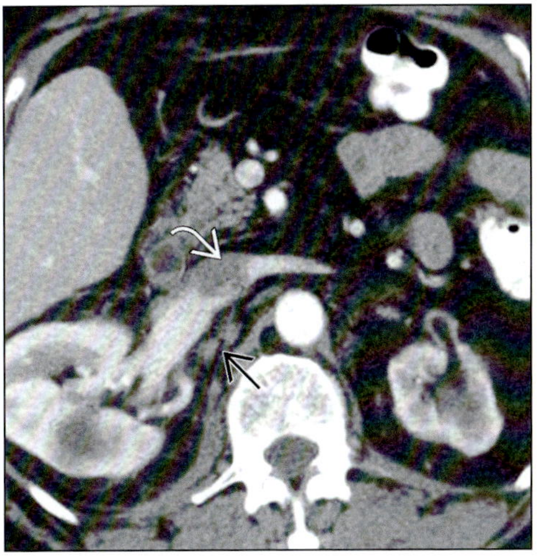

(Left) Axial CECT in the same patient shows the infiltration of fat ➡ between mass and kidney. Additionally, intraluminal tumor thrombus ➡ is seen within the inferior vena cava. *(Right)* More caudal axial CECT in the same patient demonstrates inferior extension of intraluminal tumor thrombus ➡ within the inferior vena cava. Small nodes ➡ do not meet CT criteria for pathologic enlargement.

ADRENAL CARCINOMA

Stage IV (T3 N1 M0)

Stage IV (T3 N1 M0)

(Left) Scout image from CT demonstrates calcifications ➡ in a right upper quadrant mass. Hepatic flexure is inferiorly displaced ➡ by the inferior displacement of the right kidney ➡. (Right) Axial arterial phase CECT demonstrates the very large, well-circumscribed right adrenal mass with central calcifications ➡. An enlarged paraaortic lymph node ➡ is consistent with N1 disease, upstaging this patient's disease to stage IV.

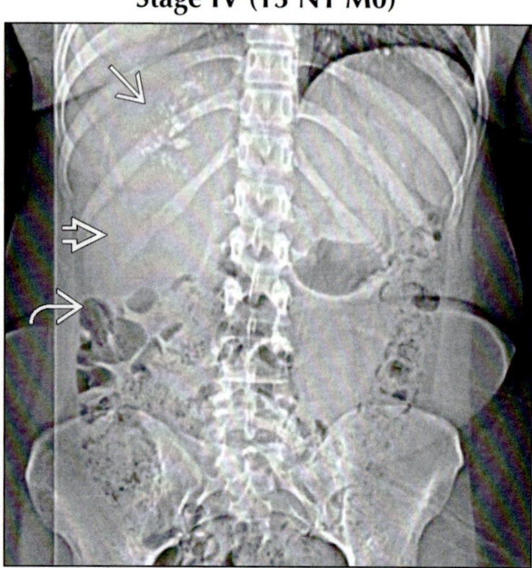

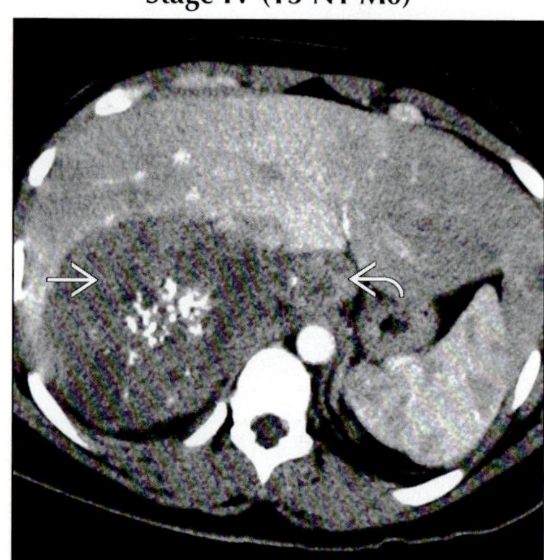

Stage IV (T3 N1 M0)

Stage IV (T3 N1 M0)

(Left) Coronal MIP image in the same patient demonstrates the inferior displacement of the right kidney ➡. Intact planes are present between the mass and adjacent organs, but large local nodal metastases ➡ are present. (Right) Gross image demonstrates the clean plane between the mass and adjacent kidney ➡, as well as the metastatic lymph nodes ➡.

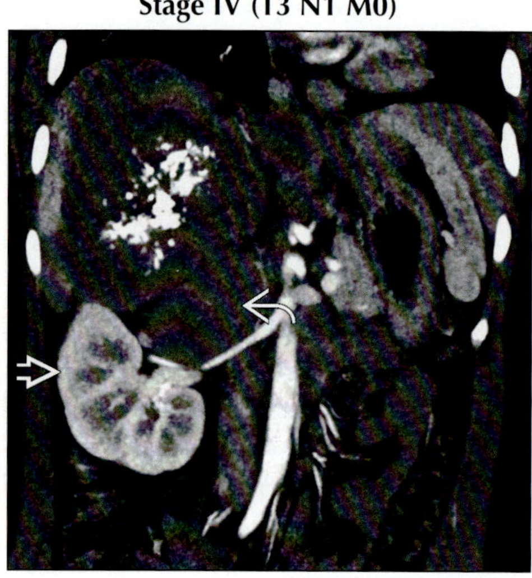

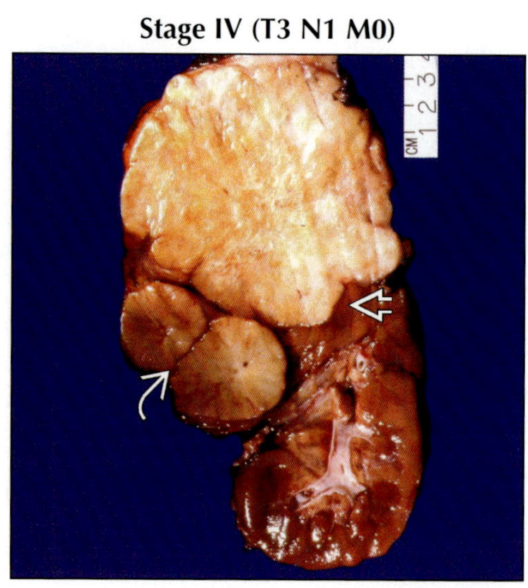

Stage IV (T4 N1 M0)

Stage IV (T4 N1 M0)

(Left) Axial CECT demonstrates heterogeneous tumor thrombus ➡ in the hepatic inferior vena cava. (Right) More caudal axial CECT in the same patient demonstrates the markedly enlarged and abnormal paraaortic lymph nodes, both ipsilateral ➡ and contralateral ➡ to the primary tumor.

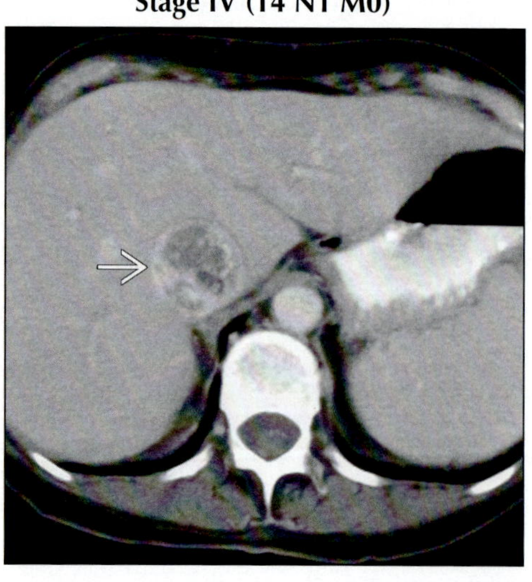

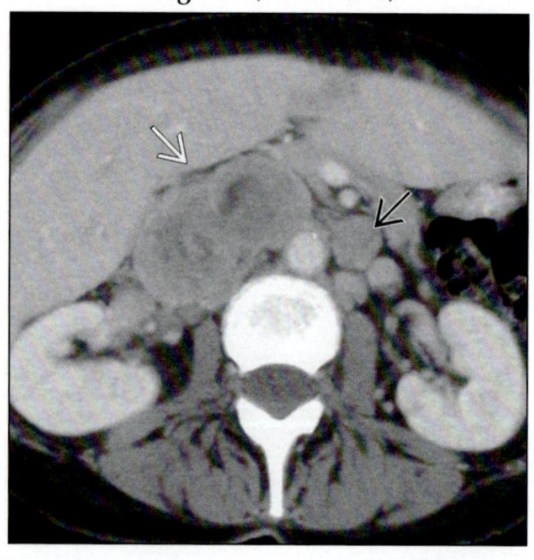

ADRENAL CARCINOMA

Stage IV (T4 N1 M0)

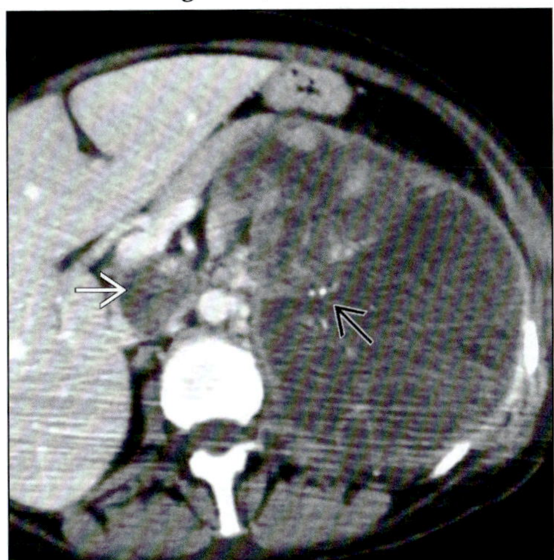

Stage IV (T4 N1 M0)

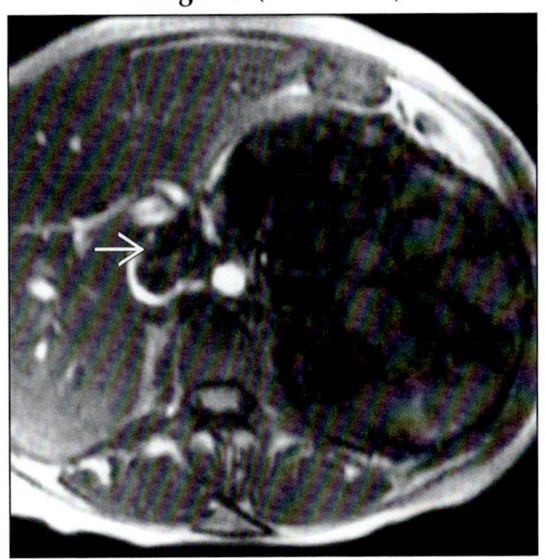

(Left) This axial CECT demonstrates a large tumor in the left pararenal space. The center of the mass is low attenuation, with calcifications ➡. Tumor thrombus ➡ in the infrahepatic inferior vena cava makes this a T4 lesion. *(Right)* Axial T1WI C+ MR in the same patient demonstrates the large, heterogeneously low T1 SI mass in the left perirenal space, with IVC thrombus ➡ of the same low signal intensity.

Stage IV (T4 N1 M0)

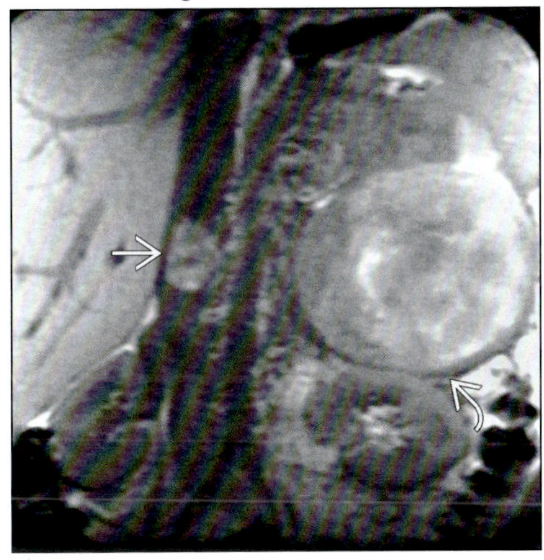

Stage IV (T4 N1 M0)

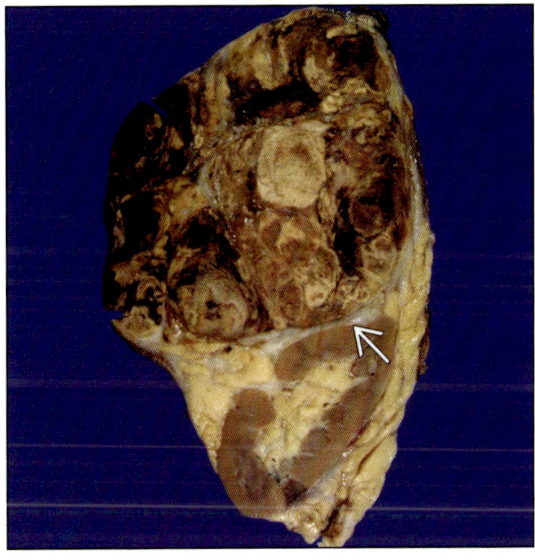

(Left) Coronal T1WI MR in the same patient shows, more convincingly, the tumor thrombus ➡ in the IVC. The left kidney is displaced inferiorly; however, there appears to be an intact plane ➡ between the mass and the kidney. *(Right)* Gross image shows the heterogeneously solid and necrotic left adrenal carcinoma. A fibrous capsule ➡ separates the mass from the adjacent kidney, corresponding to the findings on MR. The IVC invasion was confirmed at resection.

Stage IV (T4 N1 M1)

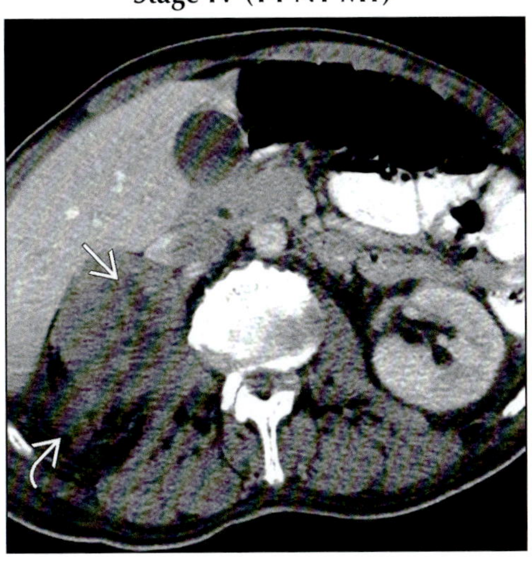

Stage IV (T4 N1 M1)

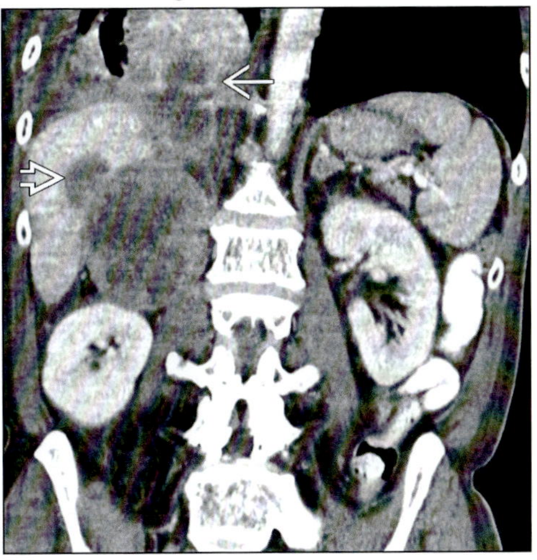

(Left) Axial CECT reveals a large, heterogeneous right adrenal mass ➡ with infiltration ➡ of the surrounding fat well demonstrated on the CT. *(Right)* Coronal image shows both the hepatic metastasis ➡ that may have arisen from direct tumor invasion and invasion of the tumor through the diaphragm to involve the right lung base ➡. This constitutes unresectable disease.

ADRENAL CARCINOMA

Stage III (T3 NX MX)

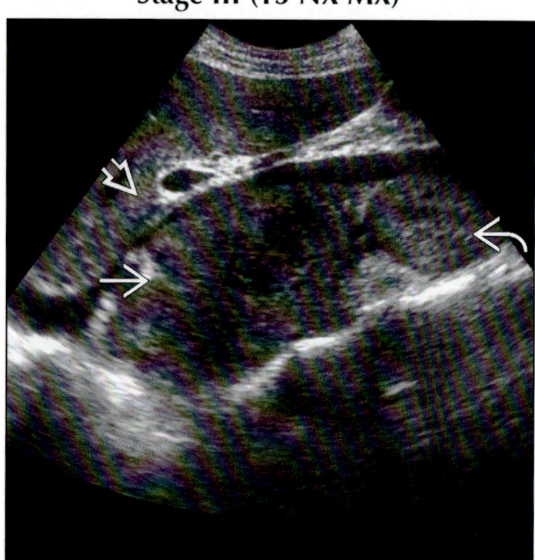

(Left) Grayscale transabdominal ultrasound shows a > 5 cm adrenal carcinoma ➡. The disruption of the adrenal capsule (local invasion/T3 disease) is not well demonstrated on US. There is no clear invasion of adjacent organs, including the inferiorly displaced right kidney ➡ and liver ➡, that would upstage the tumor to T4 disease.

Stage III (T3 NX MX)

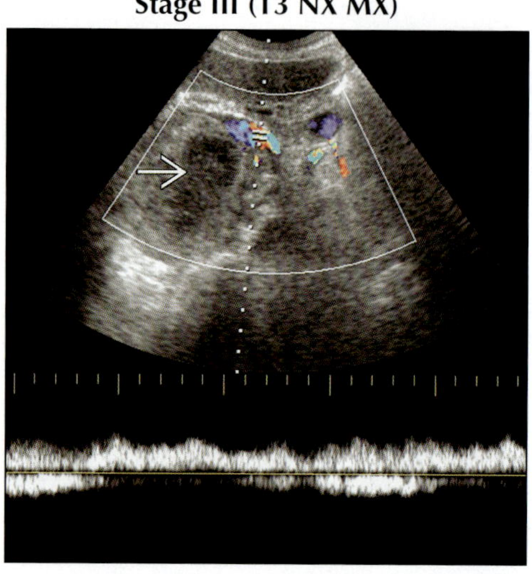

(Right) On color Doppler, the carcinoma shows an internal hypoechoic avascular component consistent with necrosis ➡.

Stage IV (T4 NX M1)

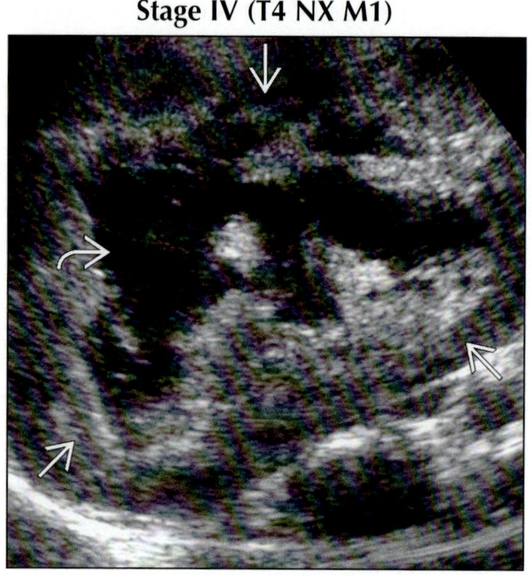

(Left) Longitudinal transabdominal grayscale ultrasound shows a large adrenal carcinoma ➡ with central necrosis ➡ mimicking an abscess. **(Right)** Transverse transabdominal ultrasound in the same patient demonstrates both the large, centrally necrotic adrenal carcinoma ➡ and a well-defined hepatic metastasis ➡ adjacent to the carcinoma.

Stage IV (T4 NX M1)

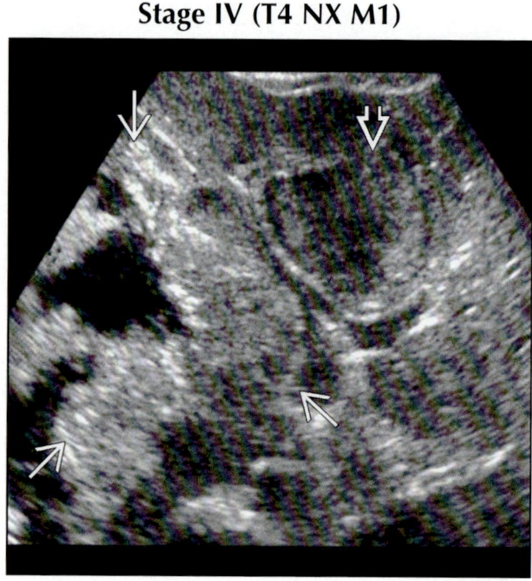

Stage IV (T4 NX M1)

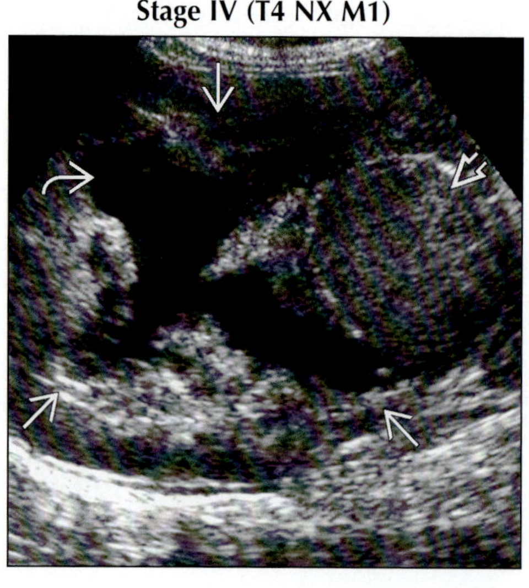

(Left) Oblique transabdominal ultrasound in the same patient shows the large, centrally necrotic ➡ adrenal carcinoma ➡. A discrete tissue plane between the primary carcinoma and the adjacent hepatic metastasis ➡ is difficult to appreciate. **(Right)** Longitudinal color Doppler ultrasound in the same patient reveals the extrinsic compression of the inferior vena cava ➡.

Stage IV (T4 NX M1)

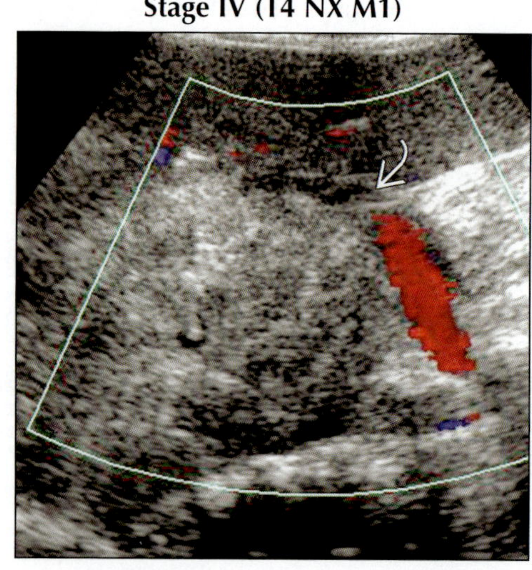

ADRENAL CARCINOMA

Local Recurrence

Local Recurrence

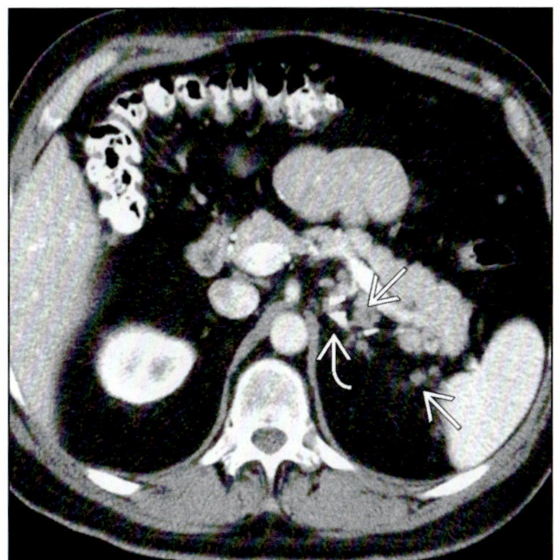

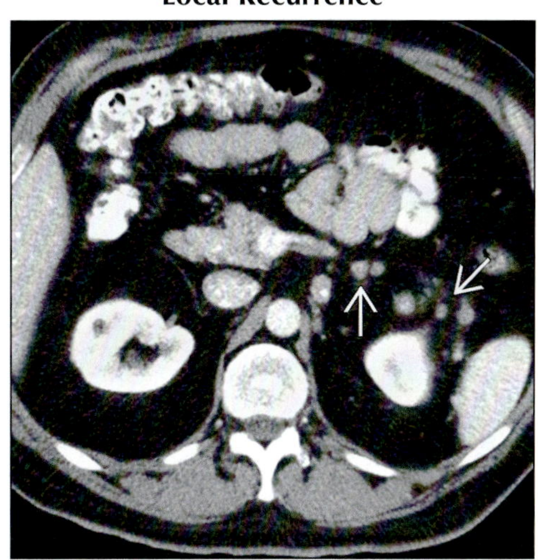

(Left) CECT demonstrates surgical clips ➡ in the region of the left adrenal gland. Soft tissue nodules stud the surgical bed and left perinephric space ➡. This patient had undergone a left adrenalectomy 1 year prior for a 3 cm lesion. *(Right)* More inferior image demonstrates numerous soft tissue nodules ➡ studding the left perinephric space. When the patient's serum cortisol began rising, repeat imaging was obtained, demonstrating the recurrence.

Local Recurrence

Local Recurrence

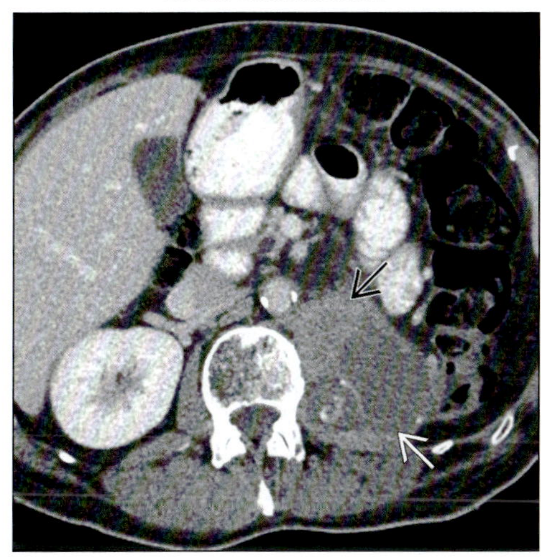

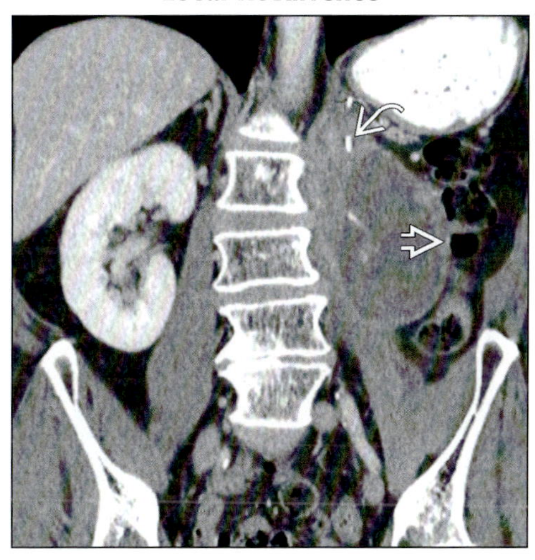

(Left) CECT in another patient shows a cystic ➡ and solid ➡ mass in the left adrenal bed. Recurrence developed 1 year after adrenalectomy for a 5 cm lesion. After an initial uncomplicated postoperative course, back pain developed and worsened, prompting further work-up. *(Right)* Coronal CECT in the same patient shows the extensive local recurrence. No discernible tissue plane is identified between the mass and the adjacent descending colon ➡. Surgical clips ➡ from adrenalectomy are present.

Local Recurrence

Local Recurrence

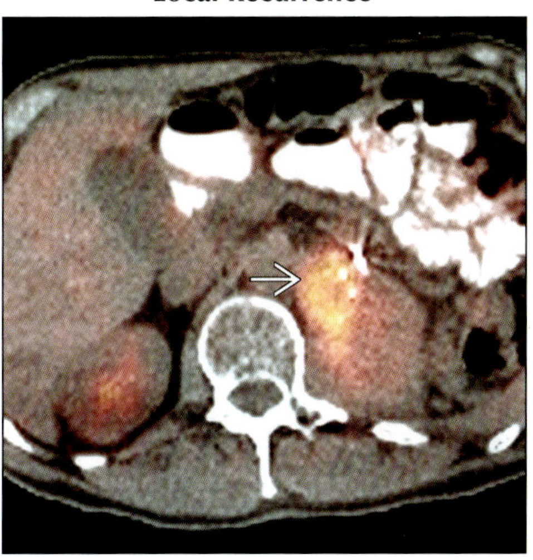

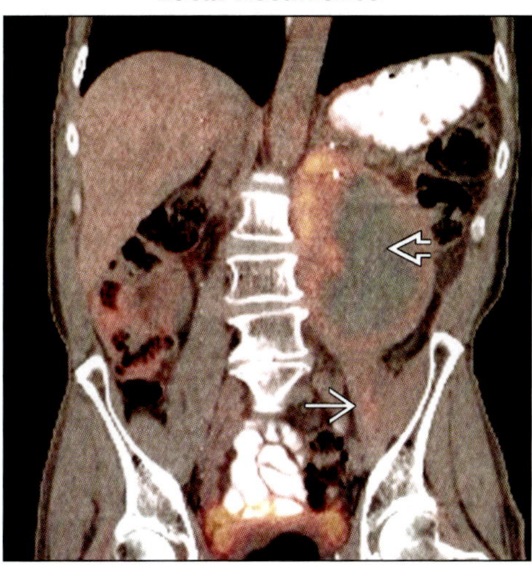

(Left) PET/CT in the same patient demonstrates high metabolic activity in the solid components of the tumor ➡. Streak artifact is present from the adrenalectomy clips. PET/CT was obtained to evaluate for metastases distant from the surgical bed, none of which were found. *(Right)* The necrotic center ➡ of the recurrent tumor is not metabolically active. There is mild increased F18 FDG activity in the left psoas muscle ➡, raising a concern for local infiltration.

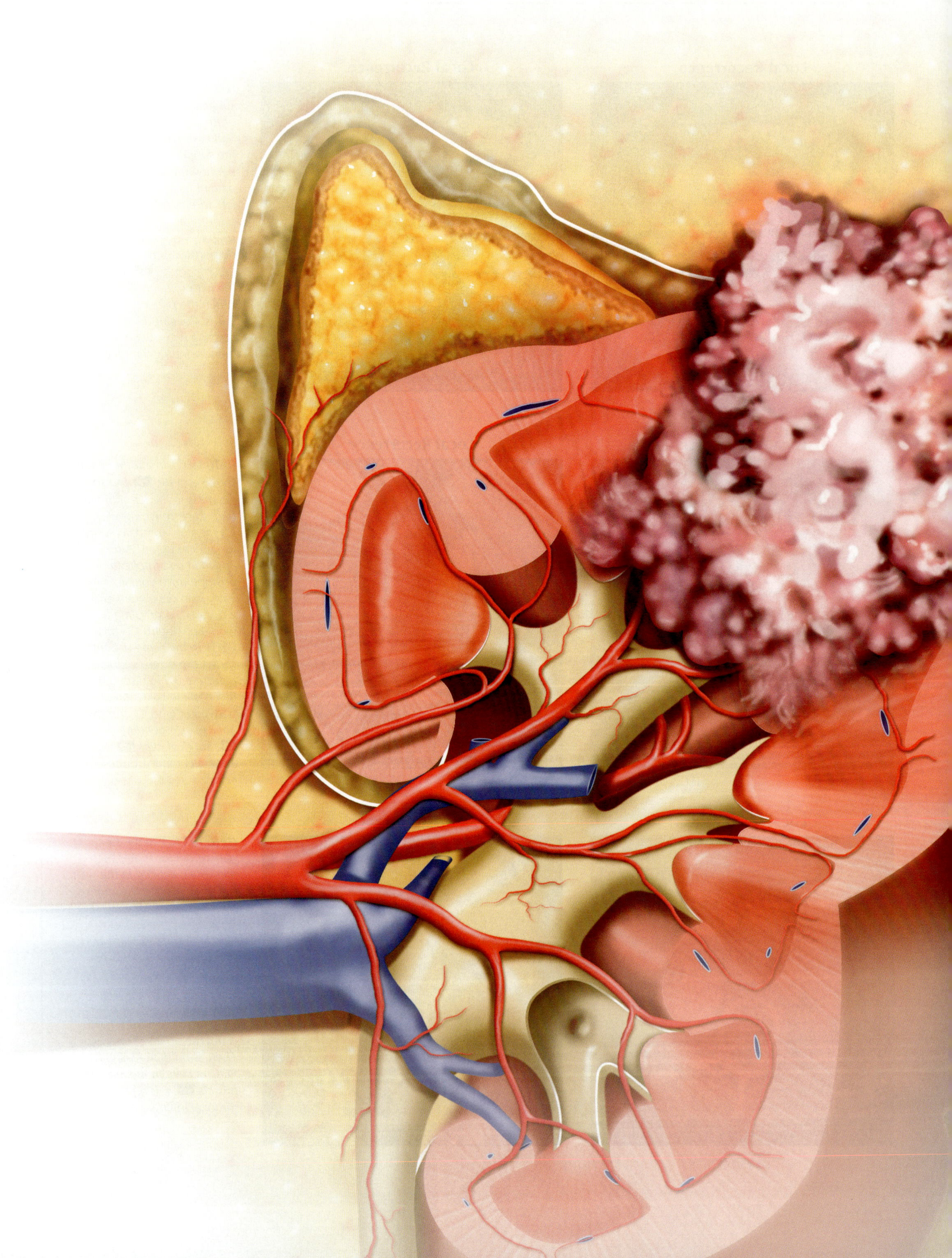

Renal Carcinoma

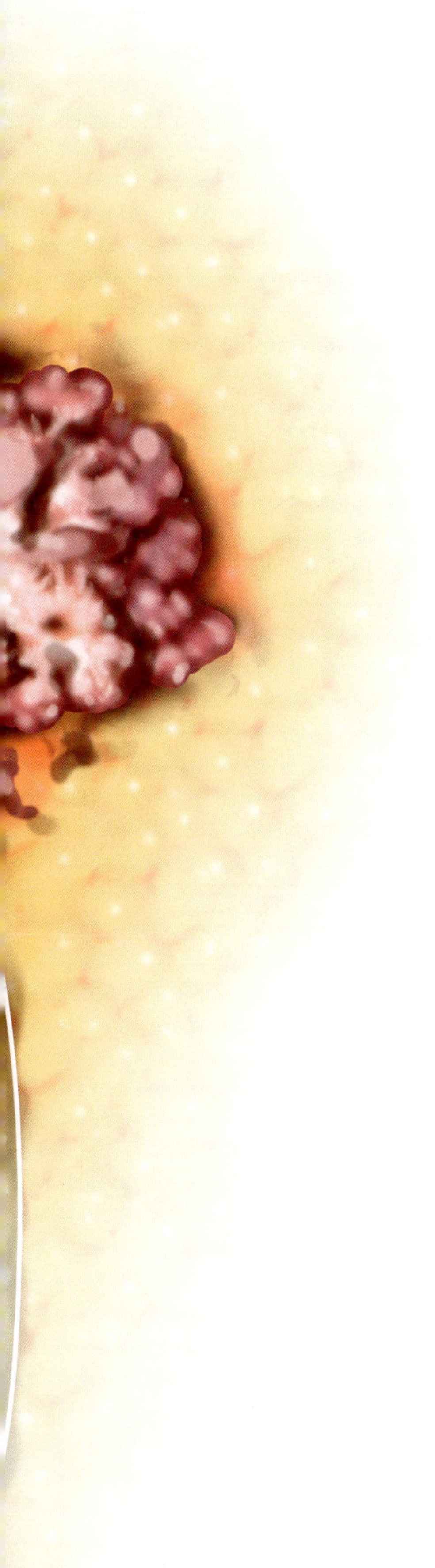

RENAL CARCINOMA

(T) Primary Tumor

Adapted from 7th edition AJCC Staging Forms.

TNM	Definitions
TX	Primary tumor cannot be assessed
T0	No evidence of primary tumor
T1	Tumor ≤ 7 cm in greatest dimension, limited to the kidney
T1a	Tumor ≤ 4 cm in greatest dimension, limited to the kidney
T1b	Tumor > 4 cm but ≤ 7 cm in greatest dimension, limited to the kidney
T2	Tumor > 7 cm in greatest dimension, limited to the kidney
T2a	Tumor > 7 cm but ≤ 10 cm in greatest dimension, limited to the kidney
T2b	Tumor > 10 cm, limited to the kidney
T3	Tumor extends into major veins or perinephric tissues but not into the ipsilateral adrenal gland and not beyond Gerota fascia
T3a	Tumor grossly extends into the renal vein or its segmental (muscle containing) branches, or tumor invades perirenal &/or renal sinus fat but not beyond Gerota fascia
T3b	Tumor grossly extends into the vena cava below the diaphragm
T3c	Tumor grossly extends into the vena cava above the diaphragm or invades the wall of the vena cava
T4	Tumor invades beyond Gerota fascia (including contiguous extension into the ipsilateral adrenal gland)

(N) Regional Lymph Nodes

NX	Regional lymph nodes cannot be assessed
N0	No regional lymph node metastasis
N1	Metastasis in regional lymph node(s)

(M) Distant Metastasis

M0	No distant metastasis
M1	Distant metastasis

AJCC Stages/Prognostic Groups

Adapted from 7th edition AJCC Staging Forms.

Stage	T	N	M
I	T1	N0	M0
II	T2	N0	M0
III	T1 or T2	N1	M0
	T3	N0 or N1	M0
IV	T4	Any N	M0
	Any T	Any N	M1

Comparison of Robson and TNM Staging

Robson Stage	Definitions	TNM
I	Tumor ≤ 2.5 cm and confined to kidney	T1
	Tumor > 2.5 cm and confined to kidney	T1-T2
II	Tumor extends into perinephric fat or adrenal	T3a if involves perinephric fat, T4 if involves ipsilateral adrenal
IIIA	Tumor invades renal vein	T3a
	Tumor extends into inferior vena cava	T3b below the diaphragm
IIIB	Lymph node involvement	N0-N1, M0
IIIC	Involvement of local vasculature and lymph nodes	T3a-c, N0-N1
IVA	Involvement of adjacent organs (except ipsilateral adrenal)	T4
IVB	Distant metastases	M1

RENAL CARCINOMA

T1a

Coronal graphic shows a typical T1a lesion ➡, defined as less than or equal to 4 cm and confined to the kidney.

T1a

Axial graphic shows a T1a renal cell carcinoma ➡, defined as less than or equal to 4 cm and confined to the kidney. Lesions may be exophytic or more centrally located, as is the T1a depicted here.

T1b

Coronal graphic shows a typical T1b lesion ➡, defined as larger than 4 cm but less than or equal to 7 cm and confined to the kidney.

T1b

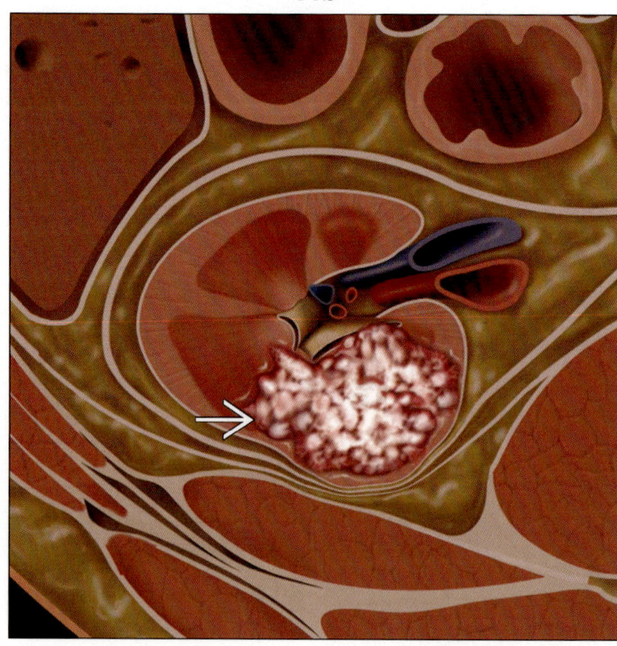

Axial graphic shows a T1b renal cell carcinoma ➡, defined as larger than 4 cm but less than or equal to 7 cm and confined to the kidney. These lesions may be exophytic but will still be categorized as T1 as long as there is no extension outside of the kidney.

T2a

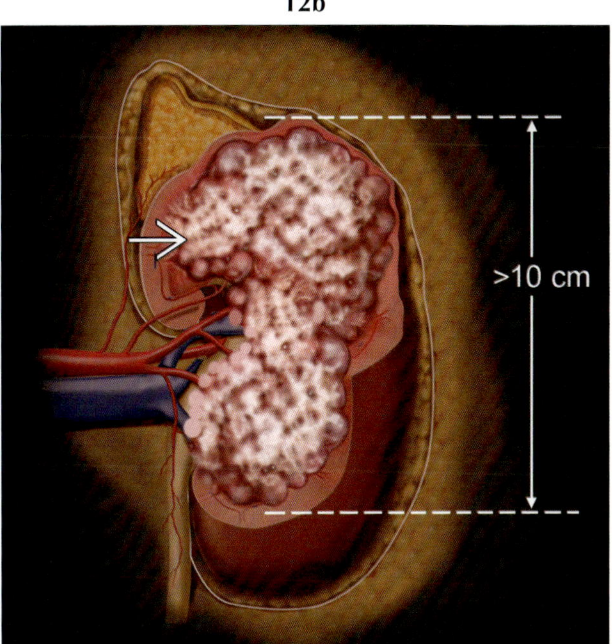

Coronal graphic shows a T2a renal cell carcinoma ➔, defined as larger than 7 cm but less than or equal to 10 cm and confined to the kidney. These lesions may also be described as exophytic but do not invade outside of the kidney.

Coronal graphic shows a typical T2b renal cell carcinoma ➔, defined as larger than 10 cm but confined to the kidney.

T3a

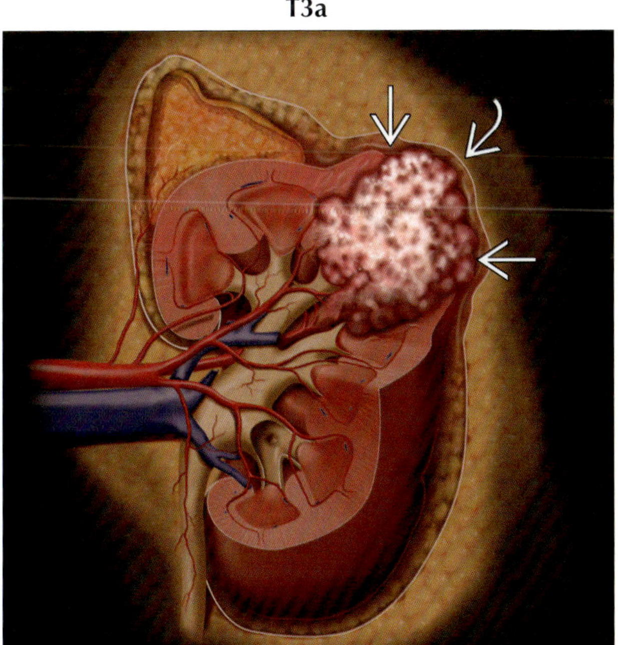

T3a

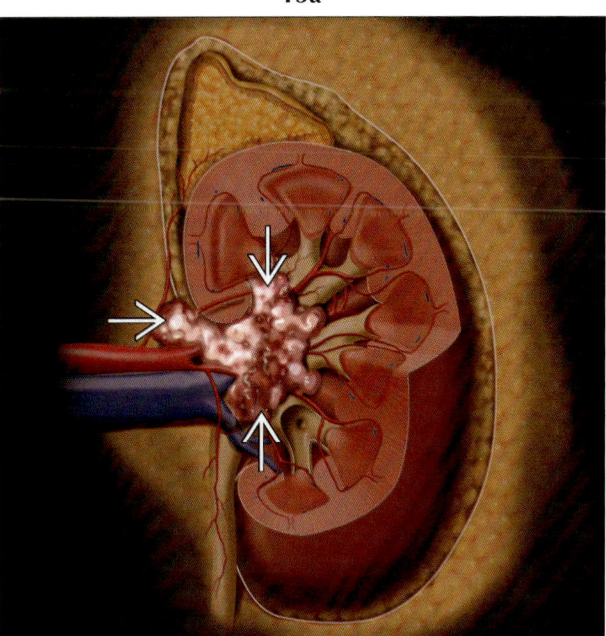

Coronal graphic shows a T3a renal cell carcinoma with tumor extension ➔ into the perirenal fat but not beyond the confines of Gerota fascia ➔.

Coronal graphic shows another example of a T3a lesion with extension into the perirenal or renal sinus fat ➔. Again, the tumor is limited by the confines of Gerota fascia.

T3a

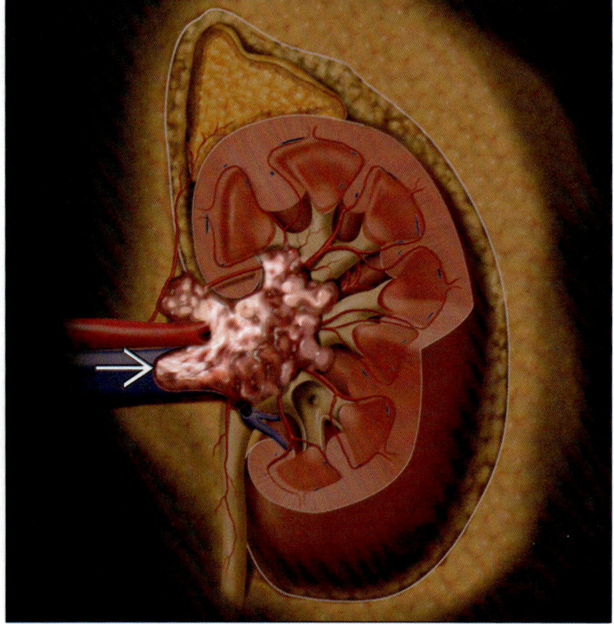

Coronal graphic shows a T3a renal cell carcinoma with extension of tumor into the renal vein ➡. Extension beyond the renal vein into the inferior vena cava would be defined as T3b lesion.

T3b

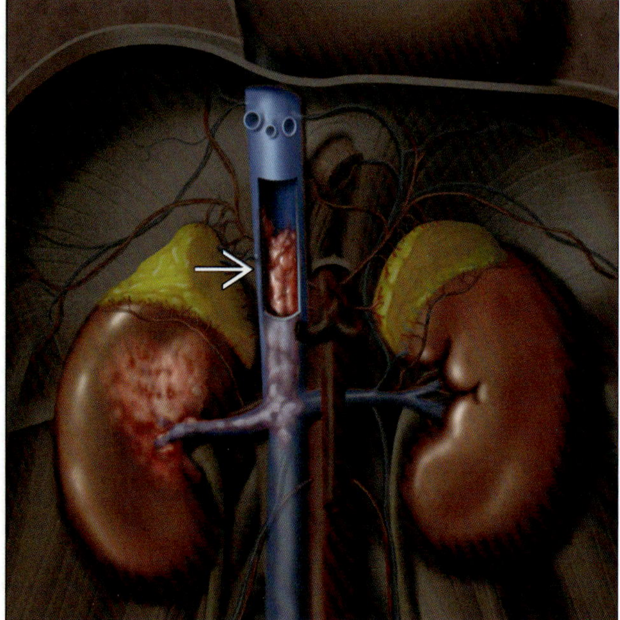

Coronal graphic shows a T3b renal cell carcinoma with extension of tumor not only into the renal vein but also into the inferior vena cava ➡. T3b lesions do not extend above the diaphragm.

T3c

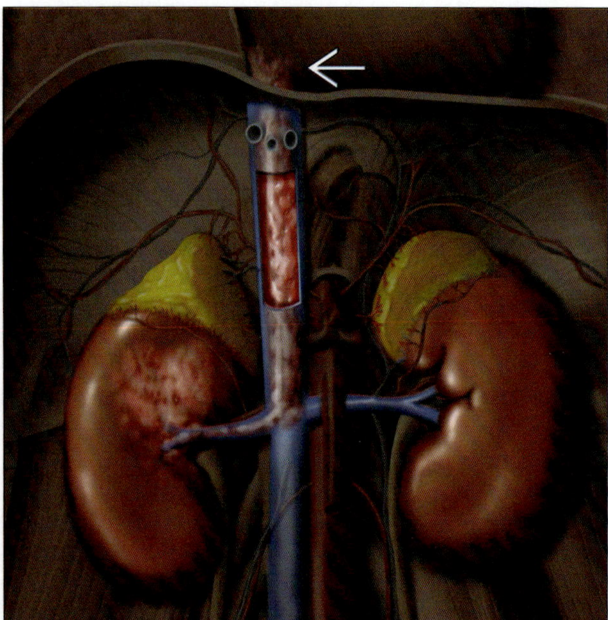

Coronal graphic shows a T3c renal cell carcinoma with involvement of tumor in the renal vein and inferior vena cava, as well as extension of tumor within the inferior vena cava above the diaphragm ➡.

T4

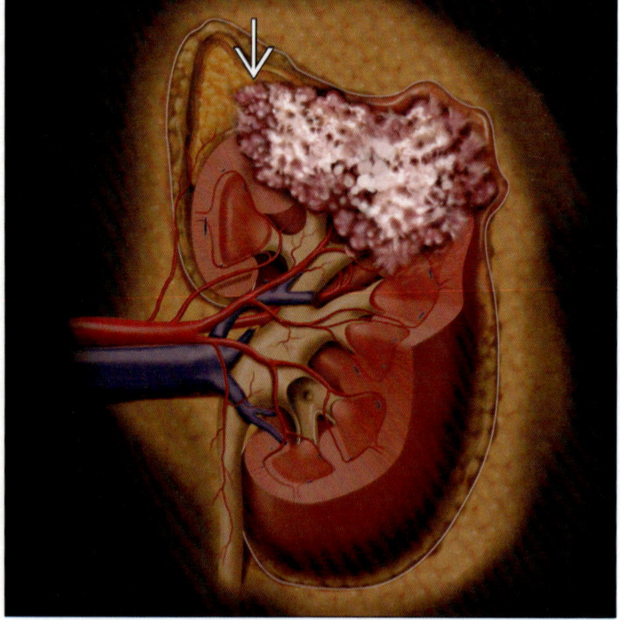

Coronal graphic shows a T4 renal cell carcinoma with extension into the ipsilateral adrenal gland ➡.

T4

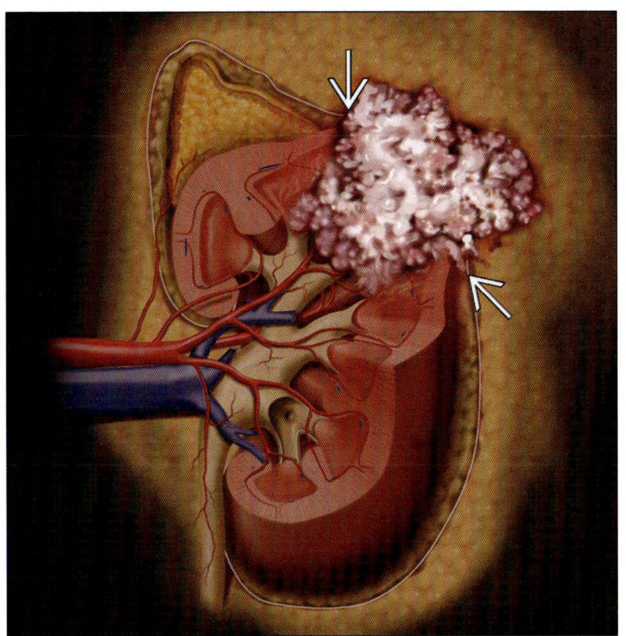

Coronal graphic shows another example of a T4 lesion with invasion into not only the perirenal fat but also with extension beyond the Gerota fascia ➡.

N1 Disease (Stage III or IV)

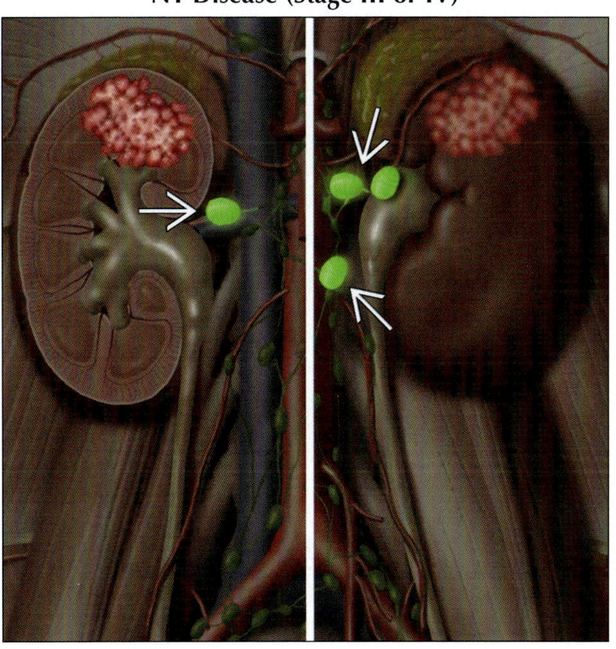

Coronal graphic shows retroperitoneal adenopathy on both sides of midline ➡. N0 disease is classified as no regional lymph node metastasis, while N1 disease is classified as metastatic disease in regional lymph nodes.

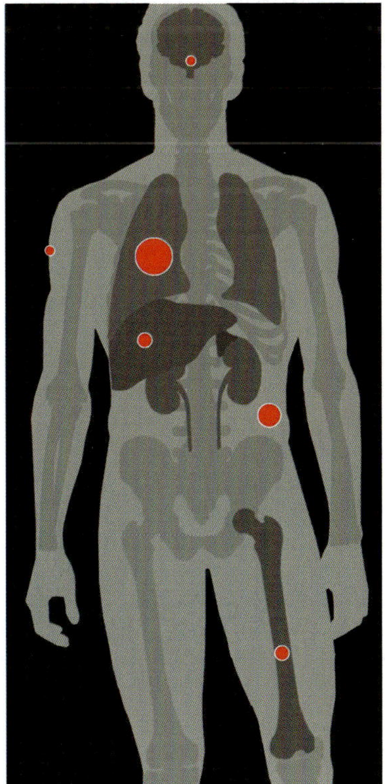

METASTASES, ORGAN FREQUENCY

Lungs	75%
Soft tissue	35%
Bone	20%
Liver	20%
Adrenal gland	19%
Cutaneous tissues	8%
CNS	8%

25-40% of patients present with metastatic disease.

OVERVIEW

General Comments
- Represents 2.6% of all cancers
- Only 2-4% occur in inherited syndromes
- Renal cell carcinoma (RCC) is most common renal cancer (85%)
- 2% bilateral involvement

Classification
- **4 major histopathologic subtypes of renal cell carcinoma**
  - Clear cell carcinoma
  - Papillary carcinoma
  - Collecting duct carcinoma
  - Chromophobe renal carcinoma

PATHOLOGY

Routes of Spread
- Hematogenous, lymphatic, &/or direct invasion
- 25% may be multifocal in the same kidney
- Found incidentally at autopsy, in some series in up to 25% of cases
- 25-40% present with metastatic disease
  - Lung (75%)
  - Soft tissue (35%)
  - Bone (20%)
  - Liver (20%)
  - Cutaneous tissues (8%)
  - CNS (8%)

General Features
- Comments
  - Renal cell carcinoma arises from renal tubular epithelium
- Genetics
  - **Hereditary papillary RCC**
    - Multiple
    - Bilateral
    - Papillary renal tumors
    - Autosomal dominant
    - C-met oncogene on chromosome 7
  - **Hereditary leiomyoma and renal cell cancer syndrome**
    - Cutaneous leiomyomas
    - Uterine fibroids
    - Renal cell cancer
    - Suspected mutation of fumarate hydratase gene
  - **von Hippel-Lindau**
    - RCC
    - Retinal angioma
    - Hemangioblastomas
    - Pheochromocytomas and others
    - Mutation of *VHL* gene on chromosome 3p25
    - RCC develops in approximately 40% of patients with von Hippel-Lindau
    - Major cause of mortality
  - **Birt-Hogg-Dubé syndrome**
    - Fibrofolliculomas on head and neck
    - Chromophobic RCC or onocytoma
    - Mutation of *BDH* gene on chromosome 17p
- Etiology
  - Genetic and environmental causes
    - Genetic
      - Tuberous sclerosis
      - von Hippel-Lindau
      - Birt-Hogg-Dubé syndrome
      - Hereditary papillary RCC
    - Environmental
      - Cigarette smoking: Dose dependent
      - Obesity
      - Hypertension
      - Acquired cystic disease from chronic dialysis
      - Chronic exposure to phenacetin
      - Benzene exposure
      - Cadmium exposure
      - Asbestos exposure
  - Other risk factors
    - Increasing age
    - Male sex
- Epidemiology & cancer incidence
  - Estimated 2008 incidence: 54,000 cases in USA
  - M:F = 2:1
  - Highest incidence in 6th to 8th decade
- Associated diseases, abnormalities
  - Multiple paraneoplastic disorders associated with RCC usually caused by tumor release of various cytokines
    - Hypercalcemia
    - Erythrocytosis
    - Polyneuropathy
    - Amyloidosis
    - Hypertension
    - Dermatomyositis
  - Syndromes may resolve after successful treatment of tumor

Gross Pathology & Surgical Features
- Varies from solid to cystic mass
- Yellow areas are due to lipid-rich tumor cells
- May have gray or black areas of necrosis or hemorrhage

Microscopic Pathology
- H&E
  - **Clear cell carcinoma**
    - Have clear or granular cytoplasm in round cells
    - Tumors may have solid, trabecular, or tubular pattern
  - **Papillary carcinoma**
    - Tumor cells are cuboidal or low columnar
    - Tumor pattern is papillary
  - **Chromophobe RCC**
    - Tumor cell morphology varies, but cells are lightly eosinophilic stained
    - Tumor pattern is solid sheets

IMAGING FINDINGS

Detection
- T staging accuracy is around 80% with noted difficulty in imaging some retroperitoneal and perinephric areas
- **General T staging imaging characteristics**
  - T1: Tumor ≤ 7 cm in greatest dimension, limited to kidney

RENAL CARCINOMA

- No evidence of perinephric fat or renal fascial involvement
- Exophytic tumors may not be reliably classified into T1a, T1b, or T2
- Solid enhancing lesion
- T2: Tumor > 7 cm in greatest dimension, limited to kidney
  - Imaging may be useful for distinguishing between T2a and T2b lesions
- T3: Tumor extends into major veins or perinephric tissues but not into ipsilateral adrenal gland and not beyond Gerota fascia
  - Ultrasound and MR very useful to demonstrate venous thrombus and to evaluate possible tumor thrombus
    - In general, thrombi that contain enhancing vessels are tumor
  - Can be used to identify thrombus in renal veins or inferior vena cava (IVC) with accuracy of 87%
- T4: Tumor invades beyond Gerota fascia or invades IVC above diaphragm
  - Chest CT is recommended for large or aggressive primary tumors
  - Brain MR and bone scans are often performed in patients with suggestive signs or symptoms
  - PET/CT may be useful for identifying possible distant metastases in patients with large primary lesions
    - Debated whether to use for primary detection of metastases or only to verify equivocal CT findings
- **Ultrasound**
  - Primary method for differentiating a cyst from a solid lesion
  - Primary tumor may be variably echogenic relative to background renal cortex
    - Isoechoic
      - May be missed on ultrasound, as tumor may be indistinguishable from background renal parenchyma
      - Look for border contour deformity
    - Hypoechoic
      - Differentiated from a cyst by lack of through transmission
    - Hyperechoic
      - Tend to be smaller
      - May look similar to angiomyolipomas
  - Large lesions often heterogeneous in echotexture
- **CT**
  - NECT and parenchymal phase CECT are necessary for all patients unless contraindicated
  - NECT
    - Variable appearance
      - Small lesions may be homogeneous in attenuation
      - Larger lesions often show central necrosis
      - May have calcifications
      - Almost never contain macroscopic fat
      - May also be primarily cystic
    - Low attenuation
      - Papillary RCCs
    - Moderate attenuation

- May be chromophobe RCC or angiomyolipoma (soft tissue component of mass, lipomatous areas will be low density)
    - High attenuation
      - Clear cell RCC lesions often have mixed pattern
      - High-attenuation regions represent soft tissue areas, while low-attenuation regions are necrotic or cystic
      - Oncocytomas may have a similar appearance on CT
    - Pseudocapsule may be seen as high-density ring surrounding tumor
  - CECT
    - Renal mass protocol includes
      - Thin slice 1.25-2.5 mm
      - Noncontrast and contrast-enhanced acquisitions
      - Arterial phase with 20 second delay helpful for evaluating arterial vessels
      - Nephrographic phase with 60-70 second delay best for evaluating parenchyma
      - Delayed phase with 5-10 minutes delay best for evaluating collecting system
      - Coronal reformatted images also helpful for better defining relationship of tumor to other structures
    - Enhancement pattern during nephrographic phase is most useful for determining type of tumor
    - Gold standard for detection and staging is CT
    - RCCs have variable enhancement patterns
      - Some will enhance briskly
      - Papillary RCCs may have very little enhancement (can be mistaken for a hyperdense cyst with pseudoenhancement)
      - Solid enhancing mass in the kidney is RCC until proven otherwise
- **MR**
  - In general, similar findings to CT
  - Variable signal characteristics and enhancement pattern
  - Typically iso- to hypointense compared to normal renal cortex on T1-weighted images
  - Typically hyperintense on T2-weighted images
  - Cystic RCCs will generally have enhancing septa or mural nodularity
- **PET/CT**
  - Similar findings on CT portion of exam as those discussed above
  - RCCs have variable FDG avidity
    - More helpful when intensely FDG avid
    - Solid mass without FDG activity can still be RCC
    - Not generally used to differentiate benign from malignant renal masses
- **Image-guided biopsies**
  - Not routinely done
  - Can be performed for problem solving
    - e.g., in a patient with a different primary malignancy for differentiating metastasis from primary renal malignancy

Staging
- **Nodal**
  - **Ultrasound**
    - Not used for nodal or metastatic evaluation

RENAL CARCINOMA

- ■ Can be used for problem solving with lesions seen in other organs, e.g., liver
- ■ Can be used to evaluate renal vessels and IVC for patency
  - – CT with contrast likely better to look for vascular invasion
- ○ CT
  - ■ Gold standard for detection of nodes and for evaluation of vascular structures
  - ■ Nodes may hyperenhance
  - ■ Smaller nodes may appear normal
  - ■ Larger nodal metastases may be heterogeneous or have central necrosis
  - ■ Best modality for looking at invasion of perinephric fat and other local structures
- ○ MR
  - ■ Typically reserved for patients with renal insufficiency or contraindications for CT contrast
  - ■ Particularly useful for determining invasion and extent of involvement into IVC
- ○ PET/CT
  - ■ For RCC metastases using FDG PET
    - – Sensitivity (63%), specificity (100%), PPV (100%)
    - – Higher than CT alone
  - ■ For identification and characterization of primary RCC tumors
    - – Sensitivity (47%), specificity (80%), accuracy (51%)
    - – Lower than CT alone
    - – False-negatives are due to urinary excretion of tracer in some tumors
  - ■ Lesions ≤ 1 cm have far lower sensitivity due to scanner limitations
- ○ CTA or MRA
  - ■ Can be helpful in establishing tumor relation to vascular supplies
  - ■ Also potentially useful for nephron sparing or laparoscopic procedures
- • Metastatic disease
  - ○ **Metastatic location frequencies**
    - ■ Lung (75%)
    - ■ Soft tissue (35%)
    - ■ Bone (20%)
    - ■ Liver (20%)
    - ■ Adrenal glands (19%)
    - ■ Cutaneous tissues (8%)
    - ■ CNS (8%)
  - ○ CT
    - ■ Tumor extension or thrombus via renal vein (23%), inferior vena cava (7%)
    - ■ Usually seen as hypervascular metastases
  - ○ MR
    - ■ On T1 post-contrast imaging, RCC usually enhances less than renal tissue
    - ■ Multiplanar capacity of MR allows ideal assessment of renal vein and IVC
    - ■ Preferred to evaluate for intracranial metastases
    - ■ Staging with MR is equal or better to CT
  - ○ PET/CT
    - ■ FDG uptake by RCC primary or metastatic lesion is variable
    - ■ PET and PET/CT are more clinically helpful when positive

- ■ Negative exam may be true negative or non-FDG-avid RCC
- ■ 80-100% specific for bony metastases

Restaging
- • **Ultrasound**
  - ○ Risk increases without clean surgical margins
  - ○ Small bowel occupying nephrectomy bed can be mistaken for recurrence
  - ○ Ultrasound is not acceptable for monitoring nephrectomy bed
- • CT
  - ○ Useful to follow patients after treatment
  - ○ 20-30% of patients with apparent localized renal cell carcinoma at time of surgery relapse following radical nephrectomy
    - ■ Majority are distant metastases
    - ■ Usually relapse within 3 years
  - ○ Lung metastases are most common late relapse finding
    - ■ May appear as hemorrhagic metastases, show lymphatic invasion, or produce consolidation
  - ○ Bone metastases are less common
  - ○ Rarely, pancreatic lesions are identified
- • MR
  - ○ MR is superior to CT in assessing venous involvement
  - ○ CT is currently preferred to MR in following patients for disease recurrence after surgery
- • PET/CT
  - ○ Nephrectomy bed has highest area of recurrence (20-40%)
  - ○ Partial nephrectomy patients should have remnant carefully evaluated
    - ■ Recurrence rates in remnant are 4-6% within 2-4 years, depending on stage
    - ■ Some recurrence may be from incomplete margins, while others represent multifocal disease
  - ○ Thoracic involvement should be evaluated by CT
  - ○ Bone scan and brain MR may be performed with appropriate clinical indications
  - ○ PET/CT has been shown useful for both local recurrence and metastases
  - ○ Metastatic frequency by tumor stage
    - ■ T1 disease (7.1%)
    - ■ T2 disease (26.5%)
    - ■ T3 disease (39.4%)

CLINICAL ISSUES

Presentation
- • "Classic" triad
  - ○ Hematuria
  - ○ Flank pain
  - ○ Abdominal mass
- • < 15% of patients present with classic triad
- • Other signs and symptoms include
  - ○ Weight loss
  - ○ Fever
  - ○ Hypercalcemia
  - ○ Night sweats
  - ○ Malaise
  - ○ Hypertension

RENAL CARCINOMA

- Roughly half of cases are identified as incidental finding on imaging
- Remainder are suspected based on
  - Various symptoms of paraneoplastic syndromes
  - Direct effects of tumor metastasis
  - Identification of palpable renal mass

Cancer Natural History & Prognosis

- 5-year survival by stage
  - T1a N0 M0 (70-90%)
  - T1b N0 M0 (80-90%)
  - T2 N0 M0 (70-80%)
  - Organ confined, T1-T2 N0 M0 (70-90%)
  - Invasion of perinephric fat, T3a N0 M0 (60-80%)
  - Venous involvement, T3b-T3c N0 M0 (40-65%)
  - Adrenal involvement, T4 N0 M0 (0-30%)
  - Locally advanced, T4 N0 M0 (0-20%)
  - Lymph involvement, any T, N+, M0 (0-20%)
  - Systemic metastases, any T, any N, M1 (0-10%)

Treatment Options

- Major treatment alternatives
  - Surgery is treatment of choice unless late stage
  - Alternatives
    - Radiofrequency ablation
    - Cryoablation
    - Ultrasound ablation
    - Microwave radiotherapy
  - Currently no recommendation for adjuvant therapy for resection of primary tumor
- Major treatment roadblocks
  - RCC typically have high levels of MDR protein, making chemotherapy difficult
- Treatment options by primary tumor stage
  - T1a: Nephron-sparing surgery preferred, radical nephrectomy in some selected patients
  - T1b-T2: Radical nephrectomy recommended, laparoscopic preferred
  - T3-T4: Radical open nephrectomy recommended

REPORTING CHECKLIST

T Staging

- Ideally, report should include bidirectional axial dimensions and coronal dimension
- Report any obvious or questionable spread outside of kidney into Gerota fascia

N Staging

- Report size and confidence level of all retroperitoneal nodes near level of renal veins
- Any nodes > 1 cm should be reported as suspicious
- Nodes ≤ 1 cm should be reported as indeterminate
- Look for additional features of central necrosis or hyperenhancement

M Staging

- Must report whether there is adrenal involvement, as this may affect whether a radical nephrectomy will be performed
  - If there is adrenal asymmetry or nodularity, consider further evaluation prior to surgery

SELECTED REFERENCES

1. American Joint Committee on Cancer: AJCC Cancer Staging Manual. 7th ed. New York: Springer, 2010
2. Bach AM et al: Contemporary radiologic imaging of renal cortical tumors. Urol Clin North Am. 35(4):593-604; vi, 2008
3. Hinshaw JL et al: Comparison of percutaneous and laparoscopic cryoablation for the treatment of solid renal masses. AJR Am J Roentgenol. 191(4):1159-68, 2008
4. Zhang J et al: Imaging of kidney cancer. Radiol Clin North Am. 45(1):119-47, 2007
5. Blitman NM et al: Renal medullary carcinoma: CT and MRI features. AJR Am J Roentgenol. 185(1):268-72, 2005
6. Ergen FB et al: MRI for preoperative staging of renal cell carcinoma using the 1997 TNM classification: comparison with surgical and pathologic staging. AJR Am J Roentgenol. 182(1):217-25, 2004
7. Reznek RH: CT/MRI in staging renal cell carcinoma. Cancer Imaging. 4 Spec No A:S25-32, 2004
8. Israel GM et al: Renal imaging for diagnosis and staging of renal cell carcinoma. Urol Clin North Am. 30(3):499-514, 2003
9. Walter C et al: Imaging of renal lesions: evaluation of fast MRI and helical CT. Br J Radiol. 76(910):696-703, 2003
10. Kim JK et al: Differentiation of subtypes of renal cell carcinoma on helical CT scans. AJR Am J Roentgenol. 178(6):1499-506, 2002
11. Ramdave S et al: Clinical role of F-18 fluorodeoxyglucose positron emission tomography for detection and management of renal cell carcinoma. J Urol. 166(3):825-30, 2001
12. Vasselli JR et al: Lack of retroperitoneal lymphadenopathy predicts survival of patients with metastatic renal cell carcinoma. J Urol. 166(1):68-72, 2001
13. Coll DM et al: 3-dimensional volume rendered computerized tomography for preoperative evaluation and intraoperative treatment of patients undergoing nephron sparing surgery. J Urol. 161(4):1097-102, 1999
14. Bechtold RE et al: Imaging approach to staging of renal cell carcinoma. Urol Clin North Am. 24(3):507-22, 1997
15. Kopka L et al: Dual-phase helical CT of the kidney: value of the corticomedullary and nephrographic phase for evaluation of renal lesions and preoperative staging of renal cell carcinoma. AJR Am J Roentgenol. 169(6):1573-8, 1997
16. Jamis-Dow CA et al: Small (< or = 3-cm) renal masses: detection with CT versus US and pathologic correlation. Radiology. 198(3):785-8, 1996
17. Curry NS: Small renal masses (lesions smaller than 3 cm): imaging evaluation and management. AJR Am J Roentgenol. 164(2):355-62, 1995
18. Newhouse JH: The radiologic evaluation of the patient with renal cancer. Urol Clin North Am. 20(2):231-46, 1993
19. Yamashita Y et al: Small renal cell carcinoma: pathologic and radiologic correlation. Radiology. 184(2):493-8, 1992
20. McClennan BL: Oncologic imaging. Staging and follow-up of renal and adrenal carcinoma. Cancer. 67(4 Suppl):1199-208, 1991
21. Fein AB et al: Diagnosis and staging of renal cell carcinoma: a comparison of MR imaging and CT. AJR Am J Roentgenol. 148(4):749-53, 1987
22. Hricak H et al: Magnetic resonance imaging in the diagnosis and staging of renal and perirenal neoplasms. Radiology. 154(3):709-15, 1985
23. Mauro MA et al: Renal cell carcinoma: angiography in the CT era. AJR Am J Roentgenol. 139(6):1135-8, 1982

RENAL CARCINOMA

Stage I (T1a N0 M0)

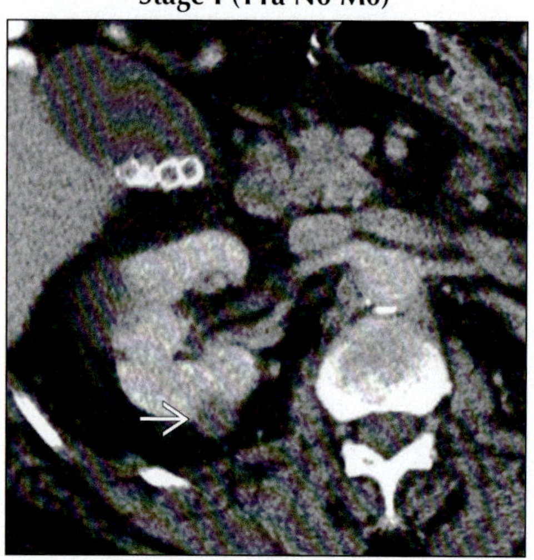

Stage I (T1a N0 M0)

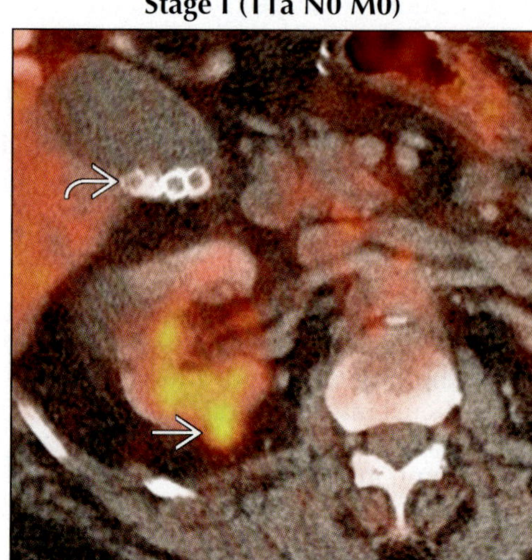

(Left) Axial CECT shows a small (just over 1 cm), low-attenuation, enhancing lesion ➡ in the posterior mid pole right kidney. Although nonspecific, the enhancement makes this suspicious for a renal cell carcinoma. *(Right)* Axial PET/CT shows focal FDG within the pathologically confirmed T1a renal cell carcinoma ➡ in the right kidney. Renal cell carcinomas have variable FDG uptake, but intensely FDG-avid lesions should be viewed as very suspicious. Note the gallstones ➡.

Stage I (T1a N0 M0)

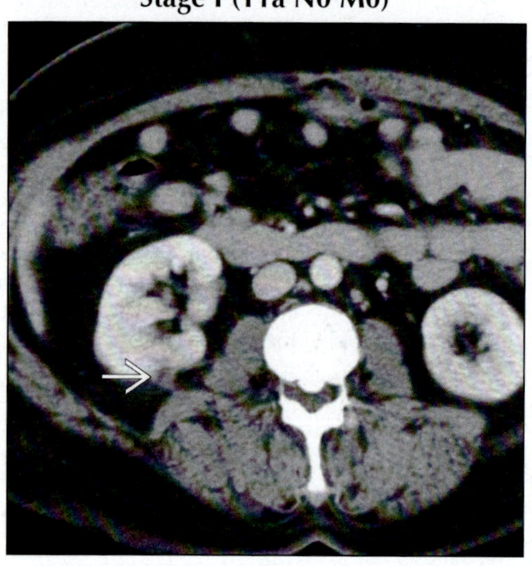

Stage I (T1a N0 M0)

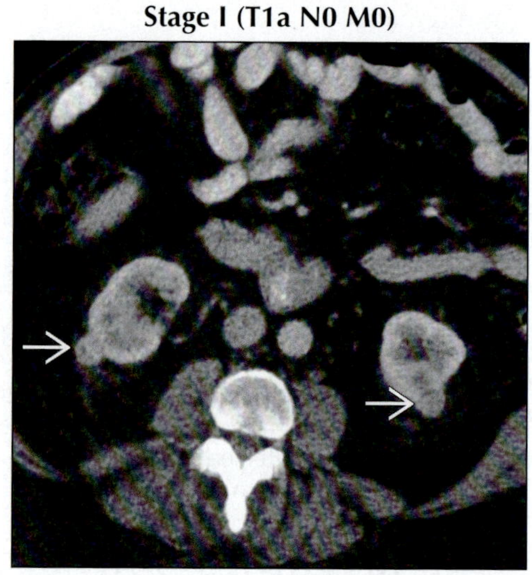

(Left) Axial CECT shows a 1 cm, incidentally discovered T1a renal cell carcinoma ➡ in the posterior mid pole right kidney, subsequently treated with radiofrequency ablation. *(Right)* Axial CECT shows bilateral enhancing renal lesions ➡ in this patient with von Hippel-Lindau, compatible with bilateral T1a renal cell carcinomas. T1a lesions are those less than or equal to 4 cm in greatest dimension and limited to the kidney.

Stage I (T1a N0 M0)

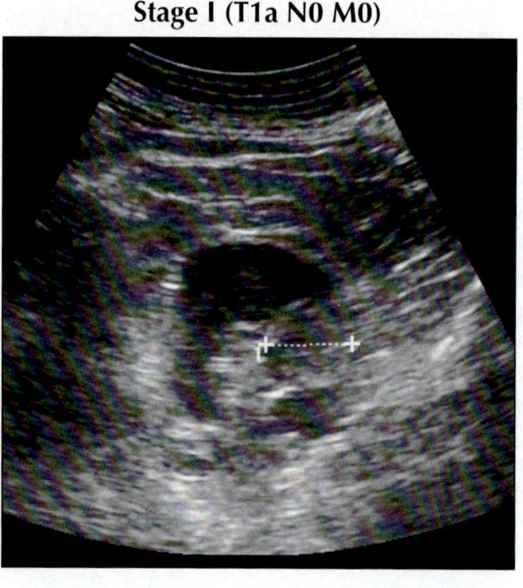

Stage I (T1a N0 M0)

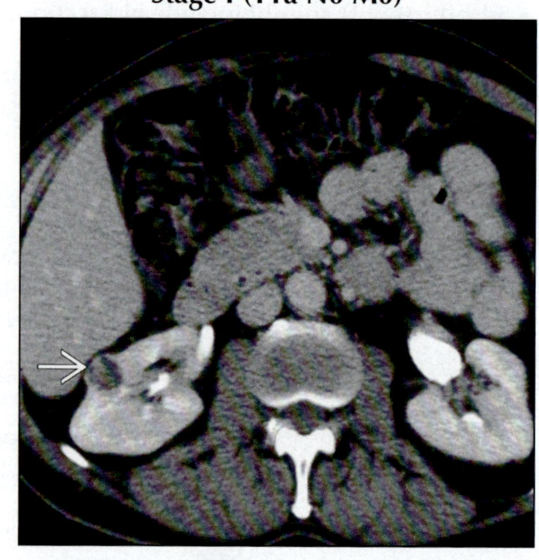

(Left) Transverse transabdominal ultrasound shows a 1.7 cm T1a renal cell carcinoma (calipers) that is iso- to slightly hyperechoic compared to normal background renal cortical tissue. *(Right)* Axial CECT shows a T1a renal cell carcinoma ➡ in the lateral aspect of the mid pole right kidney. The mass is low attenuation with areas of enhancement, characteristic of many renal cell carcinomas.

Stage I (T1a N0 M0)

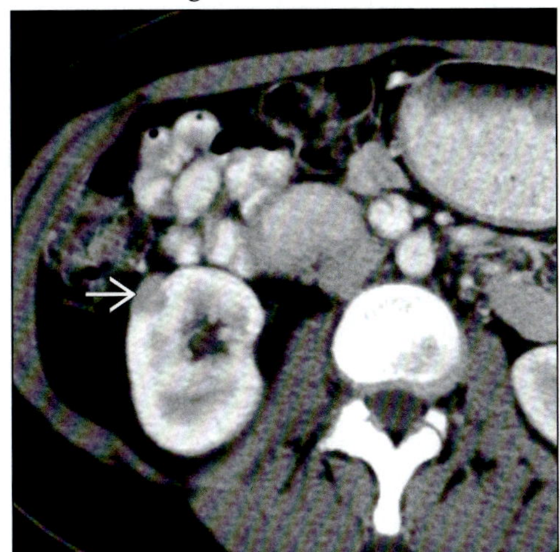

Stage I (T1a N0 M0)

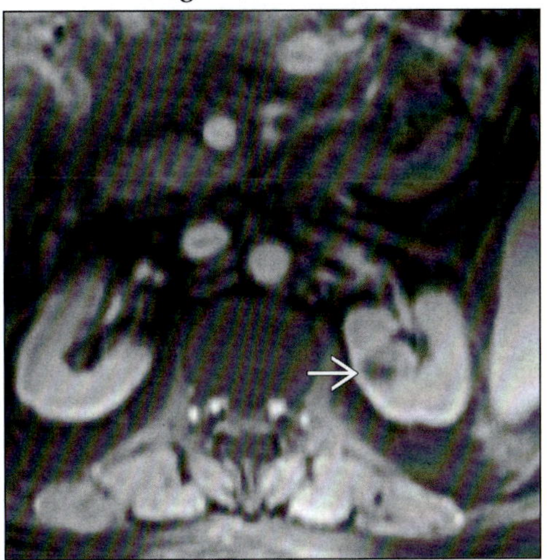

(Left) Axial CECT shows an enhancing low-attenuation lesion ➡ measuring just over 1 cm in the right kidney. The lesion was discovered incidentally and proved to be a small renal cell carcinoma (T1a) at pathology. *(Right)* Axial T1WI C+ FS MR shows a 1.5 cm mass ➡ in the medial aspect of the mid pole left kidney with heterogeneous signal characteristics and some enhancement, compatible with a T1a renal cell carcinoma.

Stage I (T1a N0 M0)

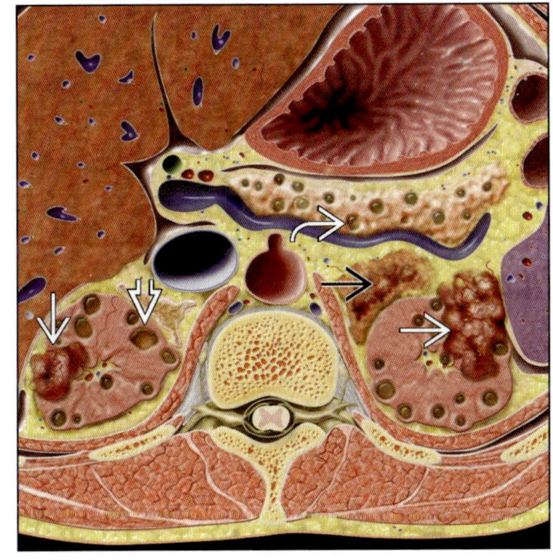

Stage I (T1a N0 M0)

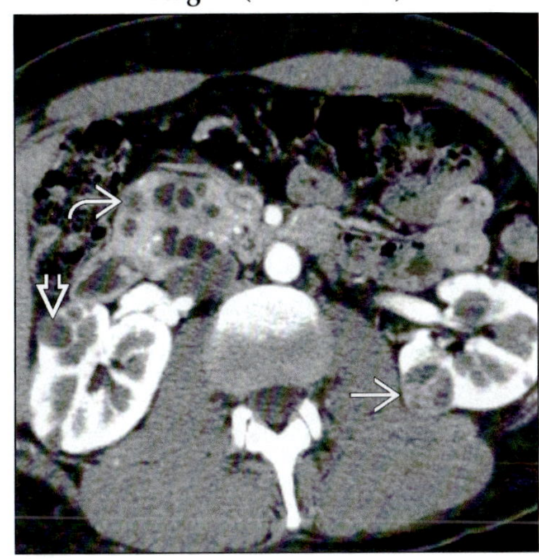

(Left) Axial graphic shows multiple renal cysts ➡, pancreatic cysts ➡, a pheochromocytoma ➡, and bilateral renal cell carcinomas ➡ in a patient with von Hippel-Lindau syndrome. As these lesions are confined to the kidney and less than 4 cm in their largest dimension, they are all T1a. *(Right)* Axial CECT in a patient with von Hippel-Lindau shows multiple renal cysts ➡, pancreatic cysts ➡, and a 2 cm renal cell carcinoma ➡, compatible with a T1a lesion.

Stage I (T1a N0 M0)

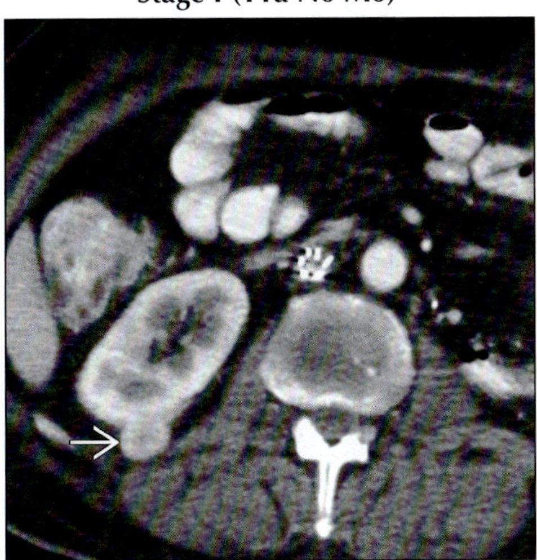

Stage I (T1a N0 M0)

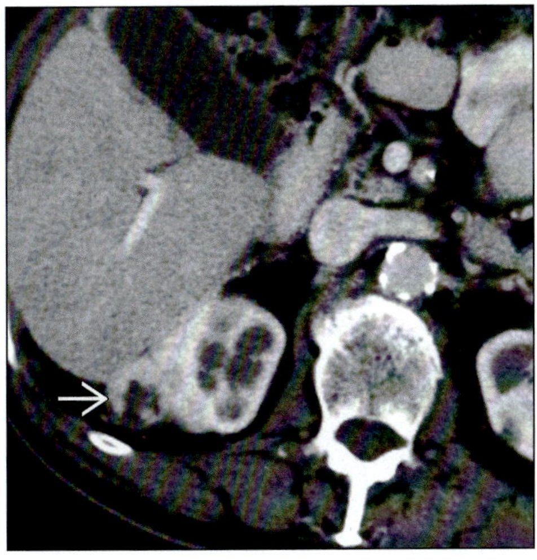

(Left) Axial CECT shows an exophytic, enhancing, solid mass ➡ in the posterior aspect of the right kidney, measuring approximately 2 cm and compatible with a T1a lesion. *(Right)* Axial CECT shows a heterogeneously enhancing exophytic mass ➡ with areas of central low attenuation or necrosis arising off the lateral aspect of the right kidney, compatible with a renal cell carcinoma.

RENAL CARCINOMA

Stage I (T1a N0 M0)

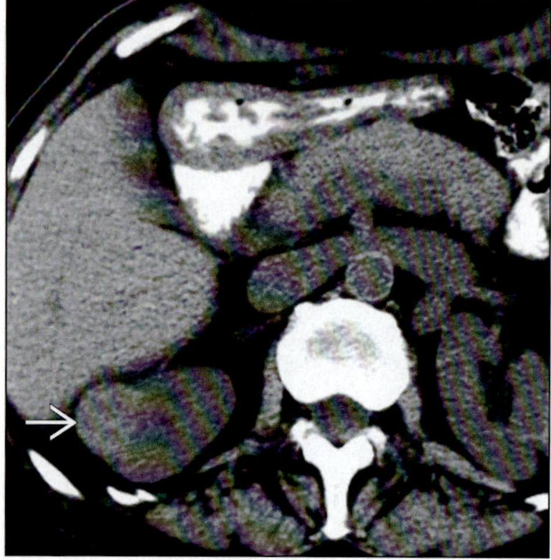

Stage I (T1a N0 M0)

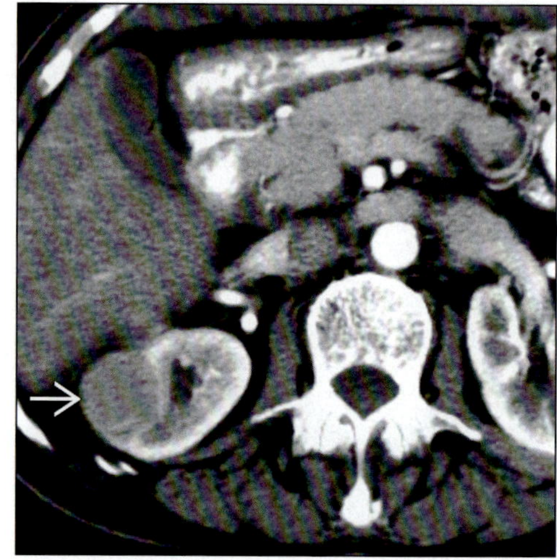

(Left) Axial NECT in a patient with a papillary renal cell carcinoma shows a solid mass ⇒ arising from the lateral superior pole of the right kidney and measuring approximately 30 Hounsfield units. *(Right)* Axial CECT in the same patient shows the region of interest post contrast at 50 Hounsfield units ⇒ indicating mild enhancement. Renal cell carcinomas generally show enhancement, though papillary cell types may enhance only mildly.

Stage I (T1a N0 M0)

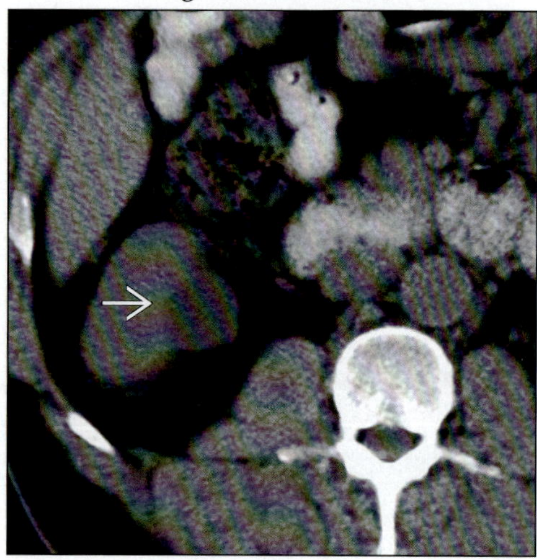

Stage I (T1a N0 M0)

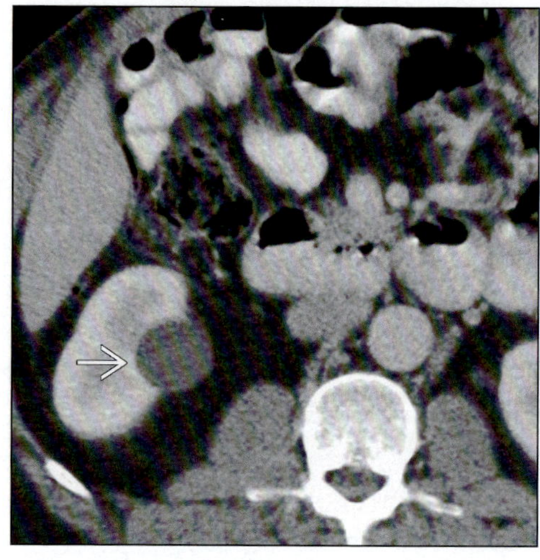

(Left) Axial NECT shows a solid mass ⇒ arising from the medial inferior pole of the right kidney and measuring 23 Hounsfield units. *(Right)* Axial CECT in the same patient demonstrates the mass ⇒ with post-contrast region of interest showing 39 Hounsfield units, indicating mild enhancement. Pathology confirmed papillary cell type. Being less than 4 cm, this lesion would be categorized T1a.

Stage I (T1a N0 M0)

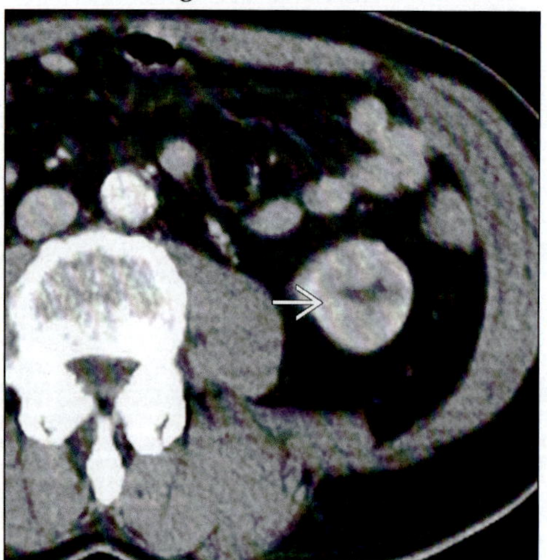

Stage I (T1a N0 M0)

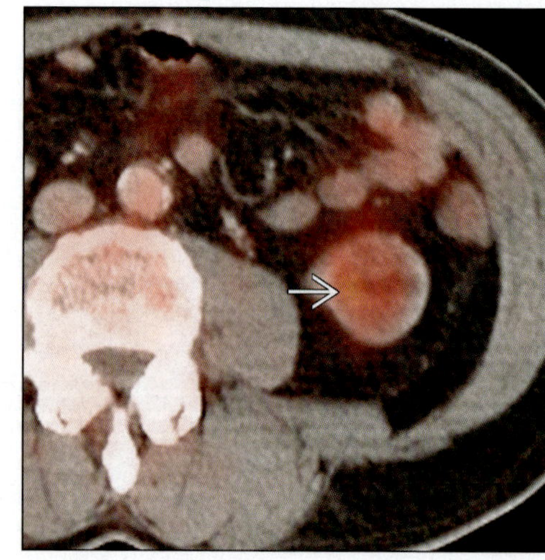

(Left) Axial CECT shows a 3.1 cm, solid, enhancing mass ⇒ in the inferior pole left kidney with areas of central necrosis, compatible with a T1a renal cell carcinoma. *(Right)* Axial fused PET/CT in the same patient shows minimal diffuse FDG activity in the mass with the exception of an area of slightly more increased activity medially ⇒. Renal cell carcinomas tend to have variable FDG activity but may have almost no increased metabolic activity.

RENAL CARCINOMA

Stage I (T1a N0 M0)

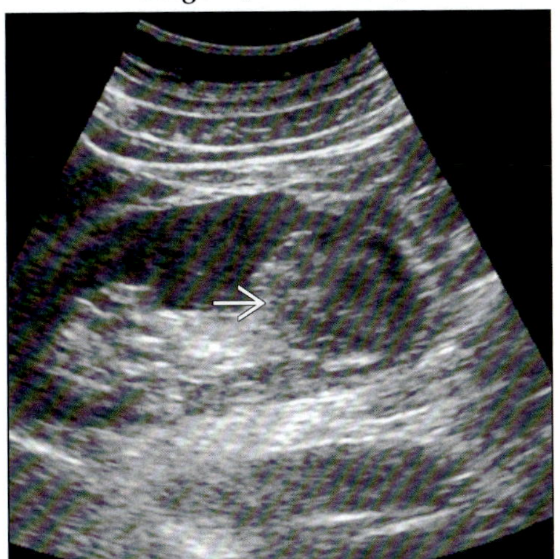

Stage I (T1a N0 M0)

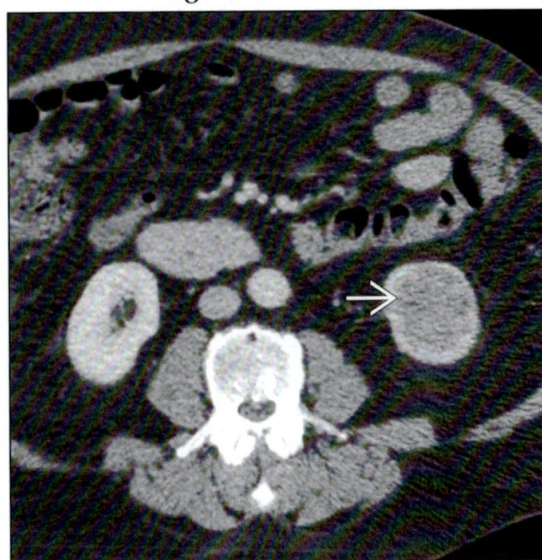

(Left) Transverse transabdominal ultrasound shows a slightly hyperechoic, almost 3 cm, solid mass ➡ in the inferior pole left kidney. The ultrasound findings are worrisome for a renal cell carcinoma. A 3 cm mass would be defined as a T1a lesion. *(Right)* Axial CECT in the same patient shows a moderately enhancing, solid renal mass ➡ compatible with a renal cell carcinoma. Pathology confirmed a T1a clear cell carcinoma.

Stage I (T1a N0 M0)

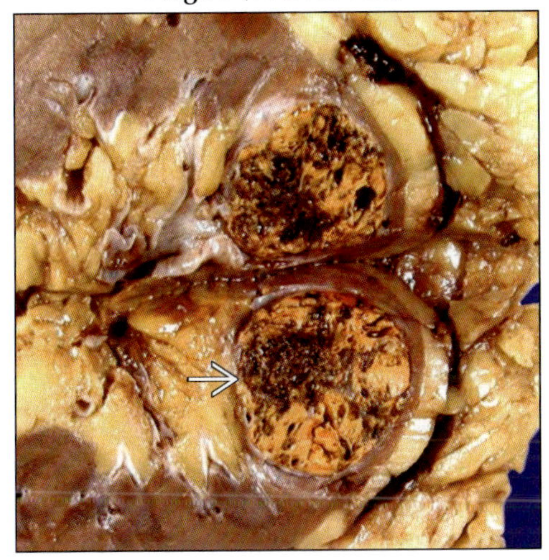

Stage I (T1a N0 M0)

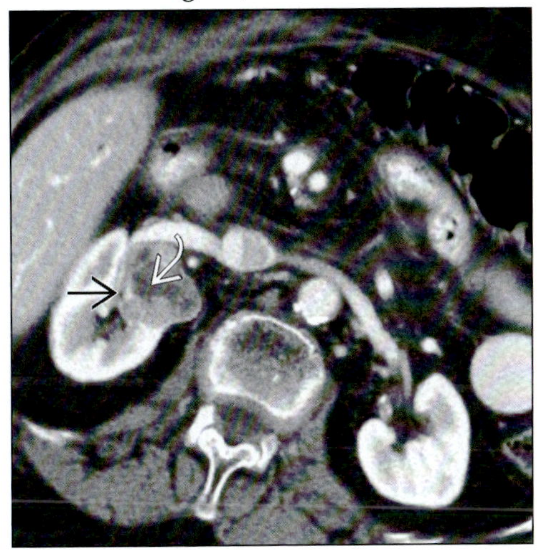

(Left) Bisected correlative pathologic specimen from the same patient shows the mass ➡ in the inferior pole left kidney to be 2.8 cm, confined to the kidney, and without positive nodes, compatible with a stage I (T1a N0 M0) lesion. *(Right)* Axial CECT in another patient shows a 3 cm mass ➡ in the medial aspect of the mid pole right kidney displaying areas of peripheral solid enhancement and central low attenuation ➡, likely indicating areas of necrosis.

Stage I (T1a N0 M0)

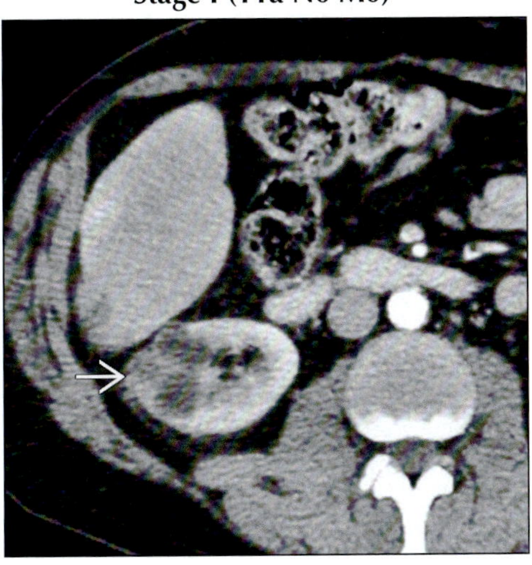

Stage I (T1a N0 M0)

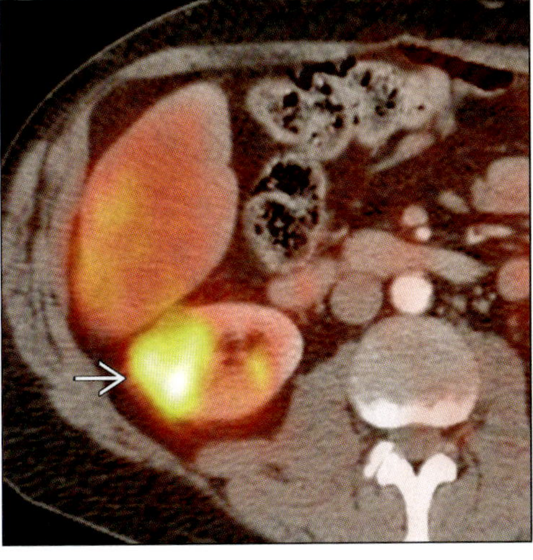

(Left) Axial CECT shows a complex mass ➡ arising from the lateral aspect of the mid pole right kidney. The low attenuation areas were solid, making this suspicious for a renal cell carcinoma. *(Right)* Axial fused PET/CT in the same patient shows intense FDG activity in the complex renal cortical mass, compatible with a T1a renal cell carcinoma. In contrast to the prior case, there is intense FDG activity ➡.

RENAL CARCINOMA

Stage I (T1b N0 M0)

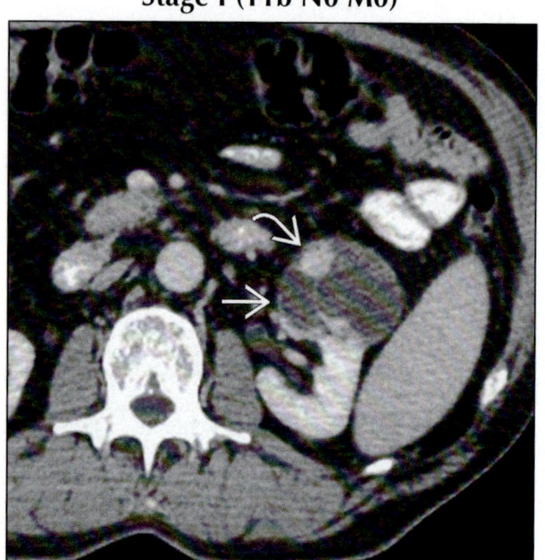

Stage I (T1b N0 M0)

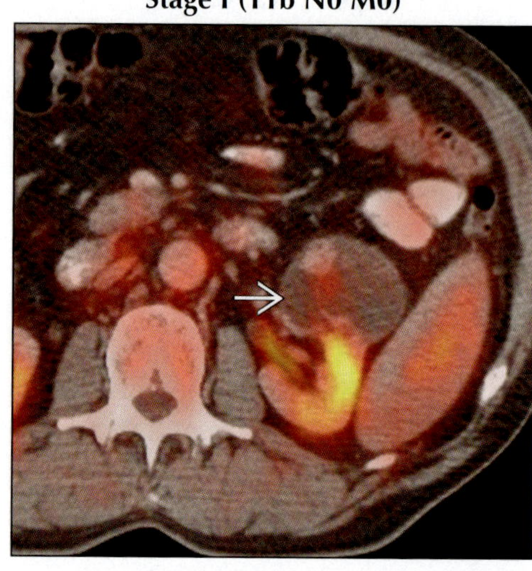

(Left) Axial CECT shows a 4.3 cm complex cystic mass ➡ arising from the anterior aspect of the mid pole left kidney with enhancing mural nodularity ➡, compatible with a T1b renal cell carcinoma. (Right) Axial fused PET/CT in the same patient shows almost no increased metabolic activity ➡ within the renal cell carcinoma, a fairly common finding identified on FDG PET in patients with renal cell carcinoma.

Stage I (T1b N0 M0)

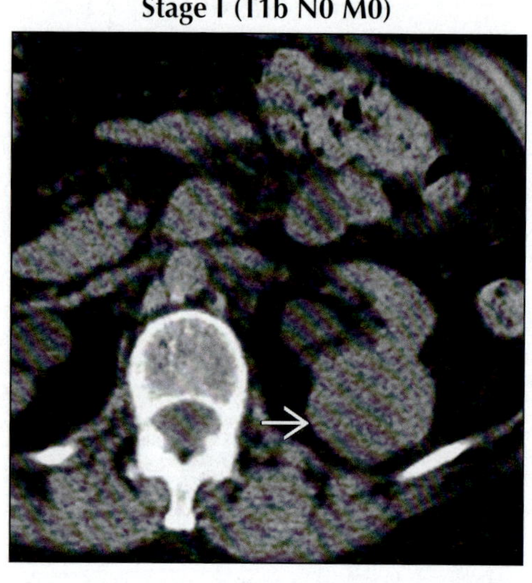

Stage I (T1b N0 M0)

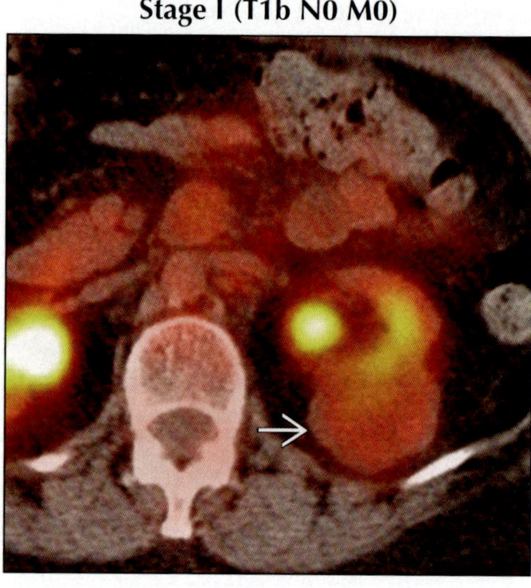

(Left) Axial NECT shows an exophytic solid renal mass ➡ in the posterior aspect of the mid pole left kidney, subsequently shown to be a 4.6 cm (T1b) renal cell carcinoma. (Right) Axial fused PET/CT in the same patient shows very little FDG activity in the renal cell carcinoma ➡. As renal cell carcinomas tend to have variable metabolic activity, the lack of increased metabolic activity does not exclude a renal cell carcinoma.

Stage I (T1b N0 M0)

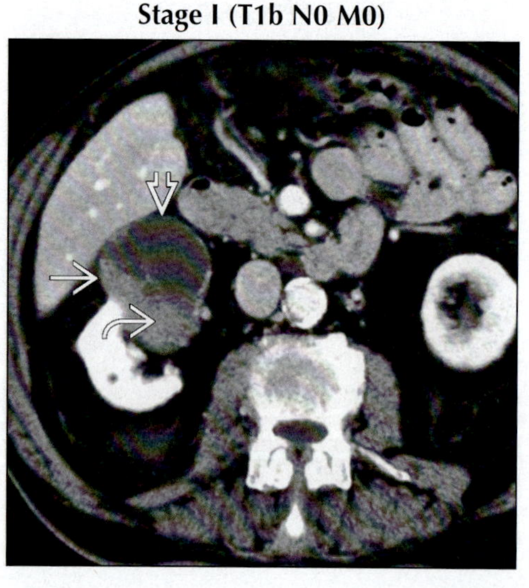

Stage I (T1b N0 M0)

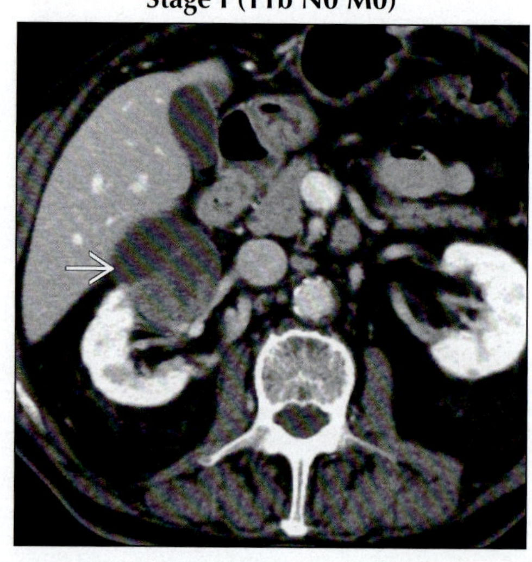

(Left) Axial CECT shows a complex cystic mass ➡ in the anterior mid pole right kidney with areas of enhancement posteriorly ➡ and more cystic areas anteriorly ➡, worrisome for a renal cell carcinoma. (Right) Axial CECT in the same patient shows similar findings of a renal mass ➡ with cystic complexity (areas of solid and cystic change). Subsequent nephrectomy showed a 4.7 cm (T1b) renal cell carcinoma.

RENAL CARCINOMA

Stage I (T1b N0 M0)

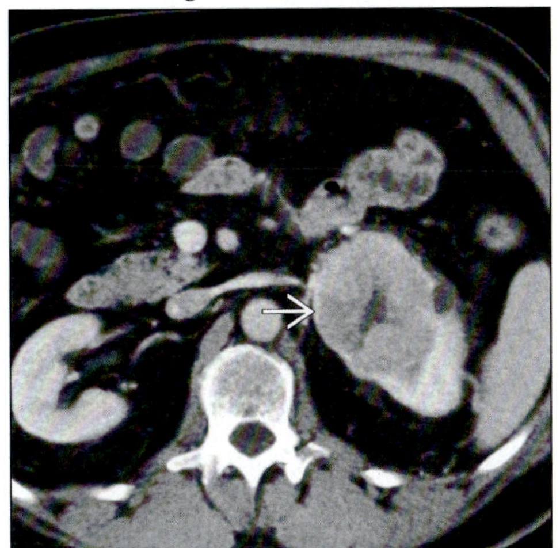

Stage I (T1b N0 M0)

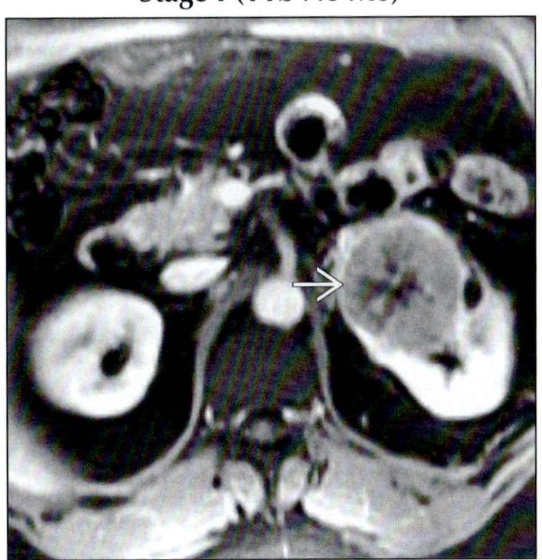

(Left) Axial CECT shows a 5 cm mass ➡ in the left kidney with heterogeneous enhancement and central low attenuation, compatible with a renal cell carcinoma. The differential diagnosis may include an oncocytoma, which also characteristically has a central scar. (Right) Axial T1WI C+ FS MR in the same patient shows a correlative MR image of an enhancing solid mass ➡ in the left kidney, most compatible with a renal cell carcinoma.

Stage I (T1b N0 M0)

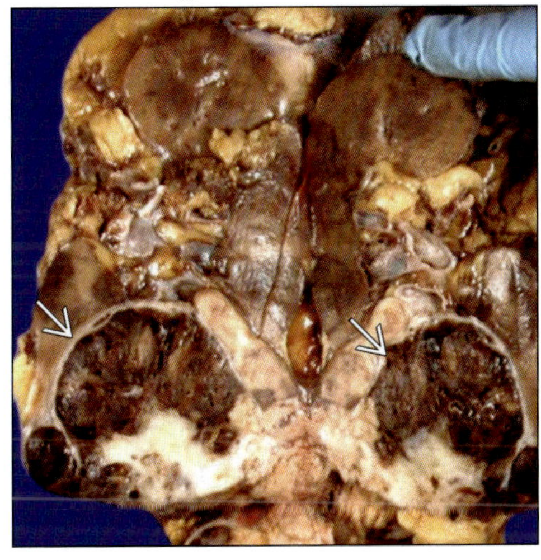

Stage I (T1b N0 M0)

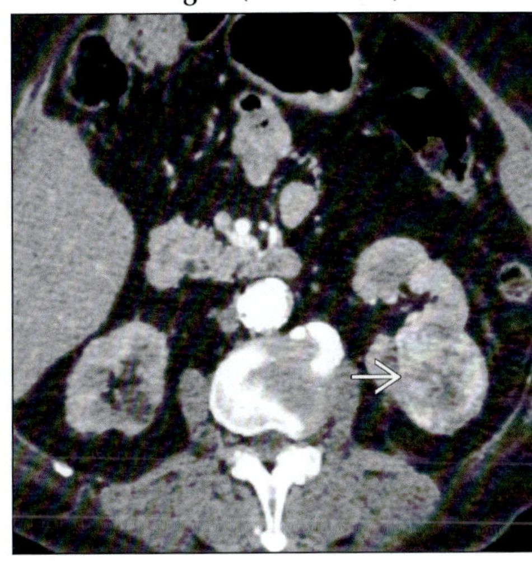

(Left) Cut gross pathologic specimen from the same patient shows the heterogeneous mass ➡ in the left kidney. This proved to be a stage I lesion (T1b). (Right) Axial CECT in another patient shows a fairly vascular mass ➡ in the posterior aspect of the midpole left kidney. The mass measures over 4 cm and is compatible with a T1b renal cell carcinoma.

Stage I (T1b N0 M0)

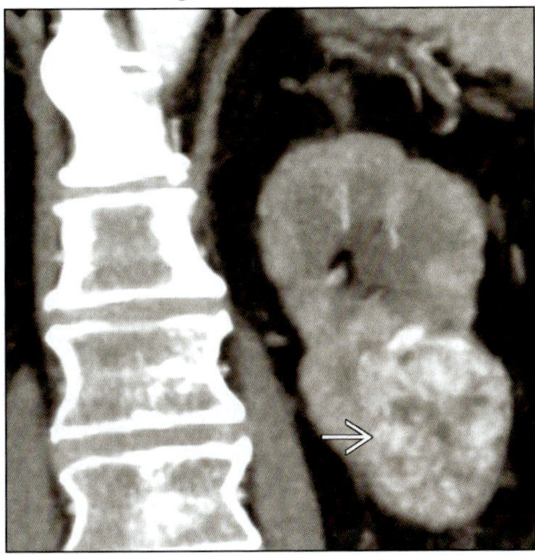

Stage I (T1b N0 M0)

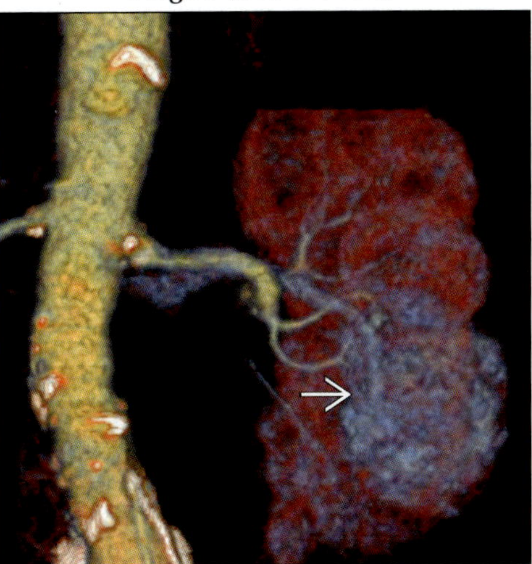

(Left) Coronal CECT in the same patient shows the renal cell carcinoma to be relatively vascular ➡ compared to the background renal parenchyma. (Right) Reconstructed image from an abdominal CTA in the same patient as the previous 2 images shows the relative vascularity of the inferior pole renal cell carcinoma ➡ compared to the background renal vascularity.

RENAL CARCINOMA

Stage I (T1b N0 M0)

(Left) Coronal T2WI FS MR shows a heterogeneous mass ➡ in the inferior pole of the left kidney, worrisome for a renal cell carcinoma. This lesion measures approximately 5.5 cm and is compatible with a T1b lesion. *(Right)* Correlative coronal cut gross pathologic specimen shows the complex inferior pole lesion ➡, which was found to be a clear cell carcinoma of the kidney.

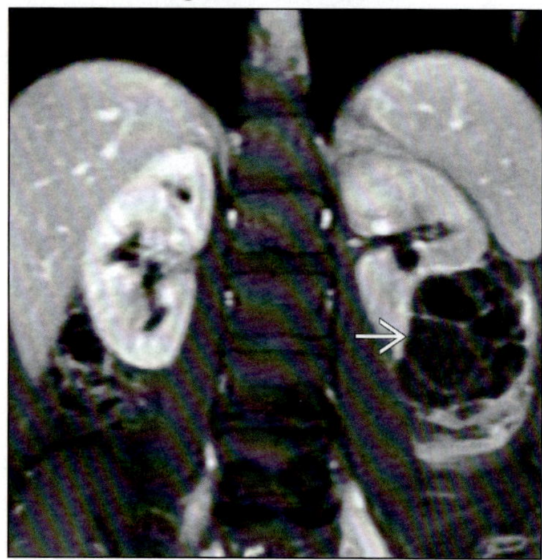

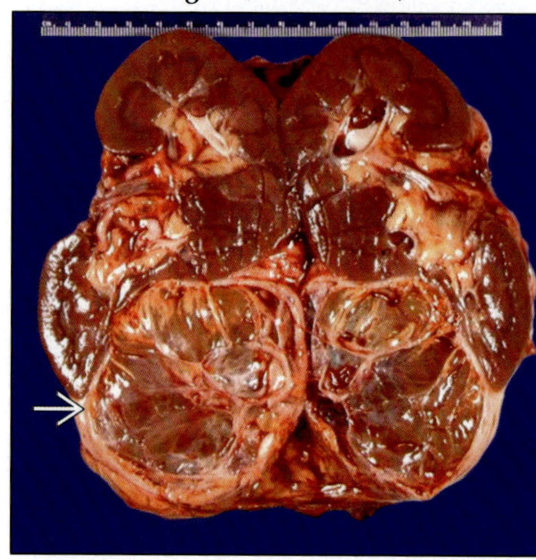

Stage I (T1b N0 M0)

(Left) Axial T1WI C+ FS MR shows an example of a T1b lesion ➡ in the posterior aspect of the inferior pole right kidney. In this case, the margins of the tumor are fairly well circumscribed, and the internal signal of the lesion is somewhat complex. *(Right)* Coronal T1WI C+ FS MR shows a 5.5 cm enhancing mass ➡ in the inferior pole of the right kidney, subsequently confirmed pathologically as a renal cell carcinoma.

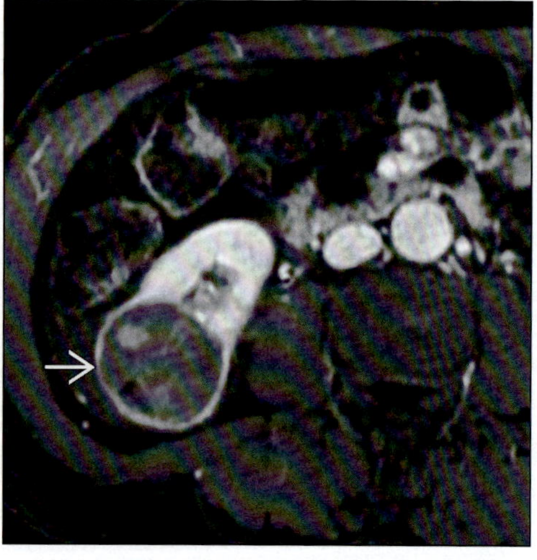

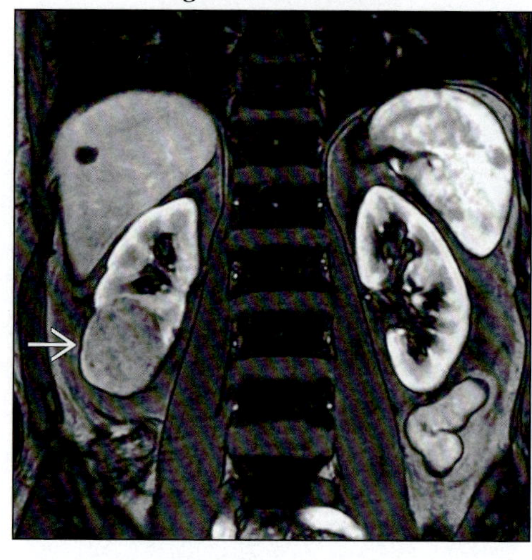

Stage I (T1b N0 M0)

(Left) Axial CECT shows a heterogeneously enhancing mass ➡ arising in the left kidney. The mass measures 5.6 cm and is compatible with a T1b lesion. The etiology of the perinephric stranding ➡ medially is unclear on this image. *(Right)* Axial CECT in the same patient with a 12 minute delay shows contrast extravasation ➡ from a ruptured calyx secondary to obstruction and possible direct tumor invasion ➡.

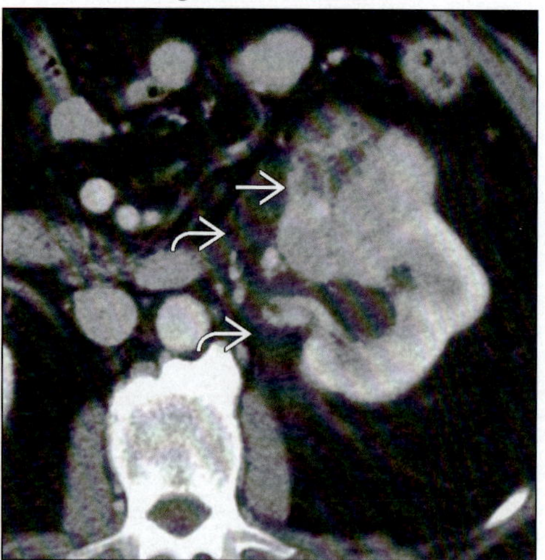

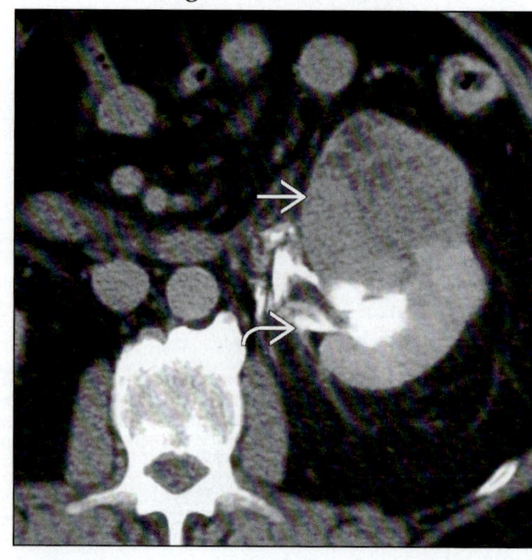

RENAL CARCINOMA

Stage I (T1b N0 M0)

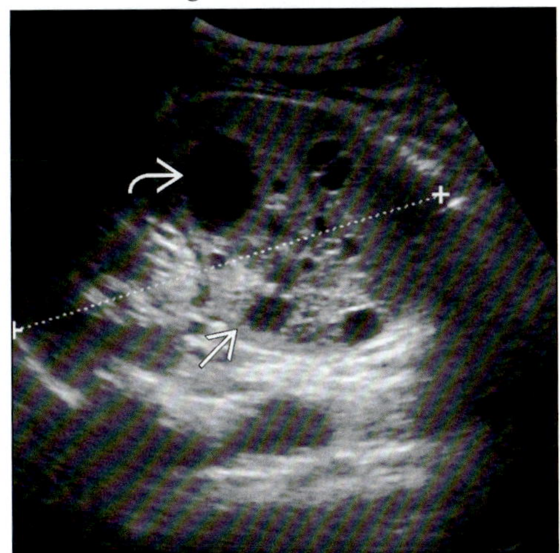

Stage I (T1b N0 M0)

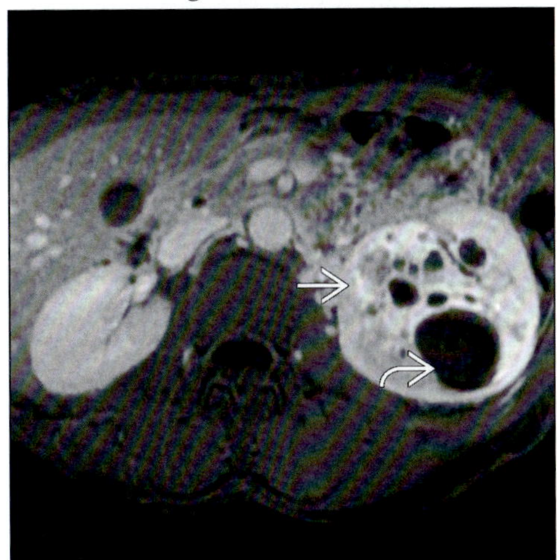

(Left) Longitudinal transabdominal ultrasound shows a 5.8 cm (T1b) mass ➡ arising from the inferior pole left kidney with heterogeneous echotexture and areas of cystic change ➡. (Right) Axial T1WI C+ FS MR in the same patient shows a correlative MR image of the complex inferior pole left kidney renal cell carcinoma ➡ with central cystic areas ➡.

Stage I (T1b N0 M0)

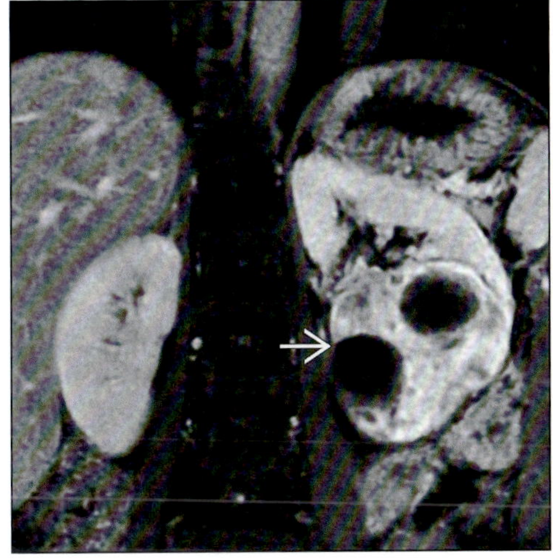

Stage I (T1b N0 M0)

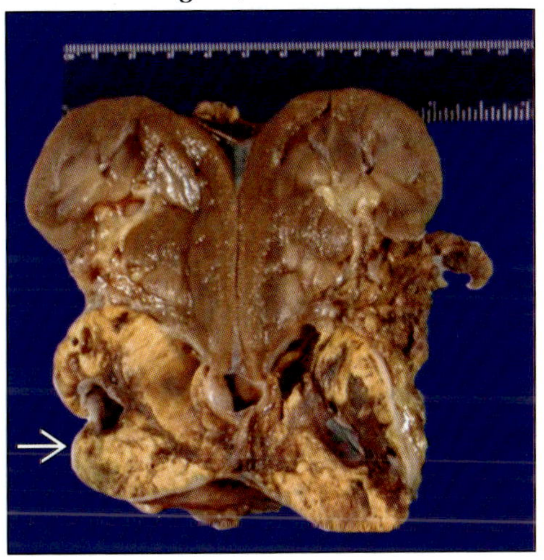

(Left) Coronal T1WI C+ FS MR in the same patient as the previous 2 images shows the mass ➡ prior to nephrectomy, again displaying complex internal signal representing areas of solid and cystic components. No regional adenopathy was identified. (Right) Cut gross pathologic specimen from the same patient shows the renal cell carcinoma as a yellowish-red lesion ➡ with areas of internal cystic change. The final pathology was stage I.

Stage I (T1b N0 M0)

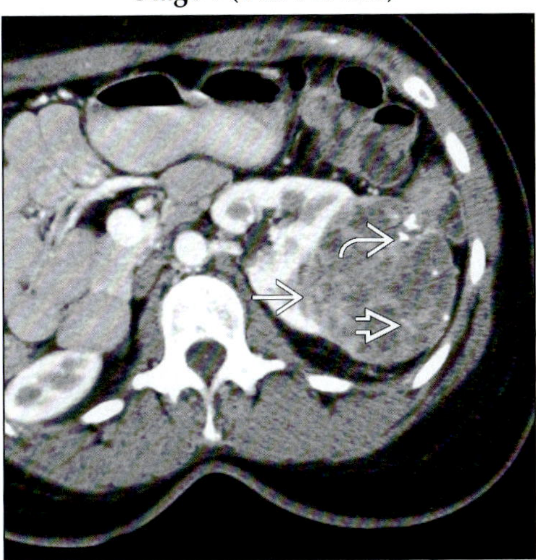

Stage I (T1b N0 M0)

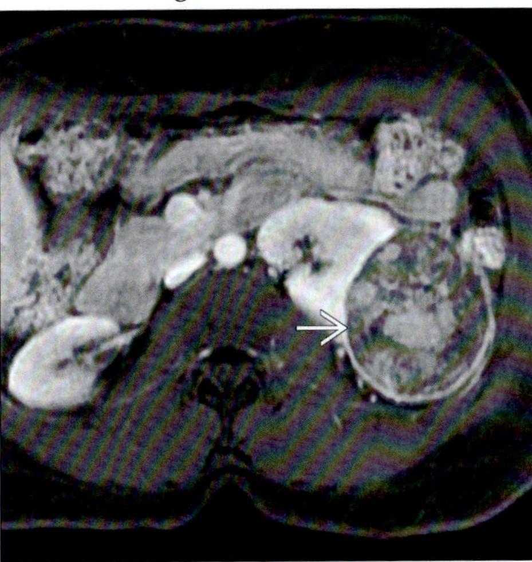

(Left) Axial CECT shows a 6 cm complex mass ➡ in the left kidney. The mass has internal components characteristic of renal cell carcinoma, including multiple enhancing septations ➡ and calcifications ➡. The size is compatible with a T1b renal cell carcinoma. (Right) Axial T1WI C+ FS MR shows a 6.2 cm solid mass ➡ arising from the posterior aspect of the mid pole left kidney with complex internal signal. These findings are compatible with a T1b renal cell carcinoma.

RENAL CARCINOMA

Stage I (T1b N0 M0)

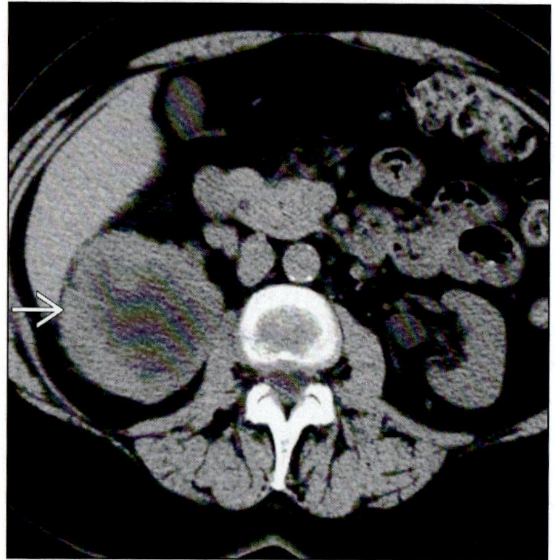

Stage I (T1b N0 M0)

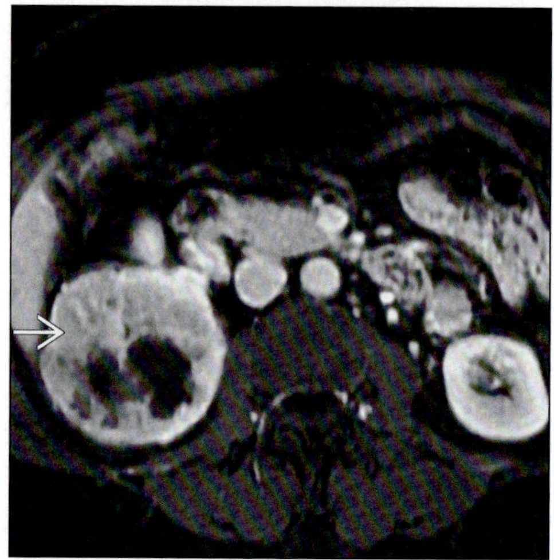

(Left) Axial NECT shows a 6.4 cm mass ➡ arising from the superior pole right kidney and suspicious for a primary renal cell carcinoma (T1b), although incompletely evaluated on this noncontrast CT. *(Right)* Axial T1WI C+ FS MR in the same patient shows a large complex mass ➡ in the right kidney with areas of abnormal enhancement, compatible with a primary renal cell carcinoma.

Stage I (T1b N0 M0)

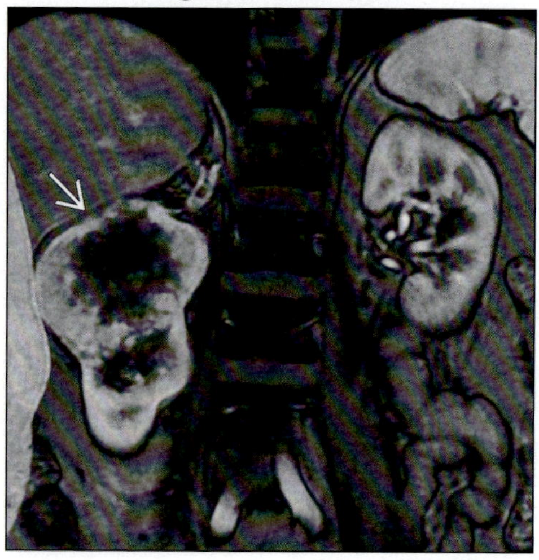

Stage I (T1b N0 M0)

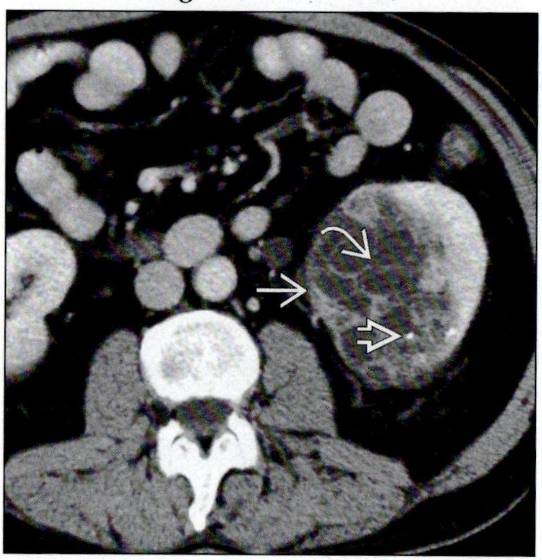

(Left) Coronal T1WI C+ FS MR in the same patient as the previous 2 images shows the complex mass ➡ arising from the superior pole right kidney. Subsequent nephrectomy demonstrated a stage I renal cell carcinoma. *(Right)* Axial CECT in another patient shows a 6.6 cm complex cystic mass ➡ arising from the medial aspect of the left kidney with multiple enhancing internal septa ➡ and focal calcifications ➡. The imaging characteristics are compatible with a renal cell carcinoma.

Stage I (T1b N0 M0)

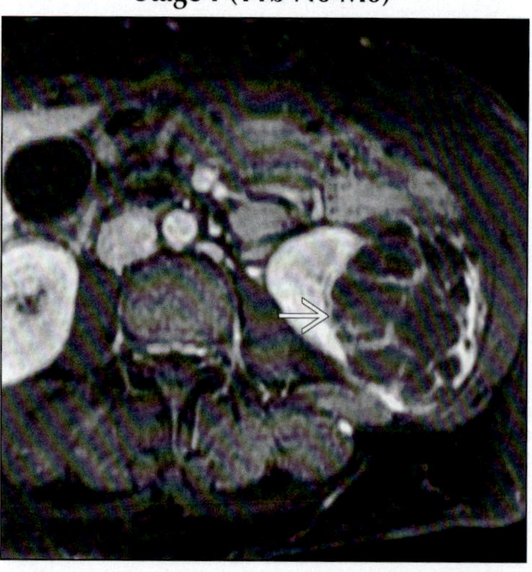

Stage II (T2a N0 M0)

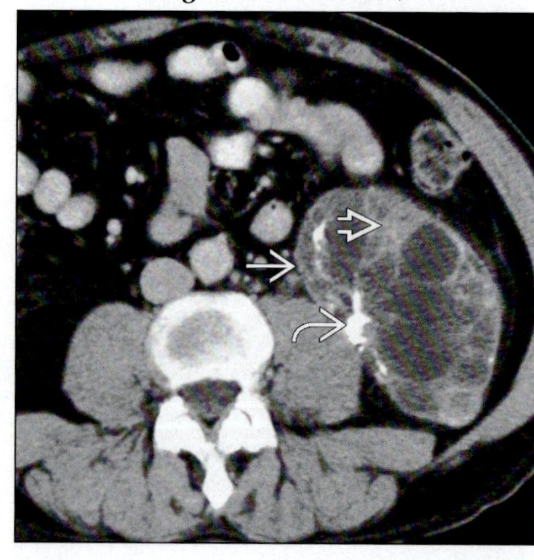

(Left) Axial T1WI C+ FS MR shows a similar-appearing, 6.7 cm, complex cystic mass ➡ with a similar appearance in the left kidney of a different patient, compatible with a T1b cystic renal cell carcinoma. *(Right)* Axial CECT shows a complex cystic mass ➡ arising from the left kidney with multiple enhancing septa ➡ and somewhat linear areas of calcification ➡. Subsequent nephrectomy proved a stage II renal cell carcinoma with a 7.3 cm (T2) lesion.

RENAL CARCINOMA

Stage II (T2a N0 M0)

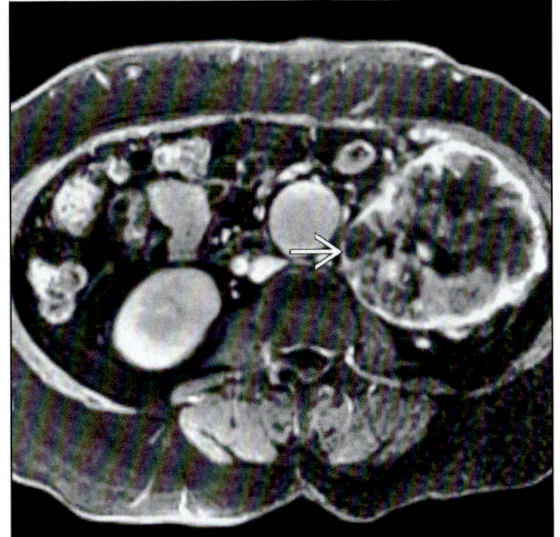

Stage II (T2a N0 M0)

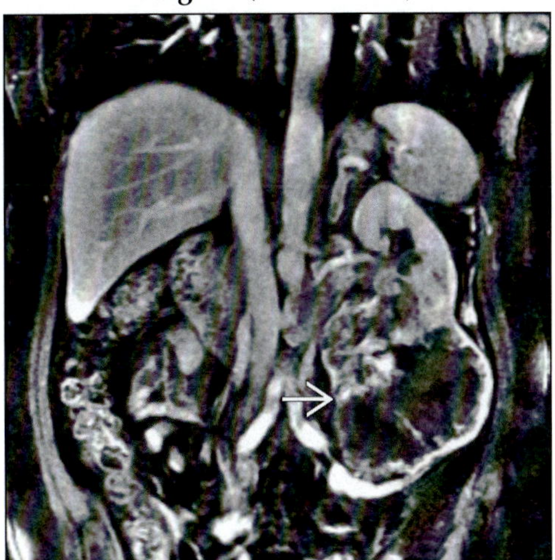

(Left) Axial T1WI C+ FS MR shows a 7.9 cm mass ⇒ in the left kidney with complex internal signal, the overall appearance of which is very worrisome for renal cell carcinoma. *(Right)* Coronal T1WI C+ FS MR in the same patient shows the large exophytic mass ⇒ arising from the inferior pole left kidney. Subsequent nephrectomy revealed a stage II (T2a N0 M0) renal cell carcinoma.

Stage II (T2a N0 M0)

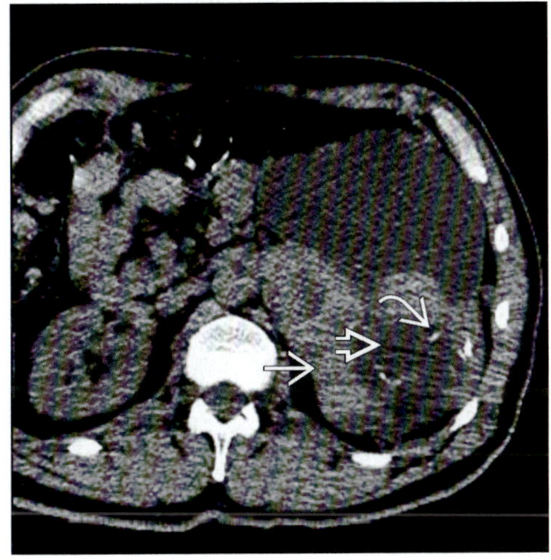

Stage II (T2a N0 M0)

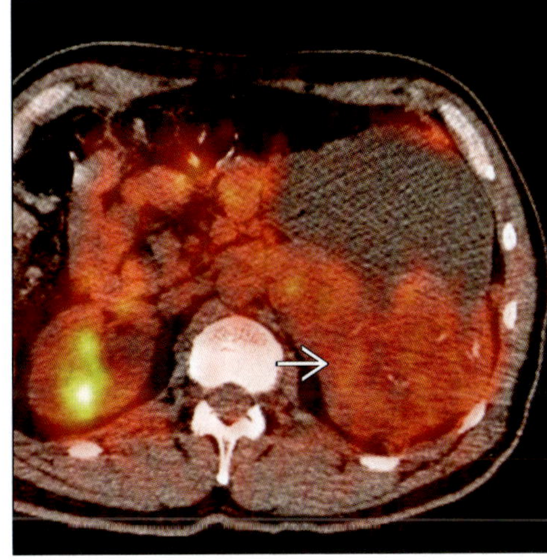

(Left) Axial NECT performed as part of a PET/CT examination shows an 8 cm complex solid mass ⇒ arising from the left kidney with internal areas of low attenuation ⇒ and focal/linear calcifications ⇒, compatible with a renal cell carcinoma. *(Right)* Axial fused PET/CT in the same patient shows almost no increased metabolic activity within the large left renal mass ⇒. At nephrectomy, this proved to be a stage II renal cell carcinoma.

Stage II (T2a N0 M0)

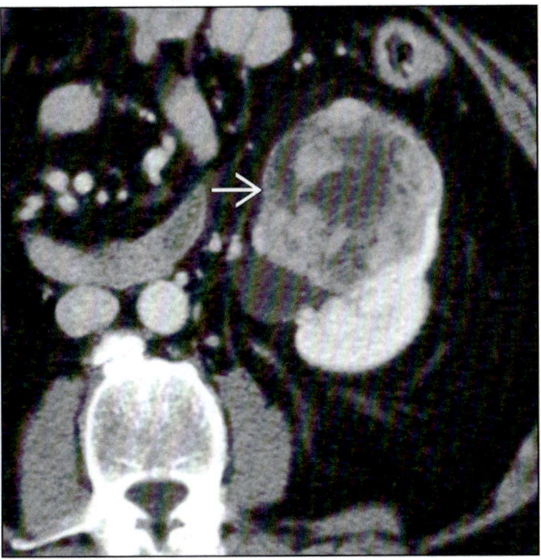

Stage II (T2a N0 M0)

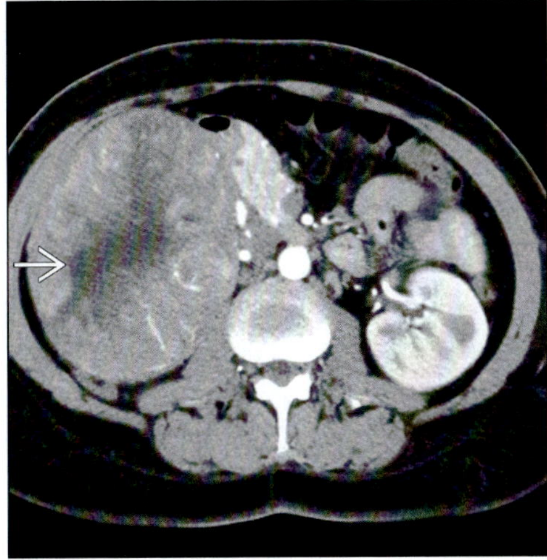

(Left) Axial CECT shows an 8.5 cm (measured in the coronal plane) enhancing mass ⇒ in the anterior aspect of the midpole left kidney. The mass was shown to be a stage II (T2a N0 M0) lesion following nephrectomy. *(Right)* Axial CECT shows a well-circumscribed large mass ⇒ arising from the right kidney with a central area of low attenuation and thick rind of peripheral enhancing tissue, compatible with a renal cell carcinoma.

RENAL CARCINOMA

Stage II (T2b N0 M0)

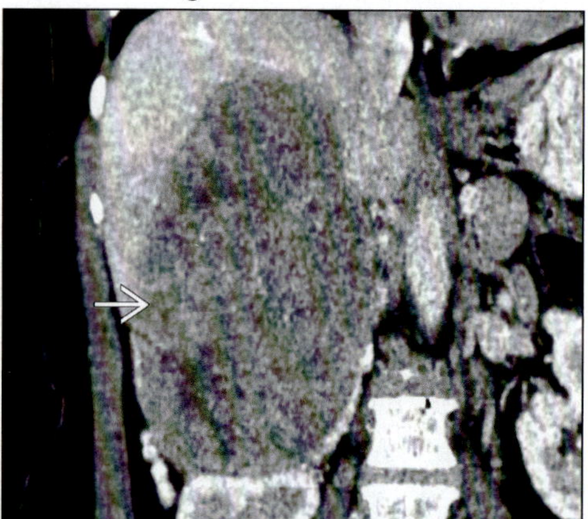

Stage II (T2b N0 M0)

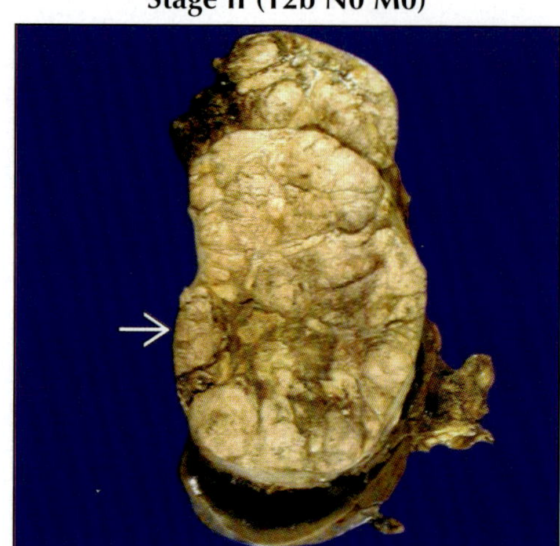

(Left) Coronal CECT in the same patient shows a 13 cm (T2b), primarily solid, enhancing mass ➡ arising from and confined to the right kidney, compatible with a renal cell carcinoma. Despite the large size of the primary lesion, no enlarged regional lymph nodes were identified. *(Right)* Gross pathologic specimen in the same patient as the previous 2 images shows the large resected mass ➡. Final pathology demonstrated a stage II (T2b N0 M0) lesion.

Stage III (T3a N0 M0)

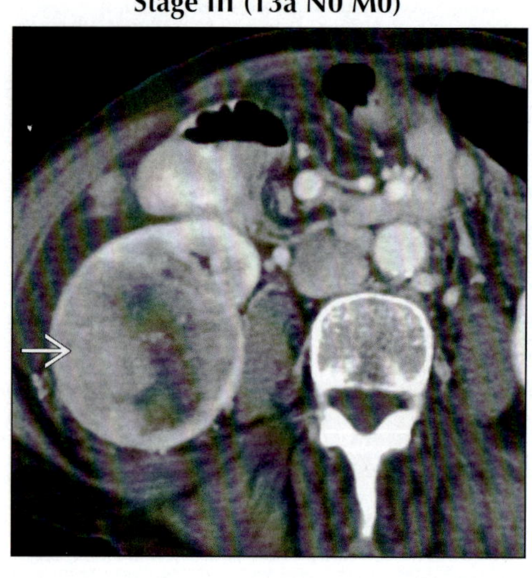

Stage III (T3a N0 M0)

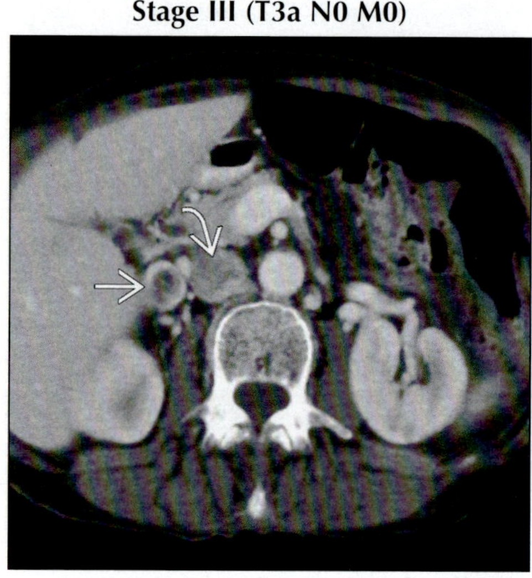

(Left) CECT shows a renal cell carcinoma ➡ in the right kidney. *(Right)* The tumor is invading the right renal vein ➡. Tumor extending into the renal vein or its segmental branches constitutes a T3a lesion; extension of tumor in the IVC is staged as T3b; and extension above the diaphragm constitutes a T3c lesion. The low attenuation within the IVC ➡ is the result of mixing of opacified with nonopacified blood and should not be mistaken for tumor invasion.

Stage III (T3a N0 M0)

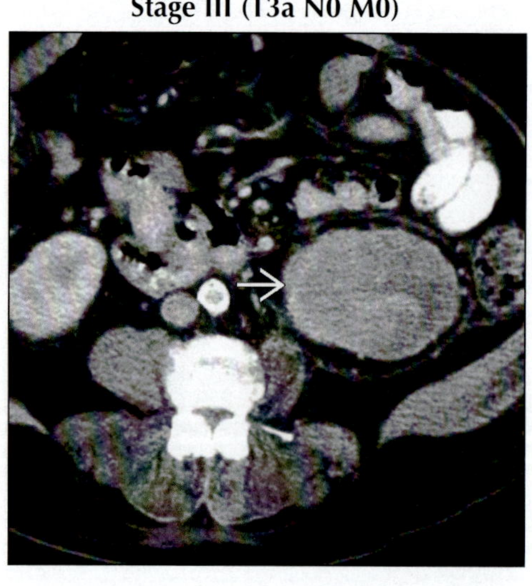

Stage III (T3a N0 M0)

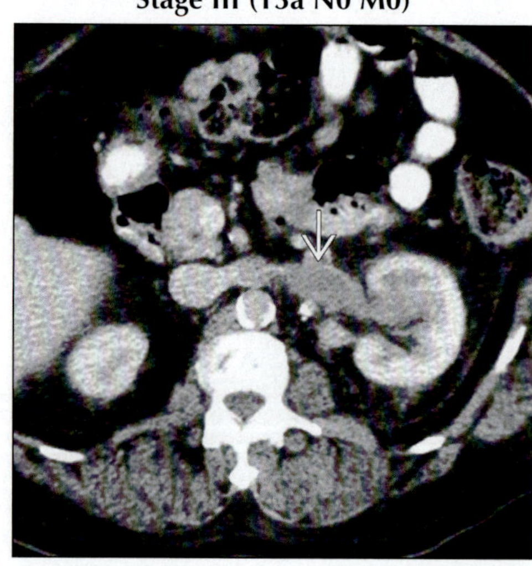

(Left) Axial CECT shows a solid enhancing renal mass ➡ in the left kidney, compatible with renal cell carcinoma. *(Right)* Axial CECT in the same patient shows enlargement of the left renal vein ➡ secondary to tumor infiltration, making this a T3a lesion.

RENAL CARCINOMA

Stage III (T3c N0 M0)

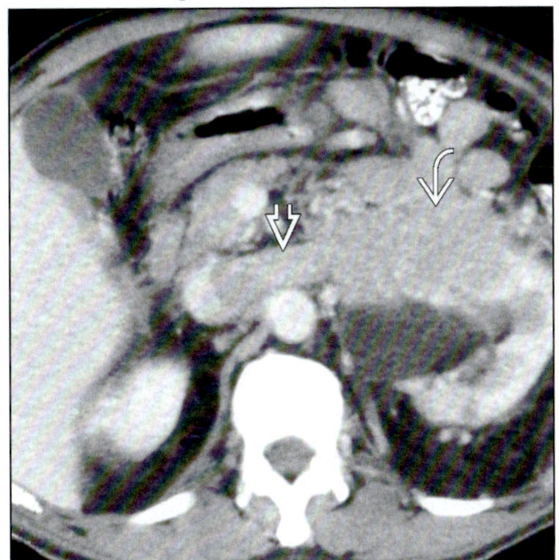

Stage III (T3c N0 M0)

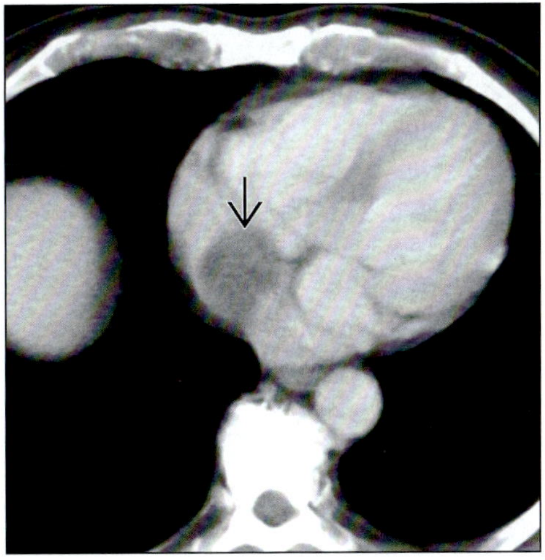

(Left) Axial CECT shows a left renal cell carcinoma ➡ with invasion of the left renal vein ➡. (Right) An image at the level of the heart in the same patient shows tumor thrombus ➡ within the right atrium. Extension of tumor thrombus above the diaphragm makes this a T3c tumor and has important implications for the surgical approach.

Stage IV (T4 N0 M0)

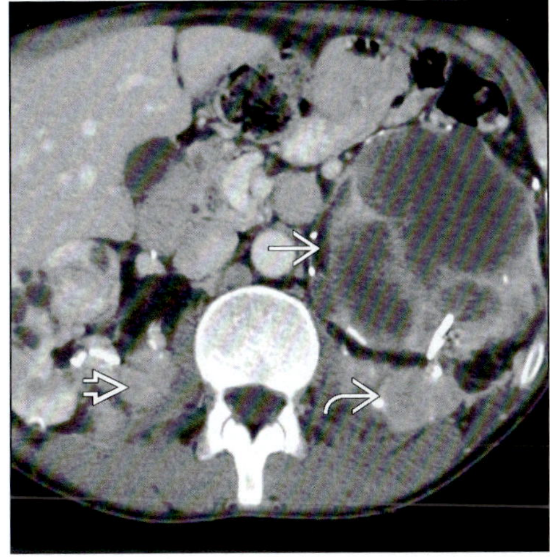

Stage IV (T4 N0 M0)

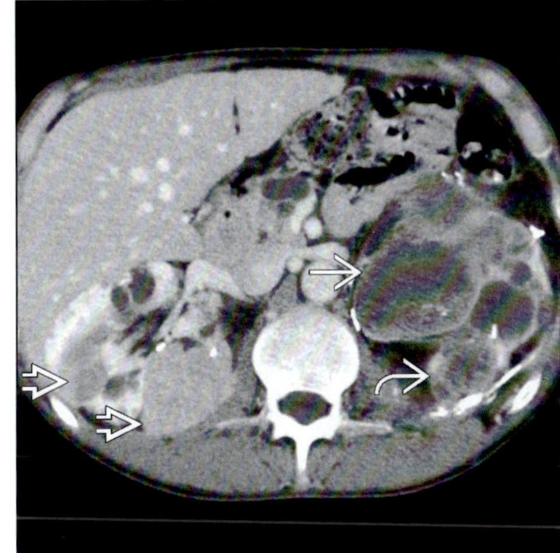

(Left) CECT in a patient with von Hippel-Lindau syndrome shows a cystic renal cell carcinoma ➡ in the left kidney with perirenal/posterior abdominal wall involvement ➡ on the ipsilateral side and tumor ➡ in the perirenal fat on the contralateral side from a another renal cell carcinoma. (Right) There are multiple contralateral renal cell carcinomas ➡, in addition to the cystic renal cell carcinoma ➡ seen on the prior image with involvement of the perirenal fat ➡.

Stage IV (T1a N1 M0)

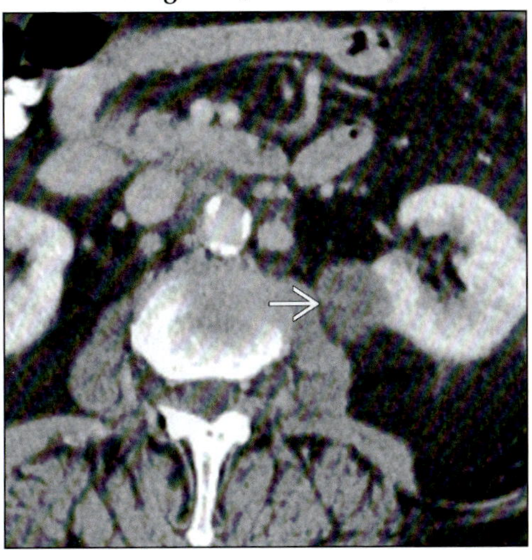

Stage IV (T1a N1 M0)

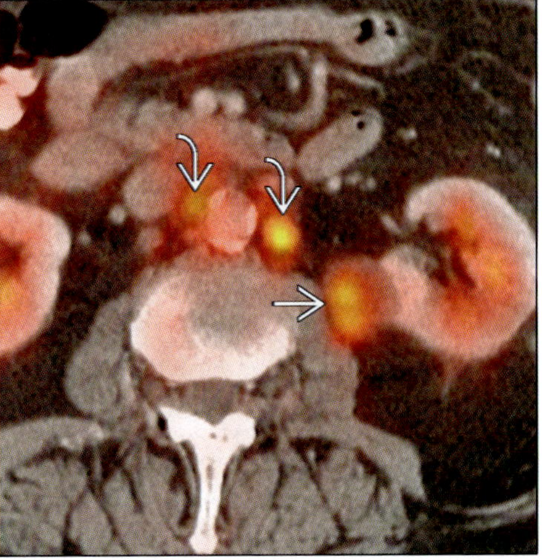

(Left) Axial CECT shows a low-attenuation but enhancing mass ➡ within the left kidney. (Right) Axial fused PET/CT in the same patient shows moderate increased FDG activity along the medial border of this renal cell carcinoma ➡. In addition, the left paraaortic and aortocaval nodes ➡ demonstrate increased metabolic activity compatible with metastatic nodes, making this N1 disease.

RENAL CARCINOMA

Stage IV (T1b N0 M1)

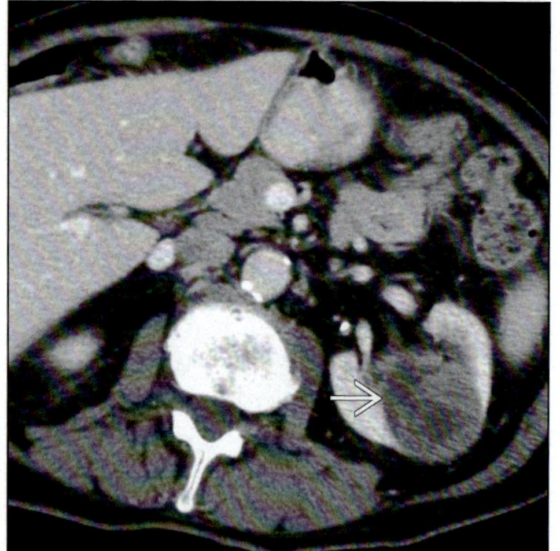

Stage IV (T1b N0 M1)

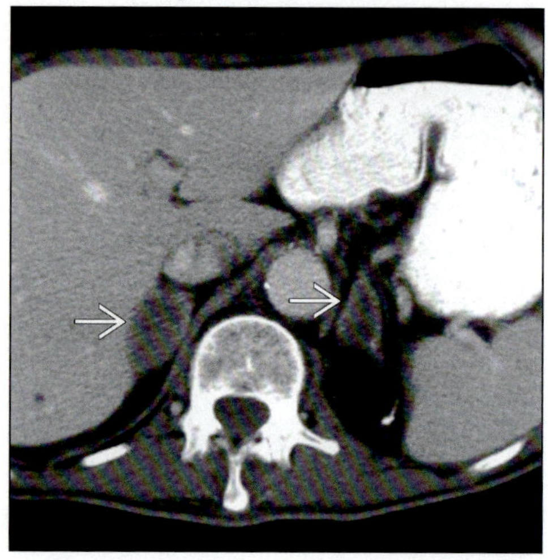

(Left) Axial CECT shows a 4.3 cm, mixed attenuation, and heterogeneously enhancing mass ➡ in the left kidney, compatible with a T1b lesion. (Right) Axial CECT in the same patient shows bilateral adrenal masses ➡. These masses are indeterminate on this single contrast-enhanced CT. The patient was referred for a CT-guided biopsy of the right adrenal gland mass, which showed metastatic renal cell carcinoma.

Stage IV (T1b N0 M1)

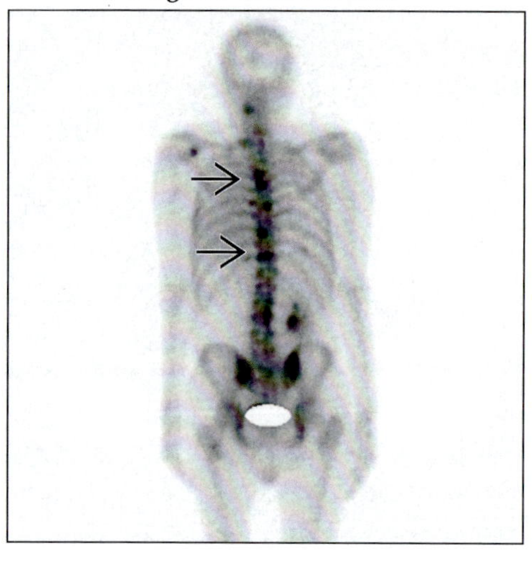

Stage IV (T3a N0 M1)

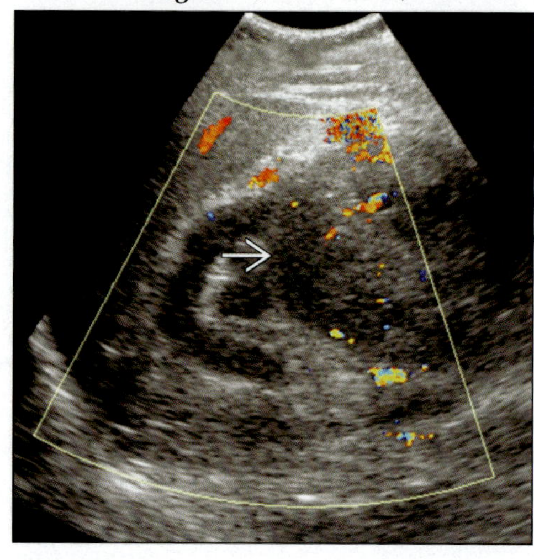

(Left) Coronal posterior bone scan in a patient who underwent a recent nephrectomy for a 6 cm renal cell carcinoma (T1b) shows multiple abnormal foci of increased tracer activity throughout the spine ➡, compatible with metastatic disease. (Right) Longitudinal color Doppler ultrasound in a patient with a stage IV renal cell carcinoma shows a fairly vascular mass ➡ within the right kidney.

Stage IV (T3a N0 M1)

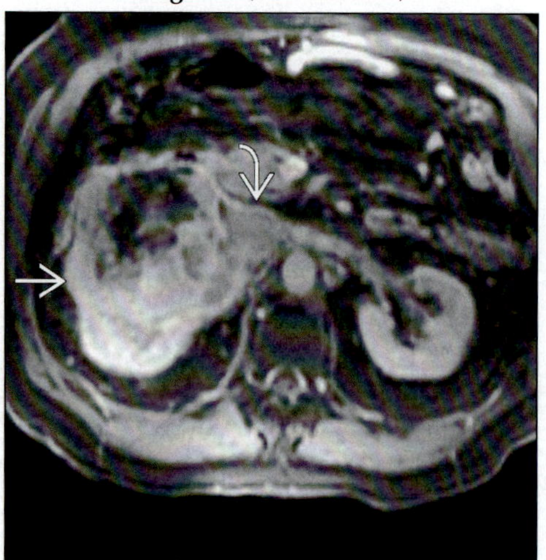

Stage IV (T3a N0 M1)

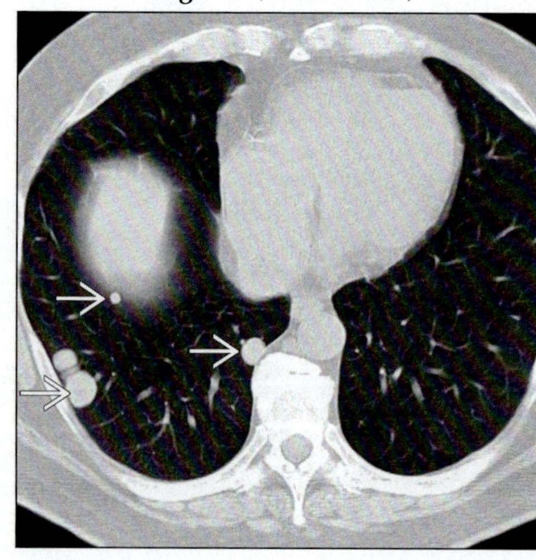

(Left) Axial T1WI C+ FS MR the same patient shows a heterogeneously enhancing mass ➡ in the right kidney with tumor extension into the right renal vein ➡. (Right) Axial CECT in the same patient shows multiple well-circumscribed, lower lobe pulmonary nodules ➡ on the right, compatible with M1 or stage IV disease.

RENAL CARCINOMA

Stage IV (T3a N0 M1)

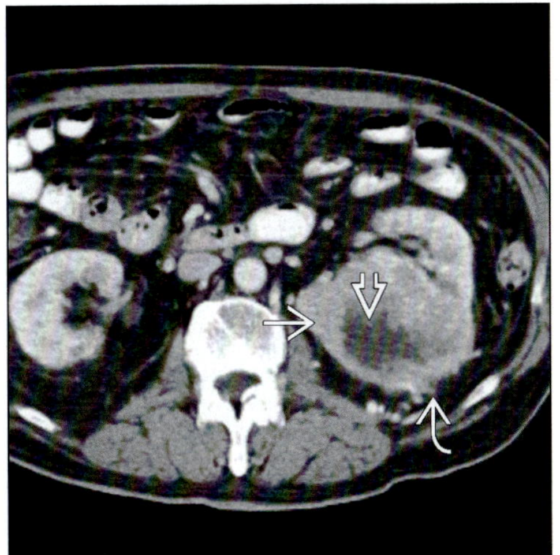

Stage IV (T3a N0 M1)

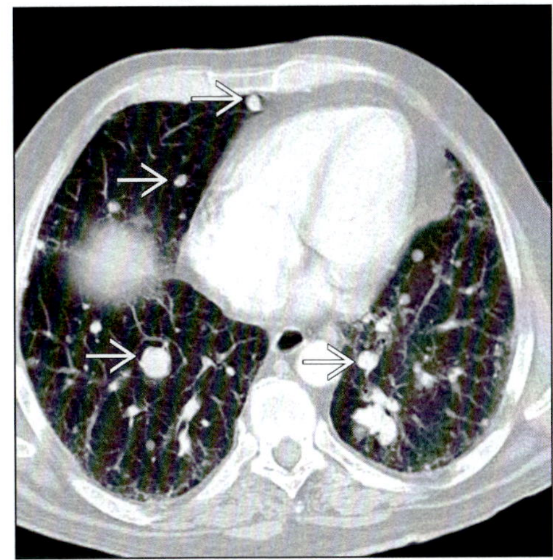

(Left) Axial CECT shows a large, diffusely enhancing mass ➡ arising from the posterior aspect of the superior pole left kidney with central necrosis ➡ and early extension of tumor into the perirenal space ➡. *(Right)* Axial CECT in the same patient shows multiple well-circumscribed, bilateral, noncalcified pulmonary nodules ➡, compatible with pulmonary metastases.

Stage IV (T3a N0 M1)

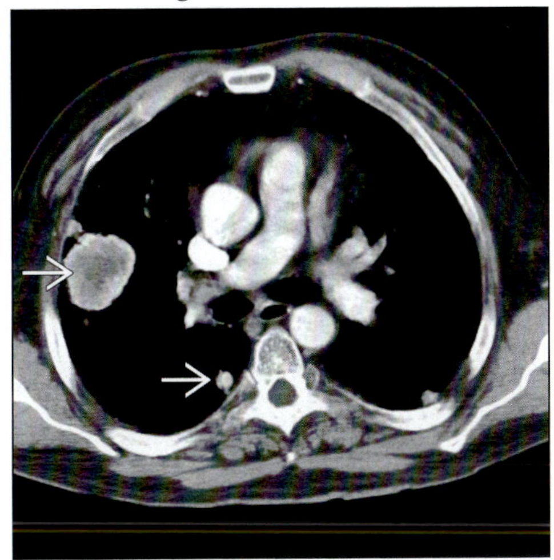

Stage IV (T4 N0 M1)

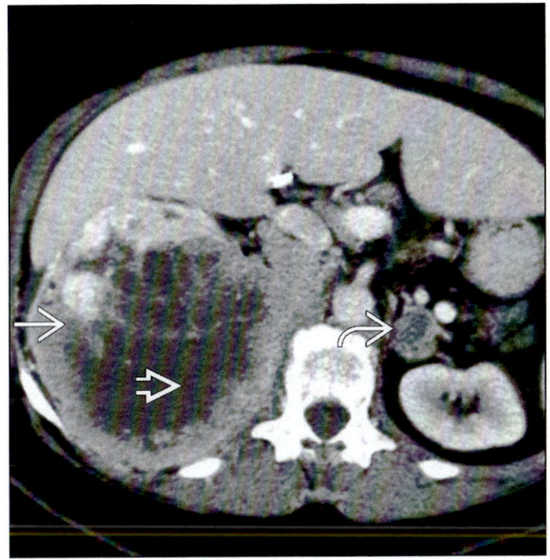

(Left) Axial CECT in the same patient as the previous 2 images shows additional pulmonary metastases ➡ with soft tissue windows. The largest lesion in the right upper lobe shows significant central necrosis. Multiple pulmonary metastases signify stage IV disease. *(Right)* Axial CECT in a different patient shows a large, enhancing, right renal mass ➡ with central necrosis ➡ and a contralateral adrenal metastasis ➡.

Stage IV (T4 N0 M1)

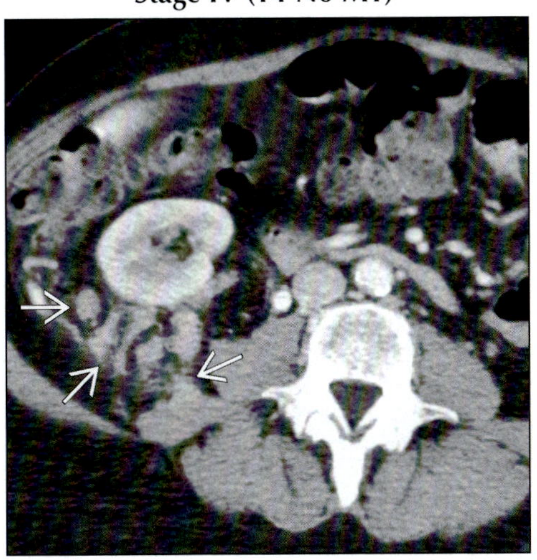

Stage IV (T4 N0 M1)

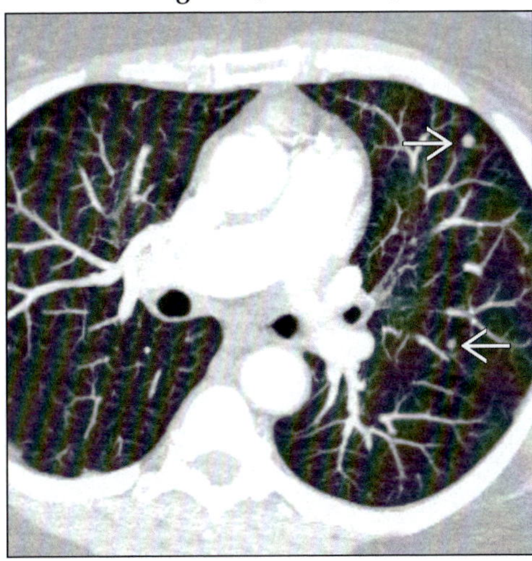

(Left) Axial CECT in the same patient shows extensive infiltration and nodularity ➡ of the perirenal fat on the right that extended beyond Gerota fascia (T4). *(Right)* Axial CECT MIP in the same patient as the previous 2 images shows 2 small, well-circumscribed, left upper lobe nodules ➡ that were not present on a CT scan of the chest 2 years earlier. These are most likely metastatic lesions. With adrenal metastasis and 2 lung nodules, this is M1 or stage IV disease.

RENAL CARCINOMA

(Left) Axial NECT shows a large heterogeneous mass arising in the left kidney with spiculated and ill-defined borders anteriorly ➡ and medially ➡ signifying extension of tumor into the perirenal fat, breeching Gerota fascia (T4). *(Right)* Axial NECT in the same patient shows a large destructive metastasis involving a right anterolateral rib ➡, compatible with M1 disease.

Stage IV (T4 N0 M1)

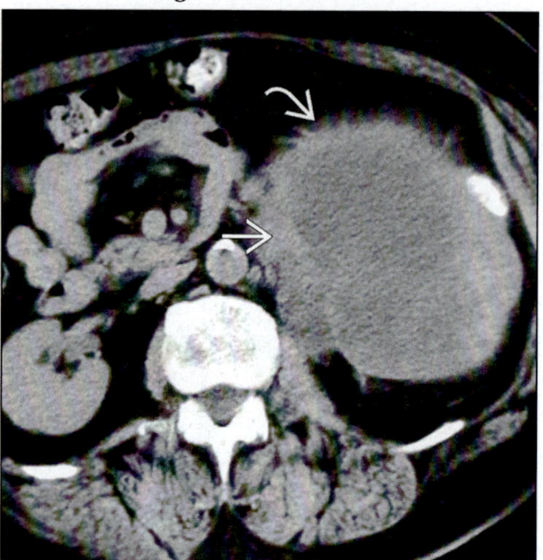

Stage IV (T4 N0 M1)

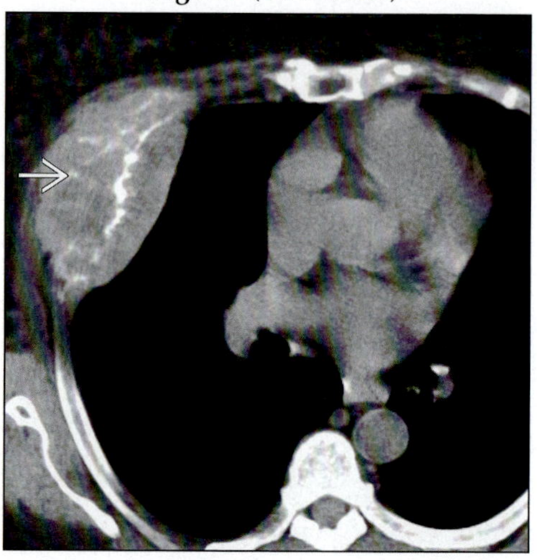

(Left) Transverse ultrasound shows a nearly isoechoic, slightly exophytic, solid mass ➡ in the mid pole left kidney. As this lesion is not completely cystic, it is worrisome for a renal cell carcinoma. *(Right)* Axial T1WI C+ FS MR in the same patient shows a primarily solid renal mass ➡, worrisome for renal cell carcinoma. The mass measures approximately 2 cm and would be compatible with a T1a lesion.

Stage IV (T1a N1 M1)

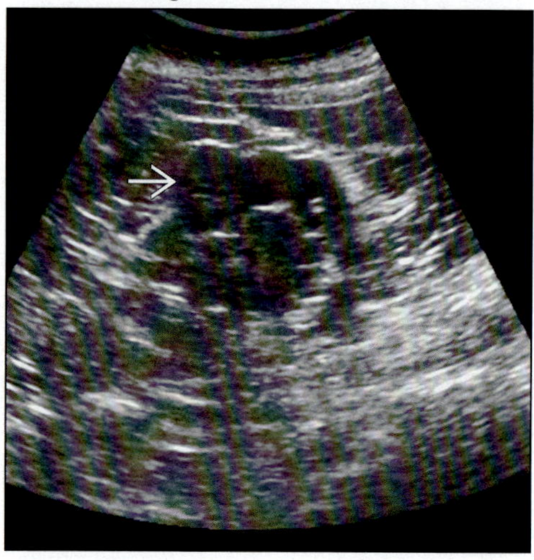

Stage IV (T1a N1 M1)

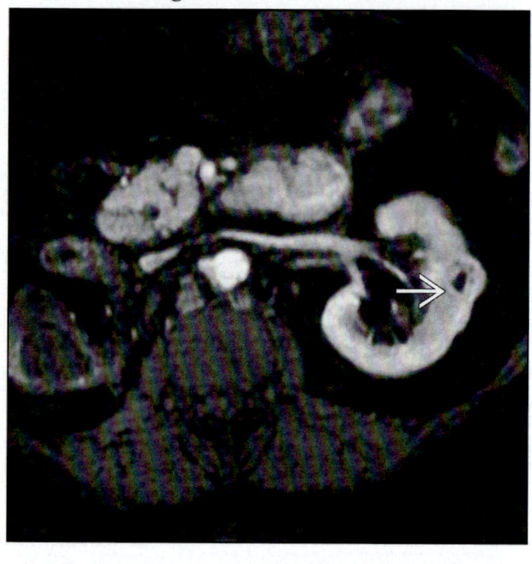

(Left) Coronal MR in the same patient shows the same primary solid left renal mass ➡ in a different plane. *(Right)* Axial T1WI C+ FS MR in the same patient as the previous 3 images shows enlarged nodal metastases ➡ to the left and to the right of the aorta despite the relatively small size of the primary tumor, compatible with N1 disease. The patient also had pulmonary metastases (M1) or overall stage IV disease.

Stage IV (T1a N1 M1)

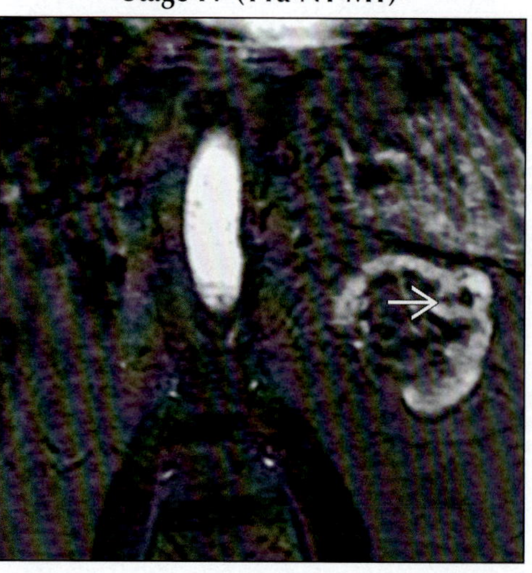

Stage IV (T1a N1 M1)

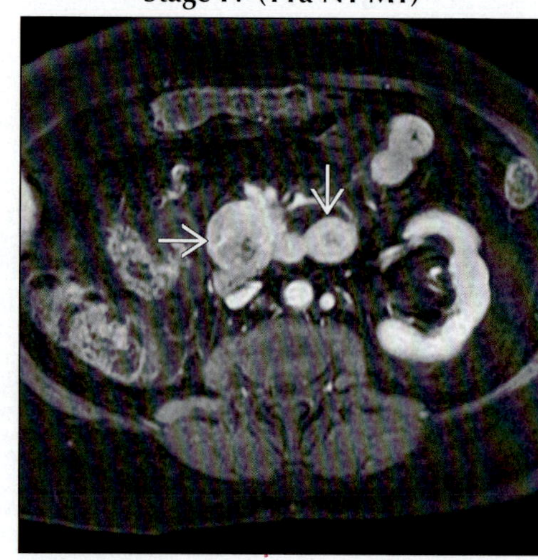

RENAL CARCINOMA

Stage IV (T3 N1 M1)

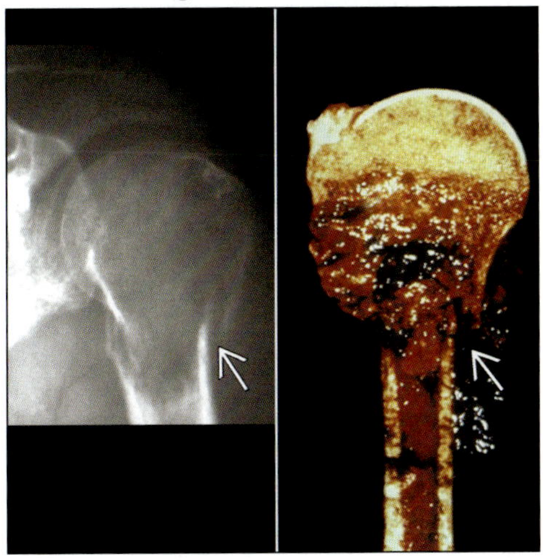

Stage IV Recurrent RCC

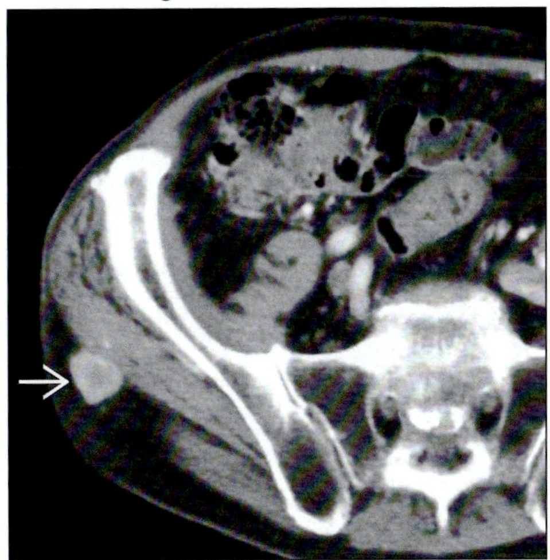

(Left) Composite image of a pathologic fracture ➜ of the humerus with the corresponding specimen at autopsy. The patient presented with acute arm pain after a minor trauma. Work up showed a T3 tumor of the kidney with extensive nodal disease and widespread metastases. *(Right)* Axial CECT shows a solid enhancing lesion ➜ in the subcutaneous fat in this patient with a history of a large renal cell carcinoma, compatible with recurrent disease.

Stage IV Recurrent RCC

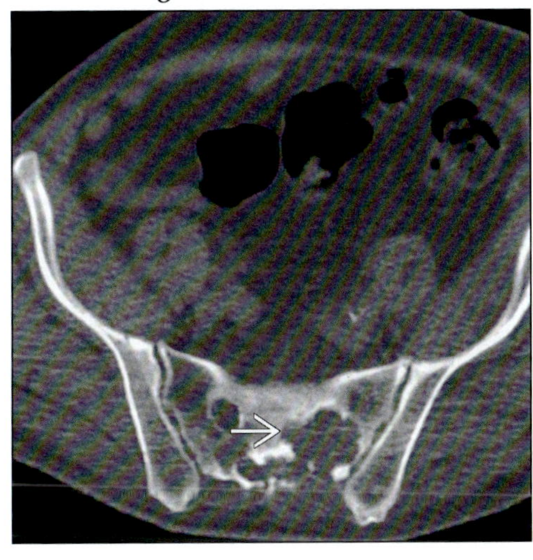

Stage IV Recurrent RCC

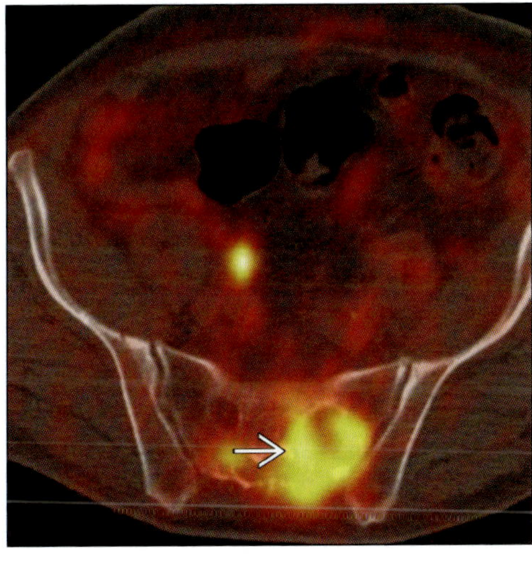

(Left) Axial NECT in this patient with a history of renal cell carcinoma shows a lytic lesion ➜ involving the left hemisacrum, worrisome for recurrent metastatic disease. *(Right)* Axial fused PET/CT in the same patient shows intense FDG activity ➜ corresponding to the lytic lesion of the left hemisacrum, compatible with recurrent renal cell carcinoma. Metastases from renal cell carcinoma may have variable FDG uptake.

Stage IV Recurrent RCC

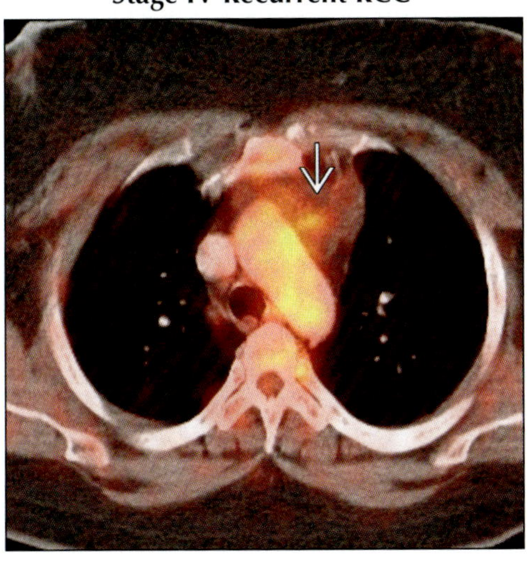

Stage IV Recurrent RCC

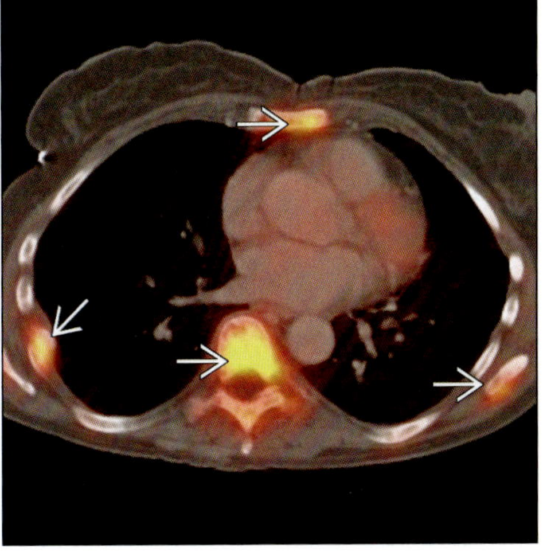

(Left) Axial fused PET/CT in a patient with a history of renal cell carcinoma shows abnormal soft tissue ➜ in the prevascular space with patchy areas of increased metabolic activity, compatible with metastatic disease. *(Right)* Axial fused PET/CT in the same patient shows multiple hypermetabolic bone lesions ➜, compatible with osseous metastases from renal cell carcinoma.

RENAL CARCINOMA

Stage IV Recurrent RCC

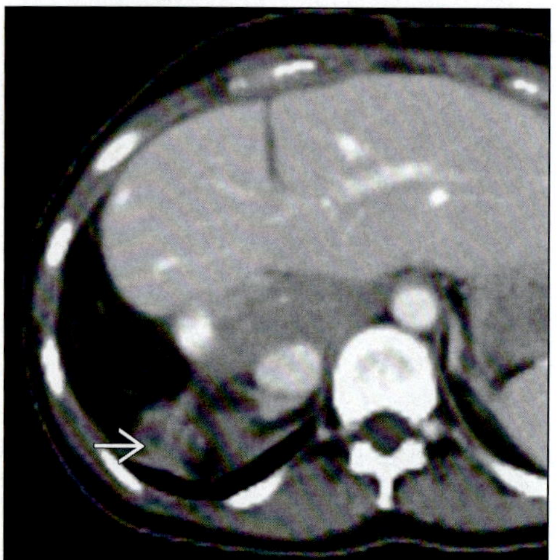

Stage IV Recurrent RCC

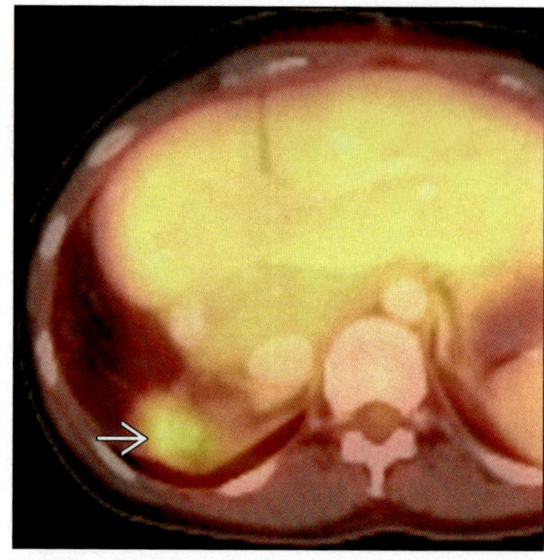

(Left) Axial CECT in a patient with a history of renal cell carcinoma shows abnormal soft tissue in the nephrectomy bed ➡ approximally 1 year following nephrectomy, worrisome for recurrent disease. *(Right)* Axial fused PET/CT in the same patient shows moderately increased FDG activity ➡ corresponding to the soft tissue in the nephrectomy bed, compatible with recurrent disease.

Stage IV Recurrent RCC

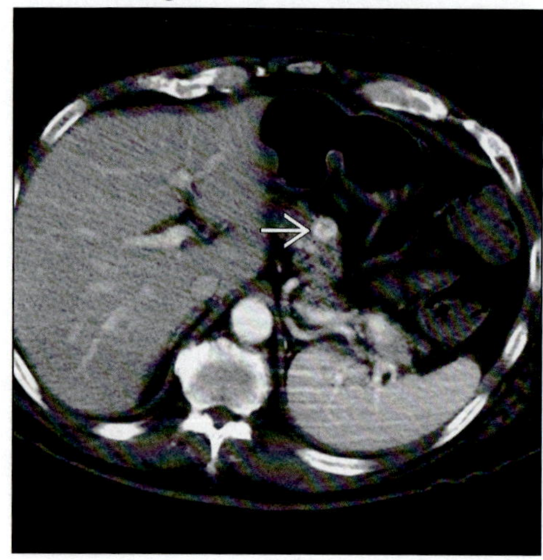

Stage IV Recurrent RCC

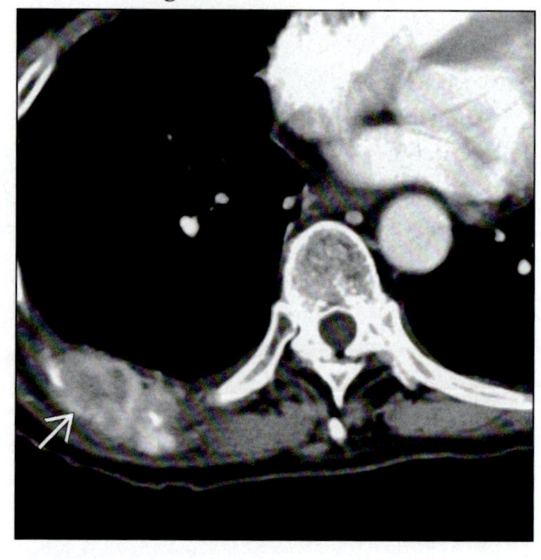

(Left) Axial CECT in this patient with a history of renal cell carcinoma shows an enhancing lesion ➡ in the body of the pancreas, compatible with recurrent metastatic disease. *(Right)* Axial CECT in this patient with a history of renal cell carcinoma shows a destructive osseous lesion ➡ involving the posterior chest wall/rib, compatible with recurrent metastatic disease.

Stage IV Recurrent RCC

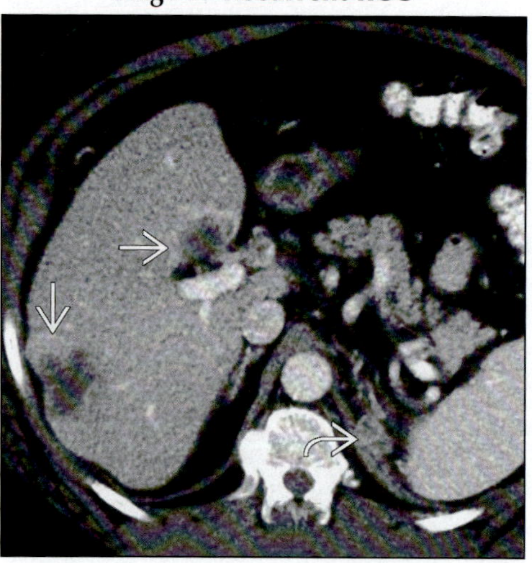

Stage IV Recurrent RCC

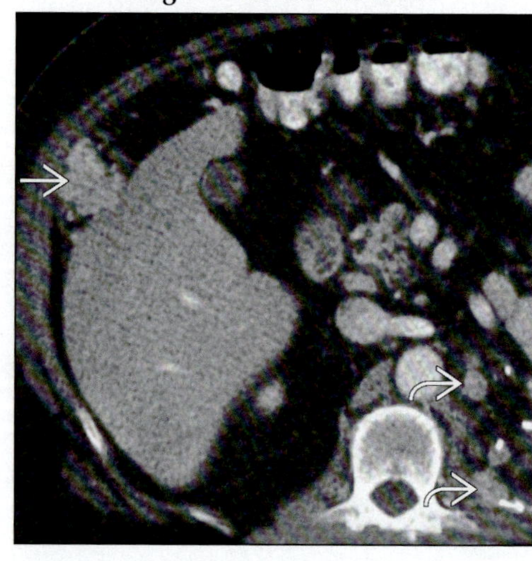

(Left) Axial CECT shows multiple low-attenuation lesions ➡ in the liver in this patient with a history renal cell carcinoma, compatible with recurrent stage IV disease. In addition, there is recurrent disease ➡ in the left renal fossa. *(Right)* Axial CECT shows a metastatic implant ➡ anterior to the liver in this patient with a history of renal cell carcinoma, compatible with recurrent disease. Also note smaller nodular implants ➡ in the left nephrectomy bed.

RENAL CARCINOMA

Stage IV Recurrent RCC

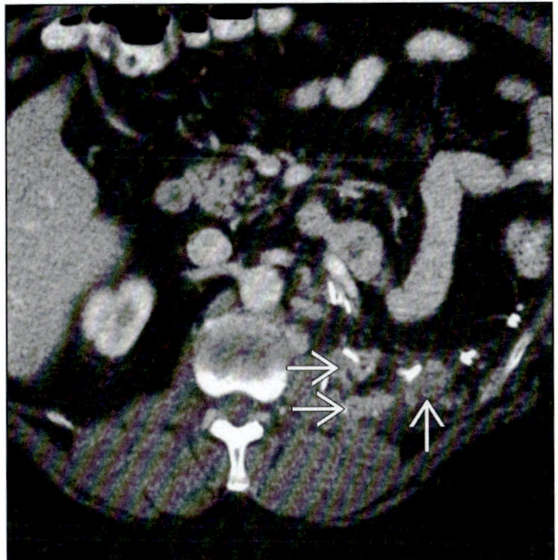

Stage IV Recurrent RCC

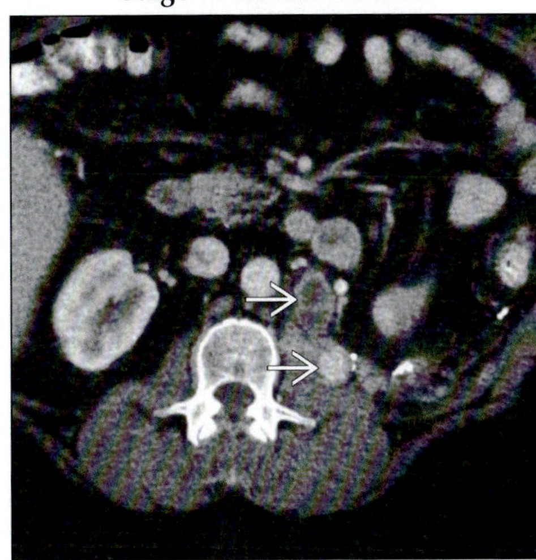

(Left) Axial CECT shows multiple soft tissue nodular implants ➡ in this patient with a history of a left-sided renal cell carcinoma status post nephrectomy, findings compatible with local recurrent disease. *(Right)* Axial CECT in the same patient shows additional nodular metastatic lesions ➡, again compatible with recurrent renal cell carcinoma.

Stage IV Recurrent RCC

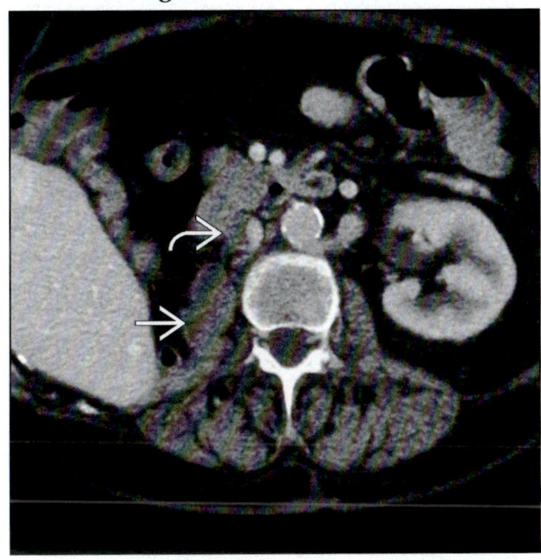

Stage IV Recurrent RCC

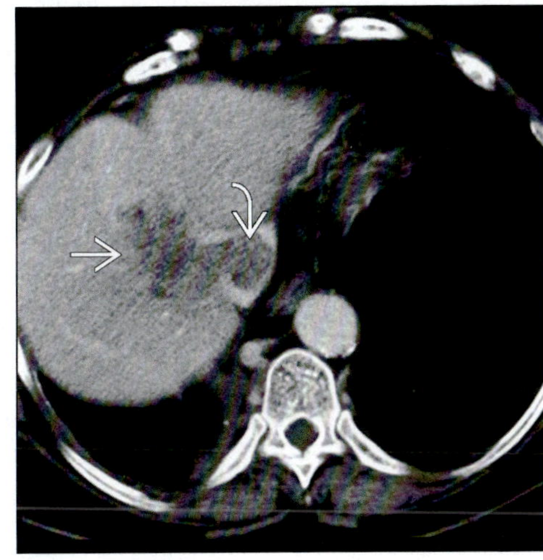

(Left) Axial CECT in a patient with right-sided renal cell carcinoma status post right nephrectomy shows multiple soft tissue nodular lesions ➡ in the nephrectomy bed, compatible with recurrent malignancy. Also note partial thrombosis of the inferior vena cava ➡. *(Right)* Axial CECT in the same patient shows extensive metastatic disease involving the liver ➡ with direct extension of tumor into the inferior vena cava ➡.

Stage IV Recurrent RCC

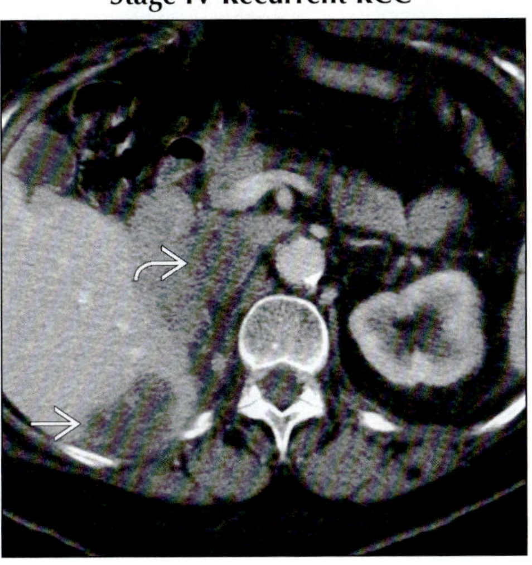

Stage IV Recurrent RCC

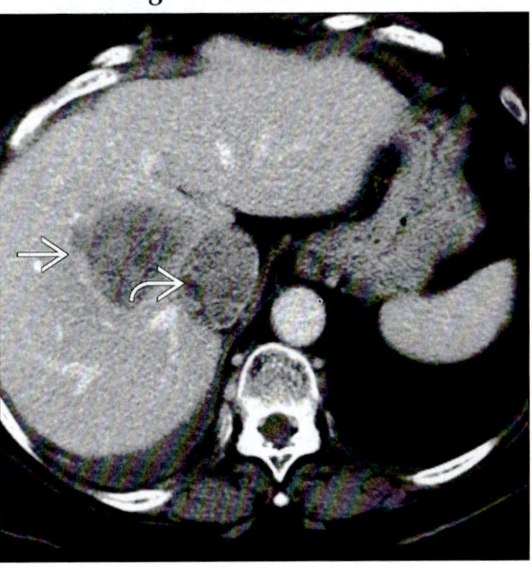

(Left) Axial CECT in the same patient shows additional areas of metastatic involvement in the posterior segment of the liver ➡ and expansion of the vena cava ➡ compatible with tumor thrombus. *(Right)* Axial CECT in the same patient shows an additional view of the expanded inferior vena cava ➡ compatible with tumor thrombus, as well as the metastatic lesion in the liver ➡.

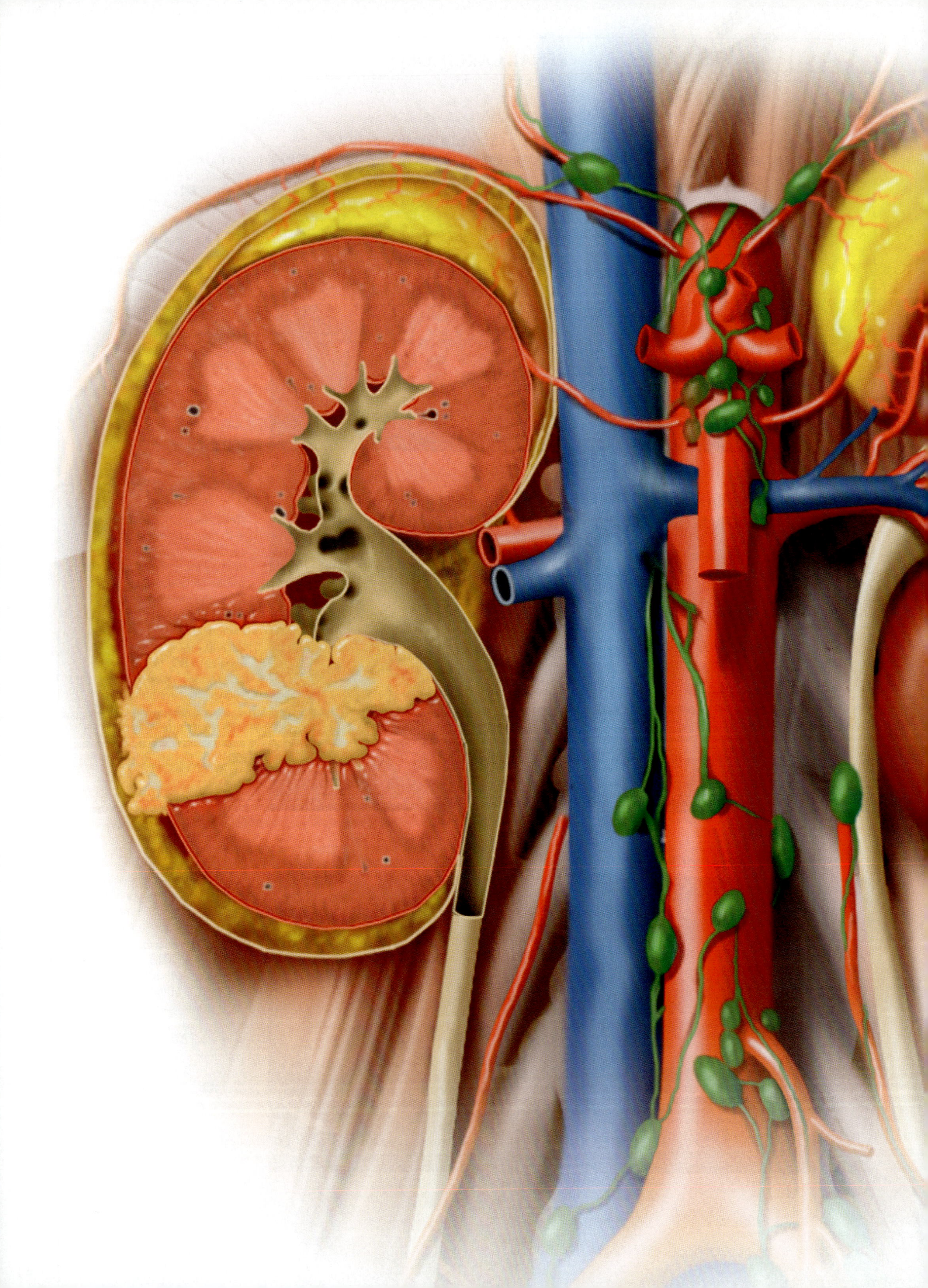

Renal Pelvis and Ureteral Carcinoma

RENAL PELVIS AND URETERAL CARCINOMA

(T) Primary Tumor

Adapted from 7th edition AJCC Staging Forms.

TNM	Definitions
TX	Primary tumor cannot be assessed
T0	No evidence of primary tumor
Ta	Papillary noninvasive carcinoma
Tis	Carcinoma in situ
T1	Tumor invades subepithelial connective tissue
T2	Tumor invades the muscularis
T3	
Renal pelvis only	Tumor invades beyond muscularis into peripelvic fat or the renal parenchyma
Ureter only	Tumor invades beyond muscularis into periureteric fat
T4	Tumor invades adjacent organs or through the kidney into the perinephric fat

(N) Regional Lymph Nodes

NX	Regional lymph nodes cannot be assessed
N0	No regional lymph node metastasis
N1	Metastasis in a single lymph node, $\leq$ 2 cm in greatest dimension
N2	Metastasis in a single lymph node, > 2 cm but $\leq$ 5 cm in greatest dimension; or multiple lymph nodes, none > 5 cm in greatest dimension
N3	Metastasis in a lymph node, > 5 cm in greatest dimension

(M) Distant Metastasis

M0	No distant metastasis
M1	Distant metastasis

Laterality does not affect the N classification.

AJCC Stages/Prognostic Groups

Adapted from 7th edition AJCC Staging Forms.

Stage	T	N	M
0a	Ta	N0	M0
0is	Tis	N0	M0
I	T1	N0	M0
II	T2	N0	M0
III	T3	N0	M0
IV	T4	N0	M0
	Any T	N1	M0
	Any T	N2	M0
	Any T	N3	M0
	Any T	Any N	M1

RENAL PELVIS AND URETERAL CARCINOMA

Ta

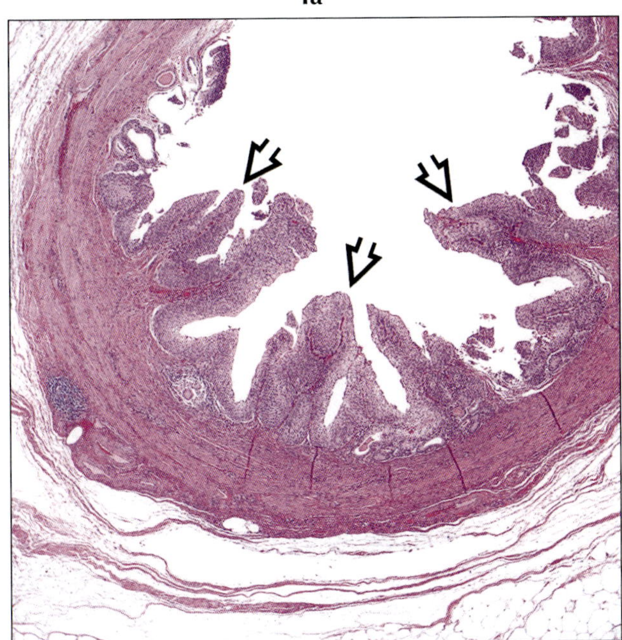

Low-power magnification (H&E stain) shows a cross section of proximal ureter with papillary noninvasive urothelial carcinoma. Note the multiple papillary fronds ▷ lined by variably thickened epithelium extending into the lumen. (Original magnification 20x.)

Ta

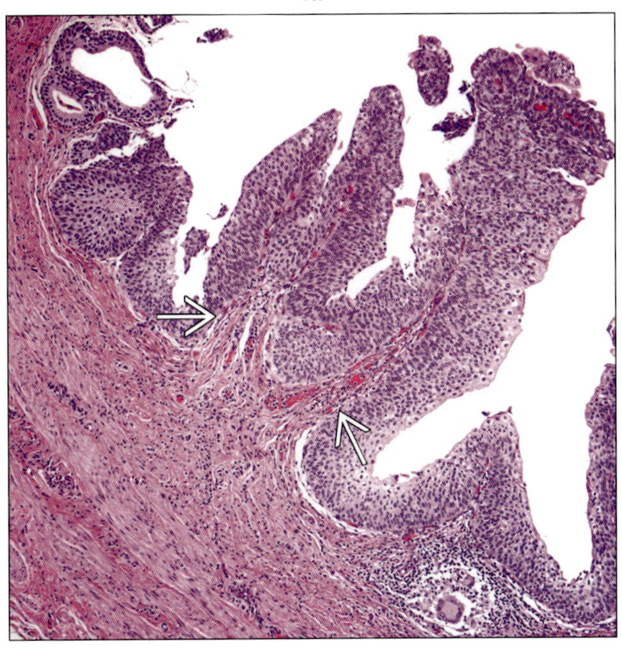

Higher power magnification of the previous image shows fibrovascular cores ➡ surrounded by an increased number of cells compared to normal urothelium. Cells are oriented in an orderly fashion perpendicular to basement membrane and lack cytologic atypia and pleomorphism. (Original magnification 100x.)

Tis

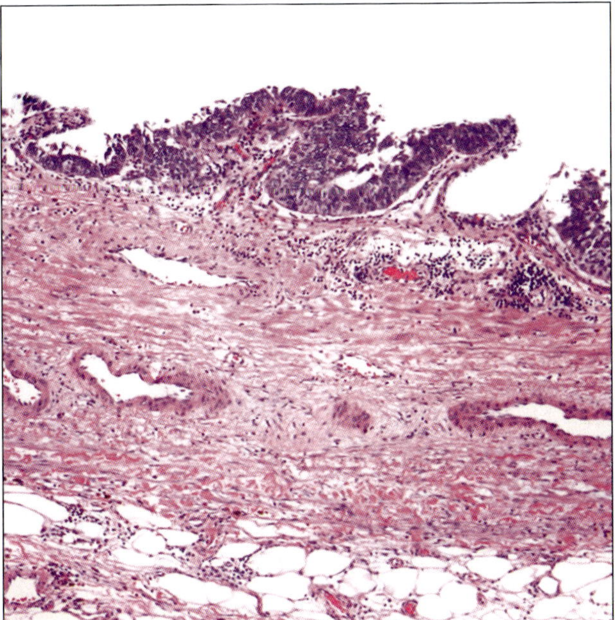

H&E shows that, in contrast to cells in the previous images, the neoplastic cells are markedly pleomorphic and hyperchromatic. The nuclei lack polarity to basement membrane. Note also the propensity of these cells to become detached from basement membrane focally. (Original magnification 100x.)

T1

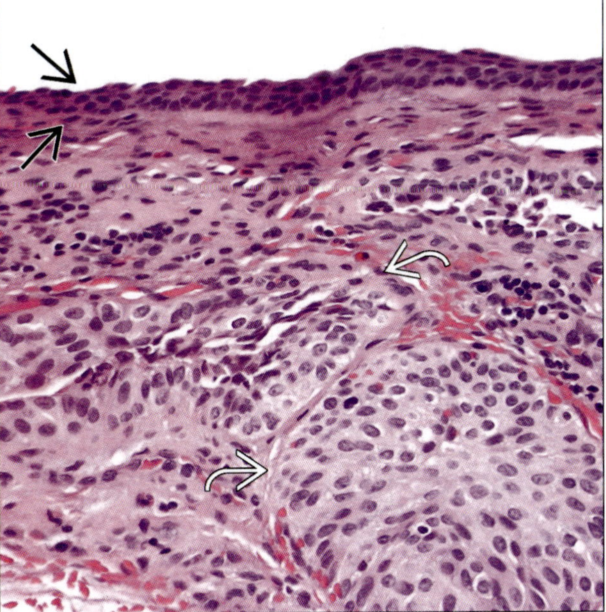

H&E stain demonstrates uninvolved superficial urothelium ➡ with underlying nests of neoplastic urothelium ➡ that invades the subepithelial connective tissue. (Original magnification 400x.)

RENAL PELVIS AND URETERAL CARCINOMA

T2

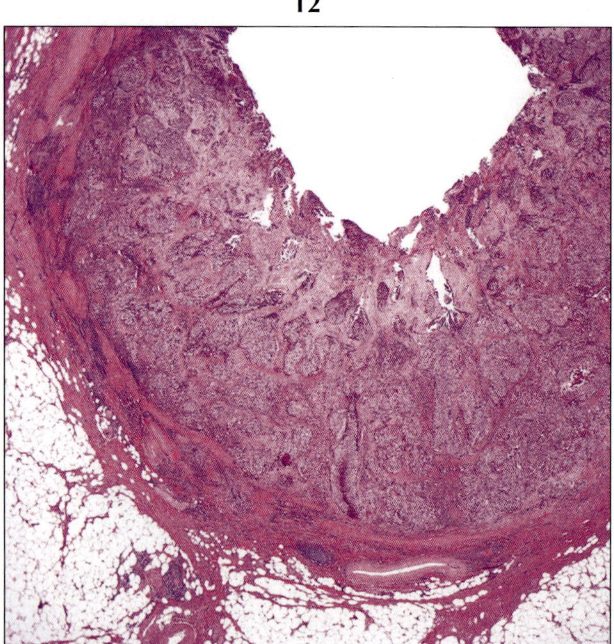

H&E stain shows a cross section of a ureter with invasive urothelial carcinoma. Tumor nests invade almost the entire thickness of the muscularis propria but do not extend into the periureteric fat. (Original magnification 20x.)

T2

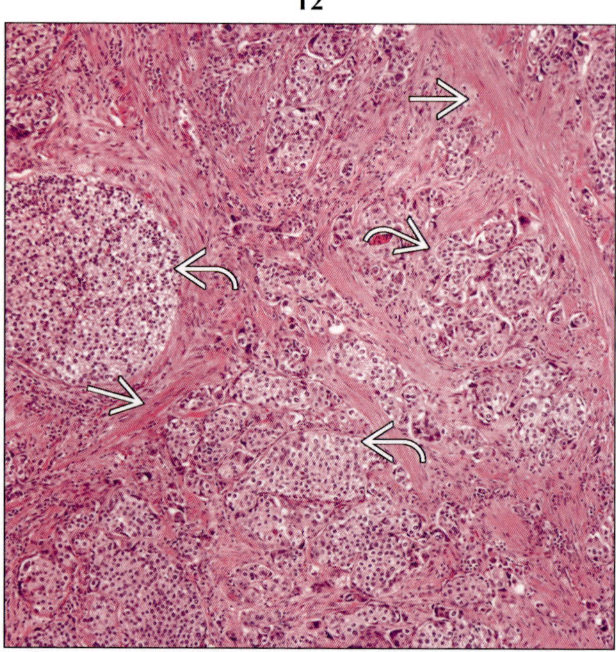

High-power magnification of the previous image shows nests of urothelial carcinoma ➔ invading and disrupting the muscularis propria (pink bundles of smooth muscles) ➔. (Original magnification 100x.)

T3

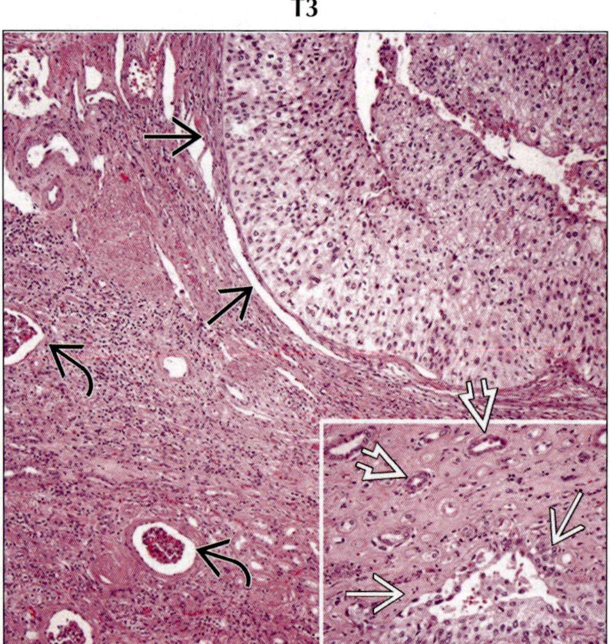

H&E stain shows a nest of urothelial carcinoma ➔ invading into renal parenchyma; note the renal glomeruli ➔. (Original magnification 100x.) The inset shows a nest of urothelial carcinoma ➔ invading renal parenchyma in proximity to renal tubules ➔. (Original magnification 400x.)

T4

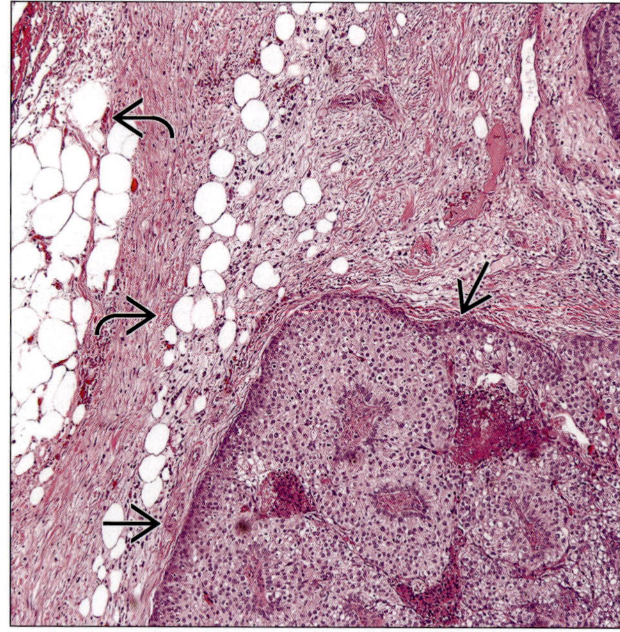

Urothelial carcinoma invades through the kidney to perinephric fat. The large nests of urothelial carcinoma ➔ infiltrate the perinephric fat (white round cells) ➔ with prominent pink desmoplastic reaction. (Original magnification 100x.)

RENAL PELVIS AND URETERAL CARCINOMA

Ta, T1, and T2

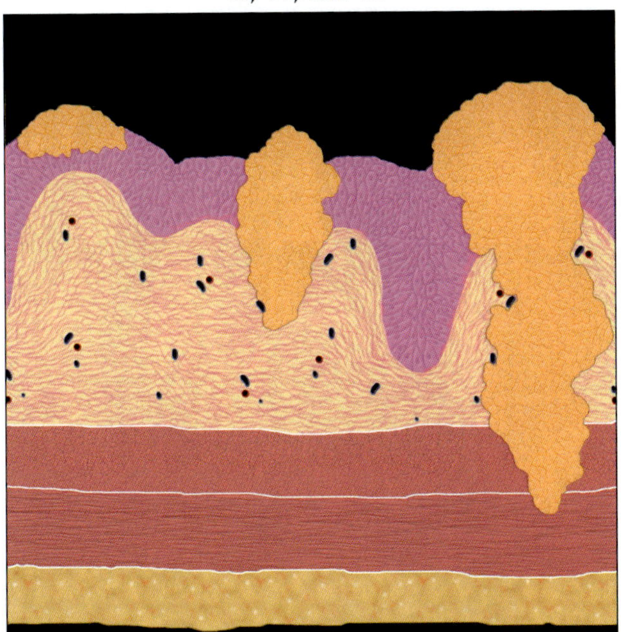

Graphic shows local extent of early stages of ureteric carcinoma: Ta is papillary noninvasive carcinoma, T1 is tumor invading subepithelial connective tissue, and T2 is tumor invading the muscularis.

T3 Renal Pelvis and Calyceal Carcinoma

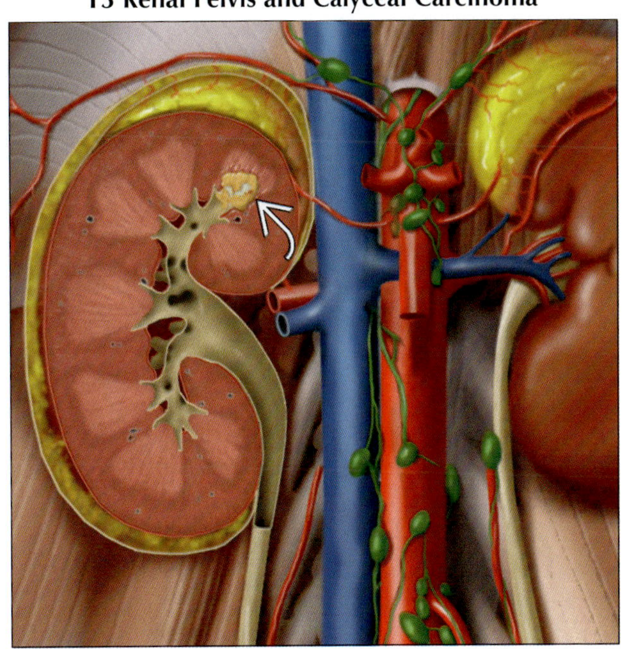

Graphic shows T3 tumor of the upper calyx ➔ with extension through the muscularis layer into the peripelvic fat or renal parenchyma.

T3 Ureteric Carcinoma

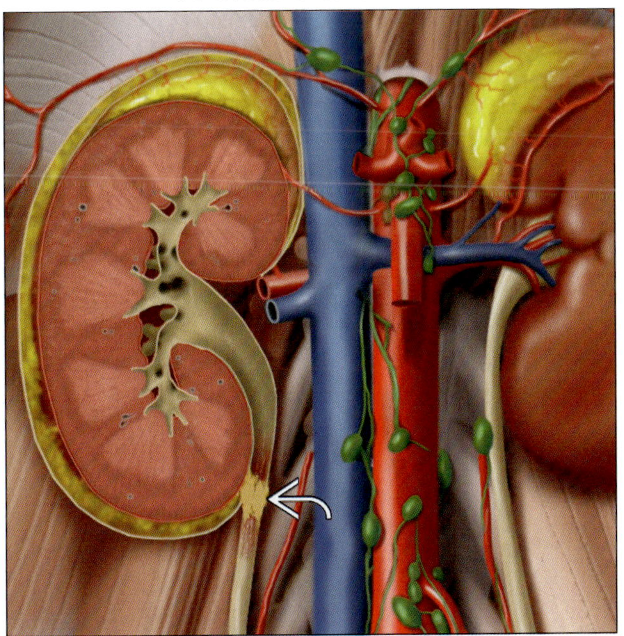

Graphic shows T3 tumor of the ureter ➔ with extension through the muscularis layer into the periureteric fat without invasion of surrounding organs or structures.

T4 Renal Pelvis and Calyceal Carcinoma

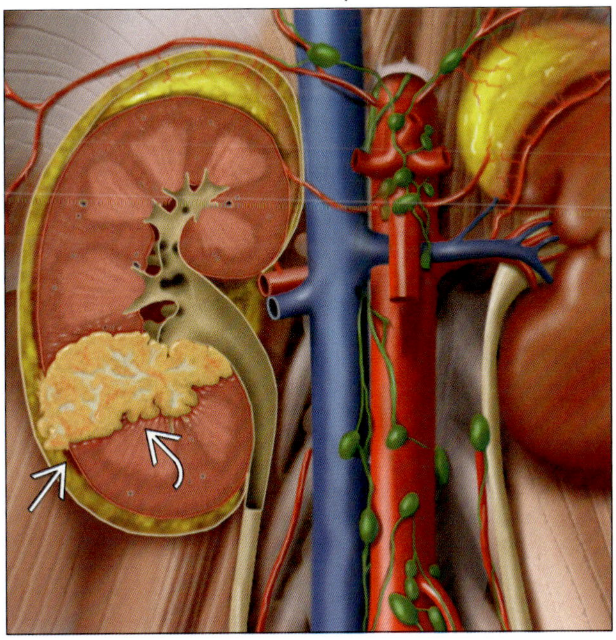

Graphic shows T4 tumor of the lower calyx ➔ with invasion through the renal parenchyma into the perinephric fat ➔.

RENAL PELVIS AND URETERAL CARCINOMA

T4 Ureteric Carcinoma

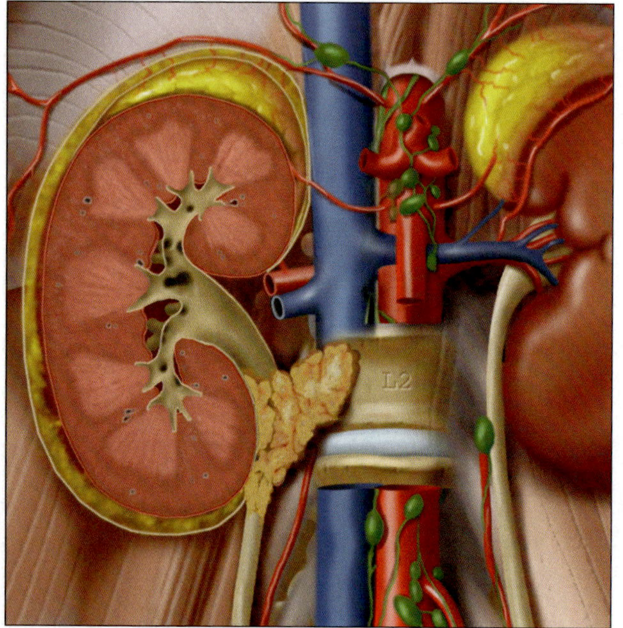

T4 ureteric tumors invade through the surrounding organs and structures. Graphic shows a T4 tumor of the upper ureter invading L2 vertebral body.

T4 Ureteric Carcinoma

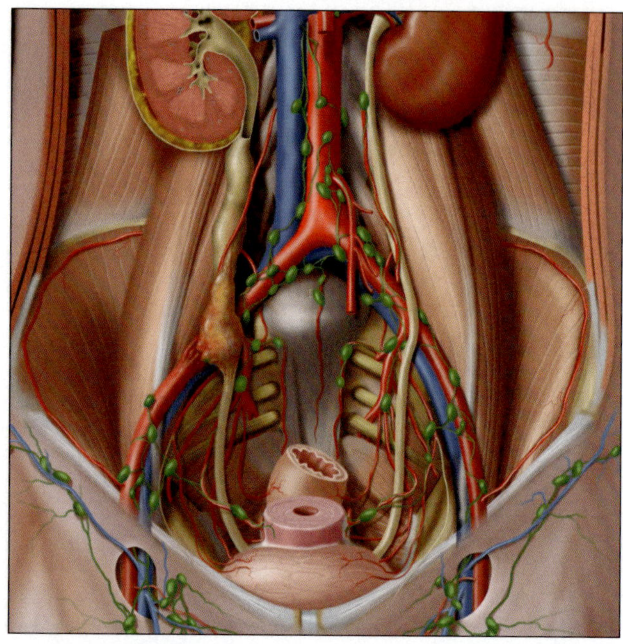

T4 ureteric tumors invade through the surrounding organs and structures. Graphic shows a T4 tumor of the middle ureter invading the right iliac vessels.

T4 Ureteric Carcinoma

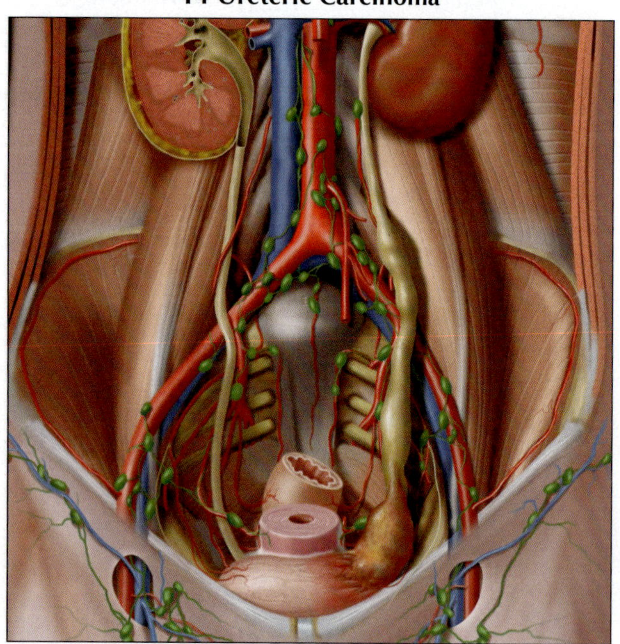

T4 ureteric tumors invade through the surrounding organs and structures. Graphic shows a T4 tumor of the lower ureter invading the urinary bladder.

Nodal Drainage of Renal Pelves and Calyces

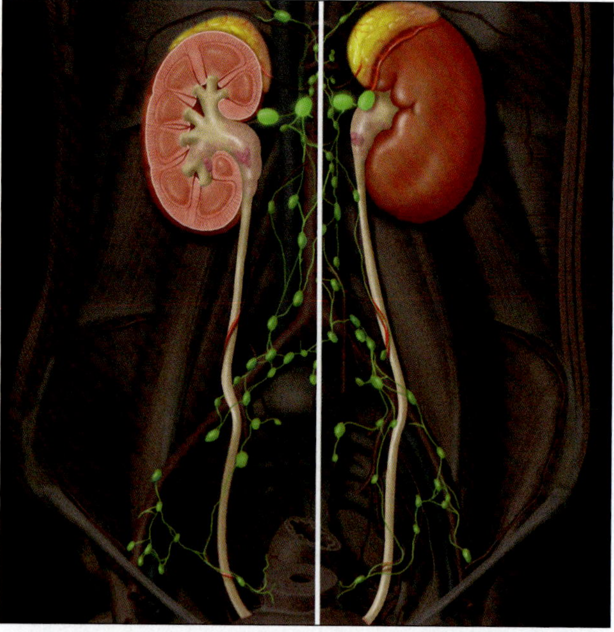

Right renal pelvis tumors spread to renal hilar, paracaval, and retrocaval nodes, whereas left renal pelvic tumors spread to renal hilar and paraaortic nodes.

RENAL PELVIS AND URETERAL CARCINOMA

Nodal Drainage of Upper 2/3 of Ureters

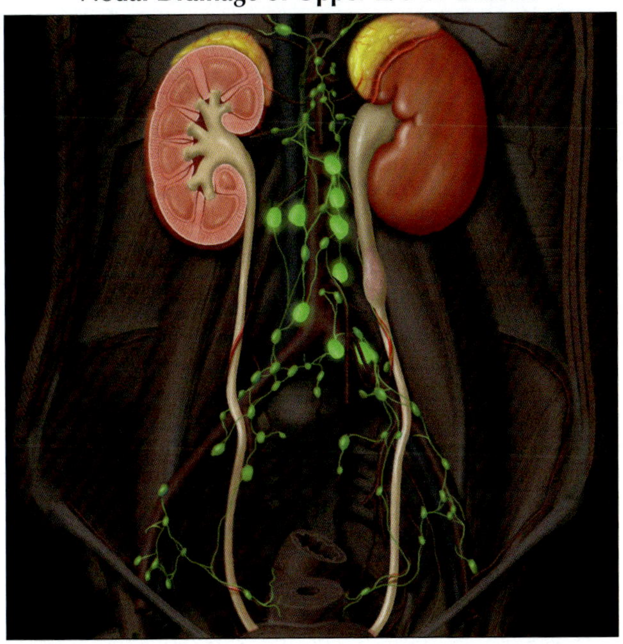

Tumors of the upper 2/3 of the right ureter spread to retrocaval and aortocaval nodes, and tumors of the upper 2/3 of the left ureter spread to paraaortic nodes, nodes at the origin of the inferior mesenteric artery, and common iliac nodes.

Nodal Drainage of Lower 1/3 of Ureters

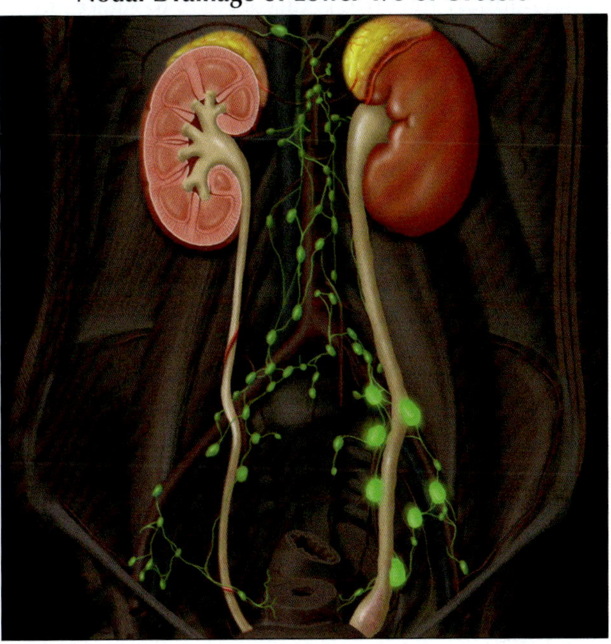

Tumors of the distal 1/3 of either ureter spread to common iliac, internal iliac, external iliac, obturator, and presacral nodes.

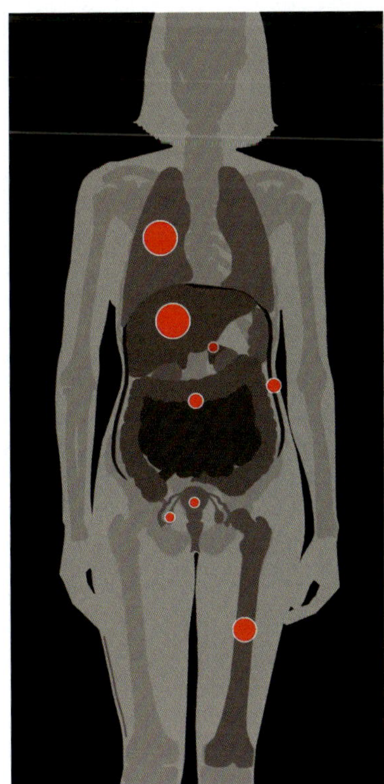

METASTASES, ORGAN FREQUENCY

Liver	63%
Lung	58%
Bone	43%
Gastrointestinal tract	20%
Peritoneum	18%
Adrenal gland	15%
Ovary	13%
Uterus	10%

Data from Batata MA et al: Primary carcinoma of the ureter: a prognostic study. Cancer. 35:1626-32, 1975.

RENAL PELVIS AND URETERAL CARCINOMA

OVERVIEW

General Comments
- Upper urinary tract (UUT) tumors refer to tumors of renal pelves and ureters
- Renal pelvic and ureteric tumors are staged together

Classification
- Transitional cell carcinoma (TCC)
  - 90% of renal pelvis tumors
  - 97% of ureteric tumors
- Squamous cell carcinoma
  - About 10% of renal pelvis tumors
  - 1% of ureteric tumors
- Adenocarcinoma
  - < 1% of upper urinary tract tumors

PATHOLOGY

Routes of Spread
- Local spread
  - Intraluminal seeding of TCC to more caudal parts of ureter
    - High rate of recurrence in distal ureteral stump in patients treated with nephrectomy and incomplete ureterectomy
    - TCC rarely recurs proximal to level of resection of ureteral lesion
  - Tumors of renal pelvis tend to spread into peripelvic fat to kidney and from there to perinephric fat
    - Invasion of renal vein and inferior vena cava (IVC) can rarely occur
  - Tumors of ureter tend to invade periureteral fat to involve adjacent organs
- Lymphatic extension
  - Likelihood of lymph node involvement is associated with increasing T disease
    - Ranges from 4% in noninvasive UUT TCC to as high as 60% in patients with T4 disease
  - Lymph nodes involved depend on site of primary tumor
    - Right renal pelvis → renal hilar, paracaval, and retrocaval nodes
    - Left renal pelvic → renal hilar and paraaortic nodes
    - Upper 2/3 of right ureter → retrocaval and aortocaval nodes
    - Upper 2/3 of left ureter → paraaortic nodes, nodes at origin of inferior mesenteric artery, and common iliac nodes
    - Distal 1/3 of either ureter → common iliac, internal iliac, external iliac, obturator, and presacral nodes and into lymphatics of urinary bladder
- Hematogenous spread
  - Common sites for metastases include liver, lung, and bone

General Features
- Genetics
  - Association with Lynch syndrome (hereditary nonpolyposis colorectal cancer) (HNPCC), type II
    - Early onset of proximal colonic nonpolyposis tumors, numerous synchronous and metachronous colon tumors, and extracolonic tumors
- Etiology
  - Cigarette smoking
    - Factor most strongly associated with UUT TCC
    - > 3x increase in risk
    - Causes 70% of UUT TCC in men and 40% in women
  - Coffee drinking causes slight increase in risk of UUT TCC
    - People who consume more than 7 cups of coffee per day
  - Analgesic abuse (phenacetin)
    - Analgesic nephropathy is associated with incidence of UUT TCC as high as 70%
  - Occupational exposure to agents utilized in petrochemical, plastic, and tar industries
  - Chronic infections, irritation, and calculi
    - Predispose patient to develop squamous cell carcinoma and, less commonly, adenocarcinoma
    - Increased risk with xanthogranulomatous pyelonephritis
  - Chemotherapeutic agents: Cyclophosphamide and ifosfamide
    - Associated tumors tend to be high grade
  - Balkan nephropathy
    - Degenerative interstitial nephritis of unknown etiology
    - 100-200x increased risk in incidence of UUT TCC in individuals from rural Balkan areas relative to that observed in individuals residing in neighboring communities
    - Tumors generally are low grade, multiple, and bilateral compared with TCC of other etiologies
  - Horseshoe kidney
    - Relative risk of TCC in patients with horseshoe kidney is increased 3-4x
- Epidemiology & cancer incidence
  - TCC of renal pelvis and collecting system represents approximately 10% of renal tumors
  - UUT TCC represents < 2-6% of all urothelial malignancies, which primarily occur in bladder
    - Ureteral tumors are even less common, accounting for about 2% of urothelial tumors
  - TCC is 3-4x more common in renal pelvis than in ureter
  - TCC is 2x more common in men than in women
  - Most common in 5th-7th decades with mean age of 65-67 years
  - Highest incidence in Balkan countries (Bulgaria, Greece, former Yugoslavia, and Romania)
- Associated diseases, abnormalities
  - UUT TCC
    - Synchronous bilateral TCC occurs in 1-2% of cases of renal pelvis lesions
    - Synchronous bilateral TCC occurs in 2-9% of cases of ureteric lesions
    - 11-13% of patients with upper tract TCC subsequently develop metachronous upper tract tumors
  - UUT TCC and urinary bladder tumors

RENAL PELVIS AND URETERAL CARCINOMA

- Up to 50% of patients initially presenting with UUT TCC will develop metachronous tumors in bladder
- 2% of patients with bladder TCC also have synchronous UUT TCC at presentation
- 6% of patients with bladder TCC will develop metachronous UUT TCC
- Squamous cell carcinoma
  - Chronic calculus disease and infection
  - Renal calculi are present in 40–80% of renal pelvis squamous cell carcinomas
  - Association with xanthogranulomatous pyelonephritis

Gross Pathology & Surgical Features

- **Renal pelvis tumors**
  - Papillary
  - Polypoid
    - Tend to distend renal pelvis without infiltration
  - Nodular
  - Ulcerative
  - Infiltrative
    - Usually high-grade tumors
    - May arise in calyx and appear as ill-defined mass within kidney
      - May be indistinguishable from renal cell carcinoma
    - Can spread massively into renal parenchyma and reach renal capsule
- **Ureteric tumors**
  - Gross appearance
    - Polypoid: Can fill ureteric lumen and lead to proximal hydroureter
    - Infiltrative: Circumferential thickening of ureteric wall leading to ureteric stricture
  - Tumor site
    - Distal ureter (73%)
    - Mid ureter (24%)
    - Proximal ureter (3%)

Microscopic Pathology

- World Health Organization/International Society of Urologic Pathology grading system
  - Low grade
  - High grade
- Grade of transitional cell cancer correlates with stage
  - Superficial tumors are generally low grade
  - Majority of infiltrative tumors are high grade
- Histological types
  - Papillary noninvasive tumor
  - Papillary invasive tumor
  - Carcinoma in situ
  - Solid invasive tumor

IMAGING FINDINGS

Detection

- Because most patients present with hematuria, initial evaluation requires assessment of kidneys and urinary tract for tumors and calculi
  - Standard work-up as recommended by American Urological Association
    - Urinalysis and cytologic analysis
    - Cystoscopy

- Excretory urography
- **Excretory urography (EU)**
  - Traditionally, noninvasive method of choice for imaging of pelvicalyceal system and ureters
  - Imaging features
    - Filling defect within contrast-enhanced collecting system, renal pelvis, or ureter
    - "Stipple" sign: Tracking of contrast material into interstices of papillary lesions
    - Calyceal amputation when there is complete calyceal obstruction
    - Stricture-like lesions of ureter or pelvicalyceal system ± hydronephrosis
    - Nonvisualization of kidney due to longstanding obstruction → hydronephrosis and nonexcretion of contrast medium
- **Retrograde pyelography**
  - Invasive procedure performed during cystoscopy
    - To further characterize abnormalities detected at EU or CT IVP
    - Allows confirmation of radiologic diagnosis
    - Facilitates ureterorenoscopy with biopsy or brushing and cytologic examination of localized urine collections
    - Particularly useful in cases of
      - Inadequate renal function with poor contrast excretion
      - Contrast allergy
  - Radiological features include
    - Intraluminal filling defect within renal pelvis or ureter, which may be smooth, irregular, or stippled
    - If TCC involves infundibulum, then amputated calyx may be seen ± focal hydronephrosis
    - Distended tumor-filled calyces are known as oncocalyces
- **Ultrasonography**
  - Most common appearance is nonshadowing hypoechoic mass within echogenic renal sinus
  - Typically infiltrative tumors that do not alter renal contours
  - May be associated with hydronephrosis, dilated infundibulum, and calyces
  - May appear as distended tumor-filled calyx (oncocalyx)
- **MDCT and CT IVP**
  - Limited value of single slice CT with detection rates of 50-90%
  - Improved performance with CT IVP for diagnosing TCC
    - Sensitivity (64-85.7%)
    - Specificity (98%)
    - Accuracy (96.3%)
  - Pyelographic phase (PP) is most useful in small tumor detection
    - Delayed imaging is helpful in patient with urinary tract obstruction and delayed contrast excretion
    - Useful to use nonstandard wide window setting for evaluation of pyelographic phase
      - Plaque-like or small lesions can be obscured by dense contrast in collecting system
  - Corticomedullary (CM) and nephrographic (NP) phases are useful in differentiating tumors from blood clots

RENAL PELVIS AND URETERAL CARCINOMA

- ▪ Difficult to assess attenuation and enhancement of luminal lesions on pyelographic phase
- ○ Imaging features
  - ▪ Renal pelvis and calyceal tumors
    - On pre-contrast images, TCC is typically hyperattenuating (5–30 HU) to urine and renal parenchyma
    - Early enhancement and de-enhancement after contrast material administration
    - More uniform enhancement compared with renal cell cancers
    - Sessile pelvic or calyceal filling defect in excretory phase
    - Pelvicalyceal irregularity
    - Focal or diffuse mural thickening
    - Oncocalyx
    - Calyceal obstruction
    - Advanced TCC preserves shape of kidney
  - ▪ Ureteric tumors
    - Short or long strictures
    - Intraluminal filling defects
    - Hydronephrosis
- **MR**
  - ○ T1WI: Isointense relative to renal medulla
    - ▪ Difficult to detect small tumors in collecting system
    - ▪ Larger renal pelvic tumors may obliterate renal sinus fat, which may be appreciated on T1WI without use of fat saturation
  - ○ T2WI: Hypointense relative to bright urine
    - ▪ Appear as filling defects within bright urine in collecting system and ureter
  - ○ Gadolinium-enhanced T1WI: Hypoenhancing mass, although avid enhancement may occur
    - ▪ Enhancement of focal filling defect in collecting system or ureter differentiates tumors from blood clots

Staging
- **MDCT and CT IVP**
  - ○ Limited value of single slice CT with staging accuracy of 36-57%
  - ○ CT does not allow distinction between stage 0–II tumors
    - ▪ It allows differentiation of early stage TCC (0-II) confined to collecting system wall from advanced disease with local extension or distant metastases, which is important for defining surgical management
    - ▪ Early stage tumors (stage 0–II) confined to muscularis are separated from renal parenchyma by renal sinus fat or excreted contrast material and have normal-appearing peripelvic fat
  - ○ Corticomedullary and nephrographic phases are more helpful in evaluation of periureteric tumor infiltration
    - ▪ Changes may be obscured by dense contrast in pyelographic phase
  - ○ Presence of hydronephrosis is associated with aggressive disease and predicts advanced pathologic stage for UUT TCC
- **MR**
  - ○ MR does not allow distinction between stage 0–II tumors

- ○ Contrast-enhanced fat-suppressed T1-weighted imaging is most useful in staging
- ○ Ureteric wall at site of tumor becomes thicker and more intensely enhancing on contrast-enhanced MR
- ○ MR can distinguish thickened noncarcinomatous ureteral walls, due to proliferation of fibrous tissue, from ureteral carcinoma
  - ▪ Fibrous tissue enhances more intensely than ureteral carcinoma
  - ▪ Periureteral fat invasion appears as disruption of intensely enhancing ureteral wall

Restaging
- Recommended imaging follow-up in patients treated for UUT TCC
  - ○ Chest x-ray every 6 months for 1st 2 years and then yearly thereafter
  - ○ Abdominopelvic CECT/CT IVP every 6 months for 1st 2 years and then yearly thereafter

CLINICAL ISSUES

Presentation
- Gross or microscopic hematuria is most common clinical presentation
- Flank pain resulting from ureteric obstruction and hydronephrosis
- Dysuria, frequency
- Some patients are asymptomatic
  - ○ 10-15% have incidental lesions detected on radiographic studies
- Weight loss, anorexia, flank mass, or bone pain are symptoms of advanced disease

Cancer Natural History & Prognosis
- TCC of ureter seems to be associated with worse prognosis compared with tumors of renal pelvis
- Median survival for patients with T1 lesions is 91.1 months compared to 12.9 months for patients with T2 (tumors involving muscularis) and beyond
- Prognosis is worse for patients with high-grade tumors than for those with low-grade tumors
- 5-year survival rates by primary tumor stage
  - ○ Ta-T1 (92%)
  - ○ T2 (78%)
  - ○ T3 (56%)
  - ○ T4 (0%)

Treatment Options
- Major treatment alternatives
  - ○ Radical nephroureterectomy (RNU) with cuff of bladder
    - ▪ Rationale for excision of entire ureter is increased risk of tumor recurrence distal to original tumor
    - ▪ Rationale for excision of bladder cuff is high rate of ureteral stump recurrence
      - Ureteral stump recurrence reported to be 30-75%
    - ▪ Open RNU still represents gold standard for management of UUT TCC
      - However, laparoscopic RNU offers advantages of minimally invasive surgery

- - Open surgery is still recommended in case of advanced tumors (pT3, N+)
  - Lymphadenectomy
  - Possible survival benefit in patients with advanced local disease (pT3 and higher)
  - ○ Segmental ureterectomy
    - Reserved to large or invasive tumor of proximal and mid ureter
  - ○ Open nephron-sparing surgery for upper tract TCC
    - Largely replaced by percutaneous antegrade renal surgery
  - ○ Distal ureterectomy with ureteric re-implantation
    - If tumor is superficial and located in distal 1/3 of ureter
    - Proximal disease must be excluded
  - ○ Endoscopic management of upper tract TCC
    - Indication
      - Patients who have anatomic or functional solitary kidneys
      - Patients with decreased renal function
      - Bilateral upper tract TCC
      - Significant comorbid diseases that preclude abdominal surgery
      - Select patients with normal contralateral kidney who have small, low-grade lesions
    - Approach
      - Retrograde ureteroscopic approach for low-volume ureteral and renal pelvic tumors
      - Percutaneous antegrade approach for larger tumors of renal pelvis and proximal ureter
- Treatment options by stage
  - ○ Stage I, II, III
    - Surgical resection as outlined above
  - ○ Stage IV
    - Palliative urinary diversion
      - Retrograde ureteral stenting
      - Percutaneous drainage ± antegrade ureteral stenting
      - Open diversions
    - Surgical resection in selected cases
    - Limited success with chemotherapy and radiation

REPORTING CHECKLIST

T Staging

- Imaging cannot differentiate early local disease (stages 0-II)
- Attention to periureteral, peripelvic, and renal parenchymal involvement
  - ○ This defines T3 (stage III) disease
- Involvement of adjacent structures or extension through kidney into perinephric fat defines T4 disease

N Staging

- Regional adenopathy depends on tumor location within ureter or renal pelvis

M Staging

- Particular attention to lung, liver, and bones

SELECTED REFERENCES

1. American Joint Committee on Cancer: AJCC Cancer Staging Manual. 7th ed. New York: Springer, 2010
2. Vikram R et al: Imaging and staging of transitional cell carcinoma: part 2, upper urinary tract. AJR Am J Roentgenol. 192(6):1488-93, 2009
3. Wang LJ et al: Diagnostic accuracy of transitional cell carcinoma on multidetector computerized tomography urography in patients with gross hematuria. J Urol. 181(2):524-31; discussion 531, 2009
4. Kawamoto S et al: Transitional cell neoplasm of the upper urinary tract: evaluation with MDCT. AJR Am J Roentgenol. 191(2):416-22, 2008
5. Maddineni SB et al: Aetiology, diagnosis and management of urothelial tumours of the renal pelvis and ureter. BJU Int. 102(9 Pt B):1302-6, 2008
6. Pedrosa I et al: MR imaging of renal masses: correlation with findings at surgery and pathologic analysis. Radiographics. 28(4):985-1003, 2008
7. Sudakoff GS et al: Multidetector computerized tomography urography as the primary imaging modality for detecting urinary tract neoplasms in patients with asymptomatic hematuria. J Urol. 179(3):862-7; discussion 867, 2008
8. Kondo T et al: Primary site and incidence of lymph node metastases in urothelial carcinoma of upper urinary tract. Urology. 69(2):265-9, 2007
9. Raman JD et al: Management of patients with upper urinary tract transitional cell carcinoma. Nat Clin Pract Urol. 4(8):432-43, 2007
10. Browne RF et al: Transitional cell carcinoma of the upper urinary tract: spectrum of imaging findings. Radiographics. 25(6):1609-27, 2005
11. Rassweiler JJ et al: Laparoscopic nephroureterectomy for upper urinary tract transitional cell carcinoma: is it better than open surgery? Eur Urol. 46(6):690-7, 2004

RENAL PELVIS AND URETERAL CARCINOMA

Stage 0a (Ta N0 M0)

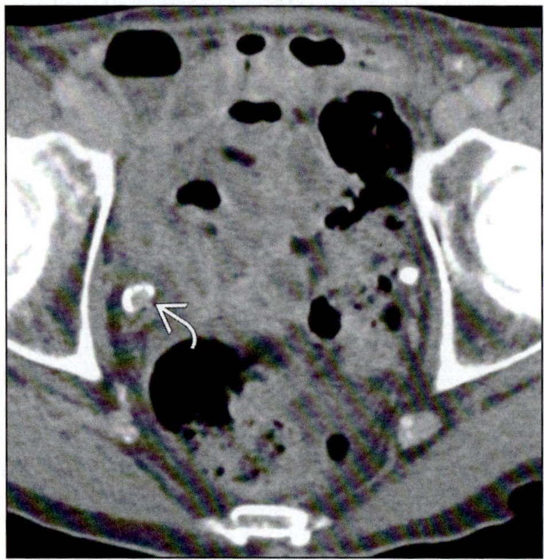

Stage 0a (Ta N0 M0)

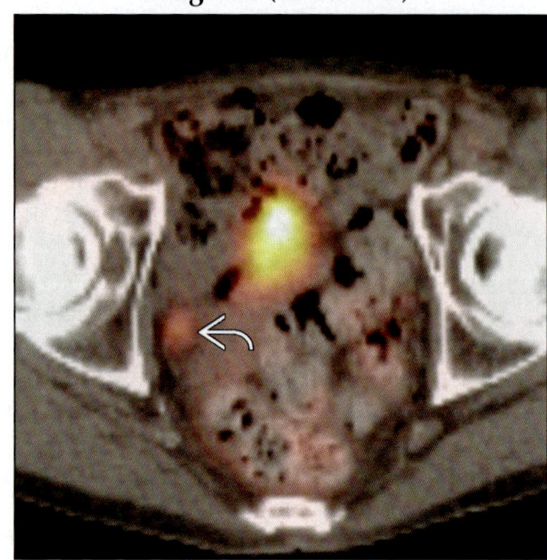

(Left) Axial CT IVP in a patient with a history of lymphoma and hematuria shows a polypoid filling defect ⮕ within the distal right ureter. At surgery, this proved to be a noninvasive carcinoma. *(Right)* Axial PET/CT in the same patient performed 2 days later for staging of lymphoma shows increased metabolic activity in the distal right ureter ⮕ due to renal excretion. It is very difficult to detect urothelial tumor on PET/CT due to urinary excretion of FDG.

Stage 0a (Ta N0 M0)

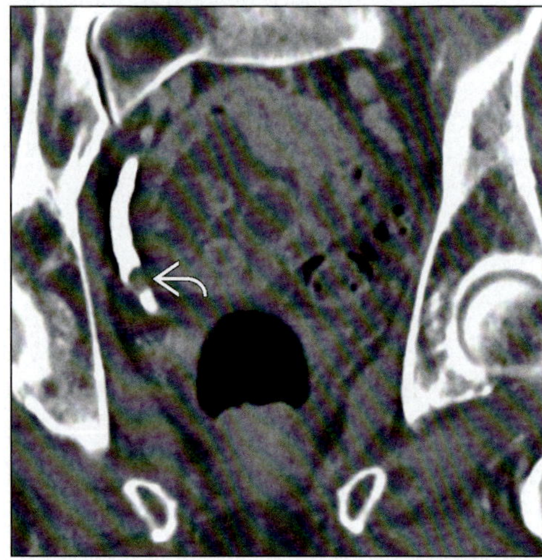

Stage 0a (Ta N0 M0)

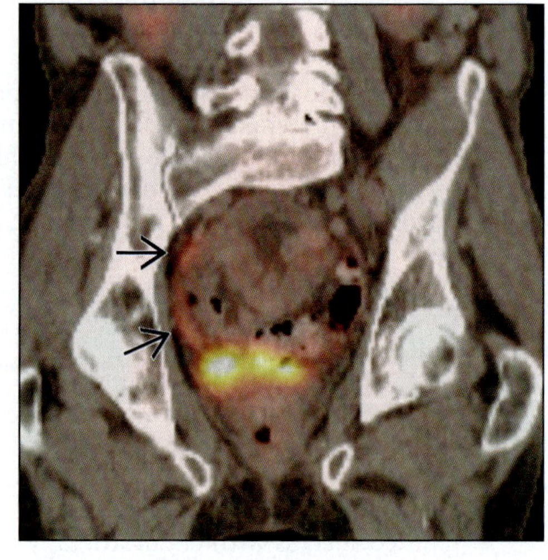

(Left) Coronal CT IVP in the same patient shows a well-defined filling defect ⮕ within the distal right ureter. *(Right)* Coronal PET/CT in the same patient shows a long segment ⮕ of increased activity within the distal right ureter. Urinary excretion of FDG masks the increased activity resulting from urothelial tumor. If a lesion is suspected, forced diuresis will help wash out excreted FDG from the ureter.

Stage 0a (Ta N0 M0)

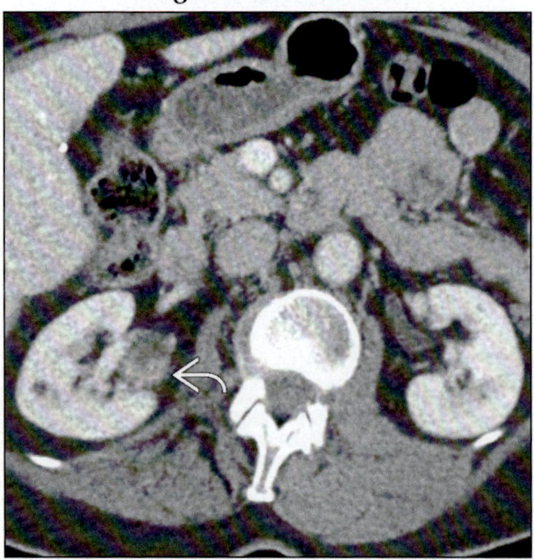

Stage 0a (Ta N0 M0)

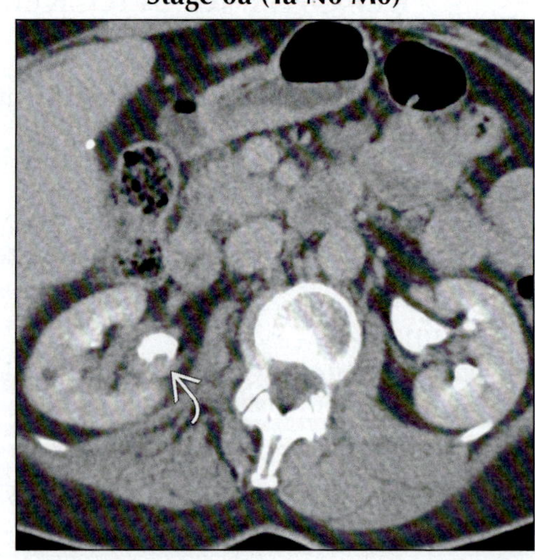

(Left) Axial CECT in another patient obtained during the nephrographic phase of contrast enhancement shows a small enhancing polypoid lesion ⮕ of the posterior wall of the right renal pelvis. *(Right)* Axial CECT in the same patient obtained during the pyelographic phase of contrast enhancement shows the right renal pelvis polypoid lesion ⮕ as a filling defect against the contrast-filled renal pelvis. This was found to be papillary noninvasive carcinoma.

RENAL PELVIS AND URETERAL CARCINOMA

Stage I (T1 N0 M0)

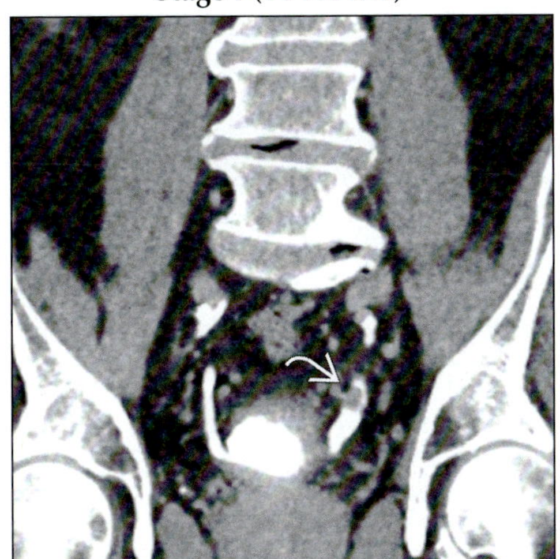

Stage I (T1 N0 M0)

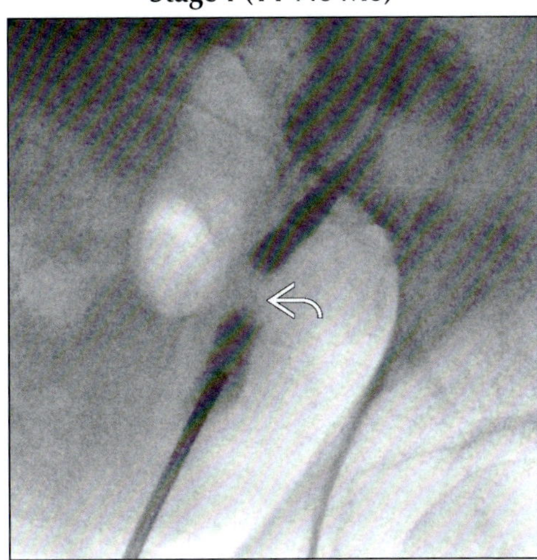

(Left) Coronal CT IVP shows an intraluminal mass ➜ *in the distal part of the left ureter. There is no evidence of periureteric invasion. CT is not helpful in differentiating early stage ureteric tumors. (Right) Frontal view of a retrograde pyelography in the same patient shows the mass* ➜ *almost obstructing the left ureter.*

Stage I (T1 N0 M0)

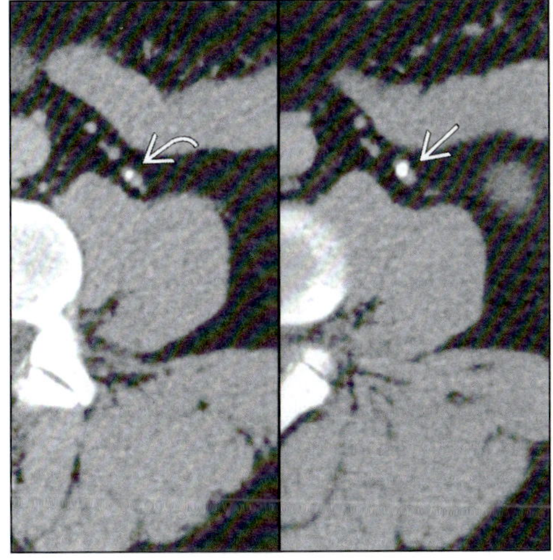

Stage I (T1 N0 M0)

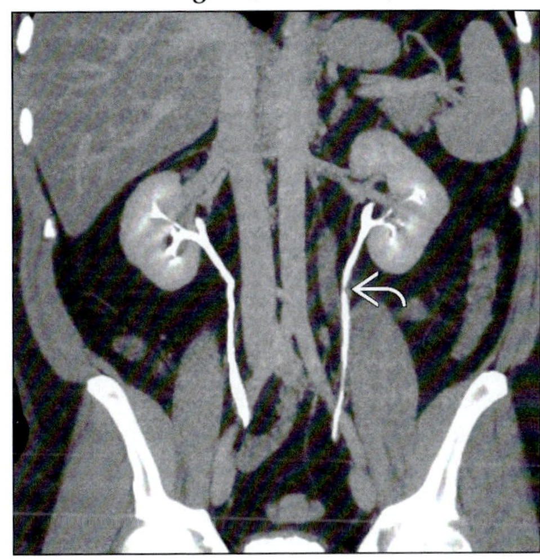

(Left) Axial CT IVP at 2 levels shows subtle narrowing of the ureter ➜ *with normal caliber above that level* ➜ *. (Right) Coronal CT IVP MIP reformatted image in the same patient shows a subtle excentric filling defect* ➜ *at the junction between the upper and middle 1/3 of the left ureter. This was found to be a TCC that invaded into the subepithelial connective tissue. The use of coronal reformats and wide window width allow detection of subtle ureteric lesions.*

Stage I (T1 N0 M0)

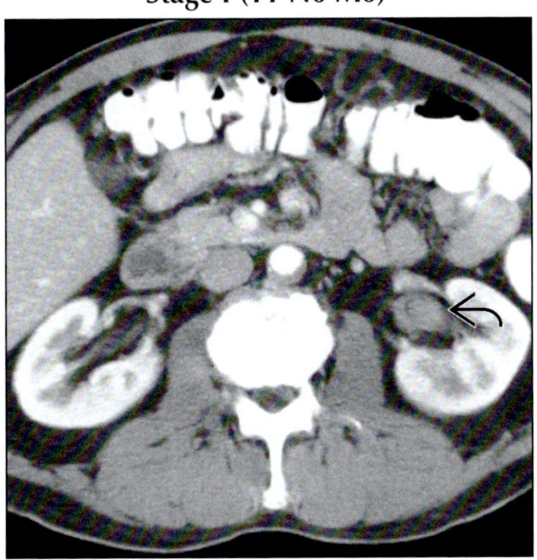

Stage I (T1 N0 M0)

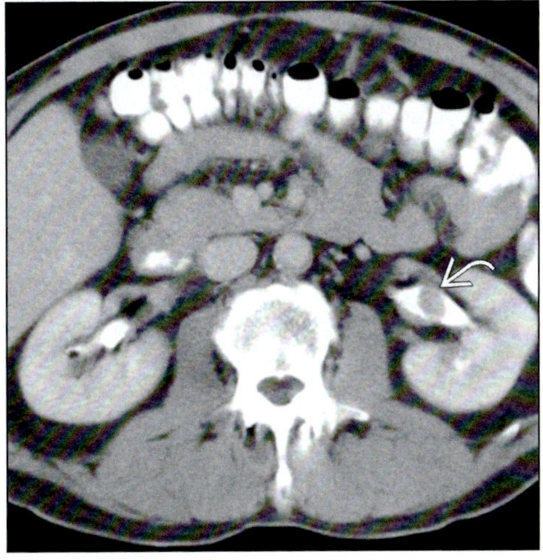

(Left) Axial CT IVP obtained during the nephrographic phase of contrast enhancement shows an enhancing mass ➜ *slightly distending the left renal pelvis. Ureteric or renal pelvis distension provides a clue to the presence of a mass, even on a nonenhanced CT. (Right) Axial CT IVP in the same patient obtained during the pyelographic phase of contrast enhancement clearly shows a filling defect* ➜ *within the left renal pelvis.*

Stage I (T1 N0 M0)

(Left) Axial CECT during the nephrographic phase of contrast enhancement shows multiple enhancing polypoid lesions ⇗ within the right renal pelvis. *(Right)* Axial CECT in the same patient during the pyelographic phase of contrast enhancement shows multiple filling defects ⇗ in the contrast-filled renal pelvis. Unilateral multicentricity does not affect staging of urothelial carcinoma.

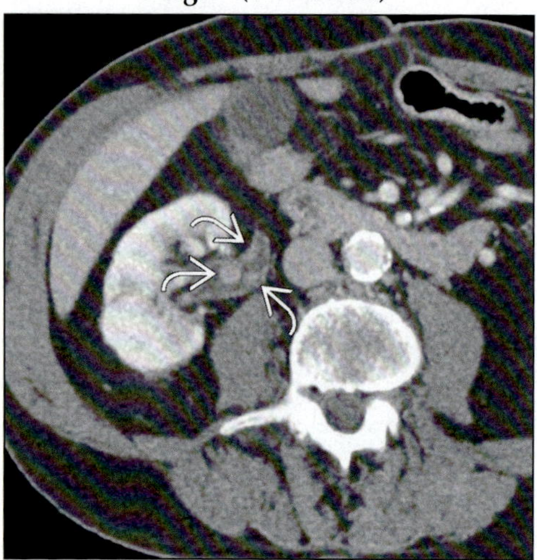

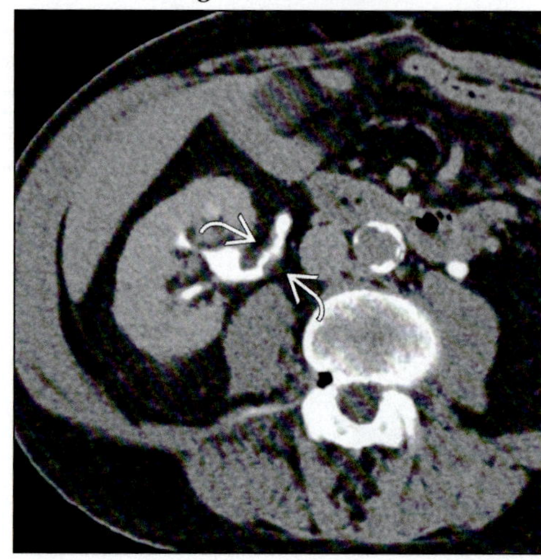

Stage II (T2 N0 M0)

(Left) Axial CECT shows an enhancing lesion ⇗ expanding the right renal pelvis. Note also focal calcifications ⇗. *(Right)* Frontal retrograde pyelogram in the same patient shows a filling defect ⇗ within the renal pelvis and extending into the superior calyx. The mass was found at surgery to invade the muscularis without invading the peripelvic fat, representing T2 tumor.

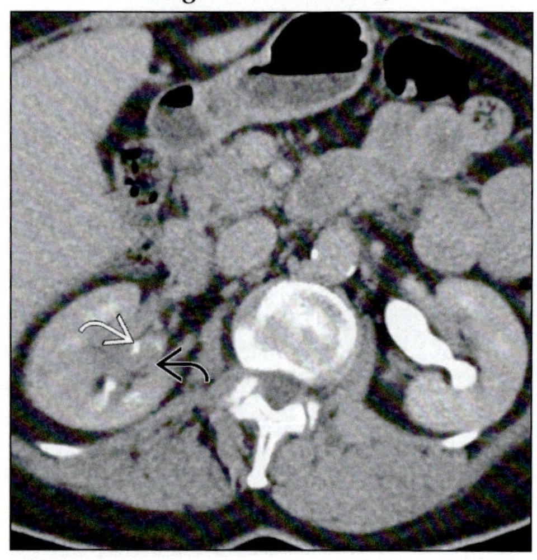

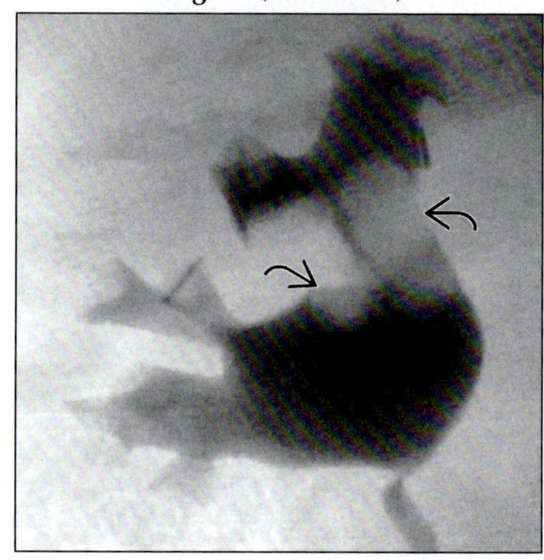

Stage II (T2 N0 M0)

(Left) Axial CT IVP shows a mass ⇗ filling the left renal pelvis and upper calyces without involvement of the renal sinus fat or renal parenchyma. *(Right)* Frontal excretory urography in the same patient shows a large stippled filling defect ⇗ involving the renal pelvis and upper calyces of the left kidney. The "stipple" sign refers to tracking of contrast material ⇗ into the interstices of a papillary lesion.

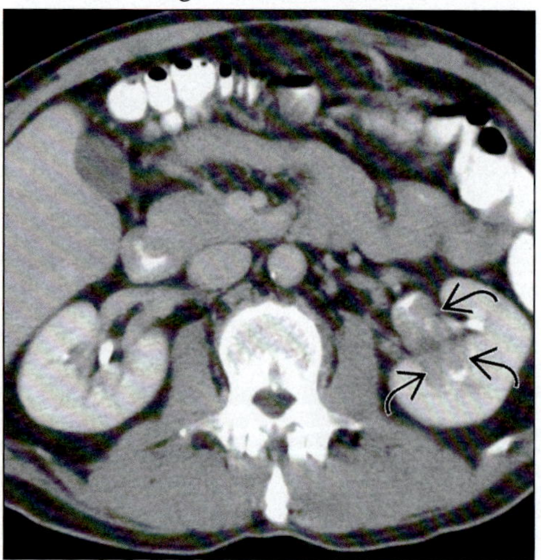

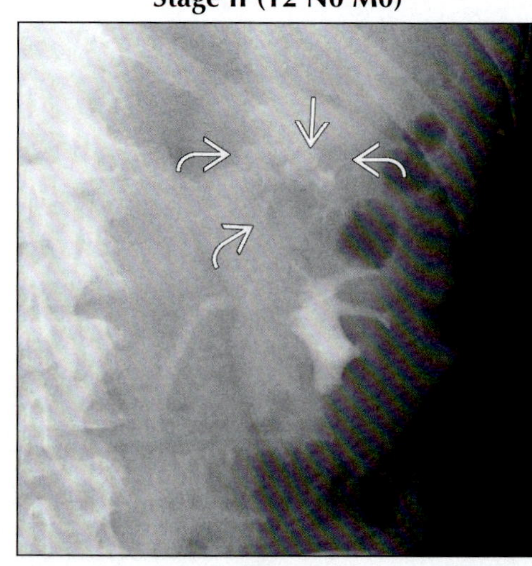

RENAL PELVIS AND URETERAL CARCINOMA

Stage II (T2 N0 M0)

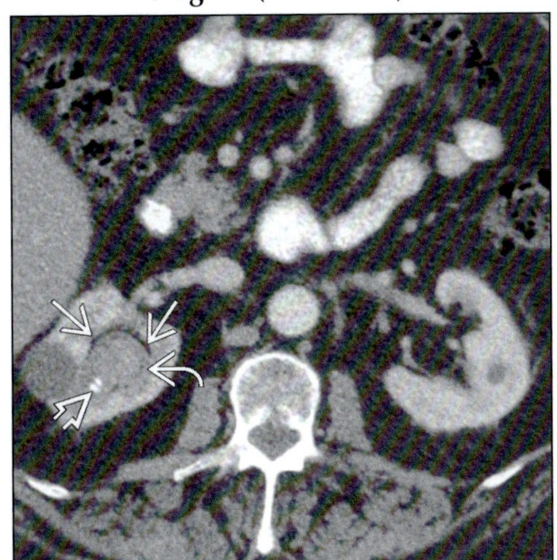

Stage II (T2 N0 M0)

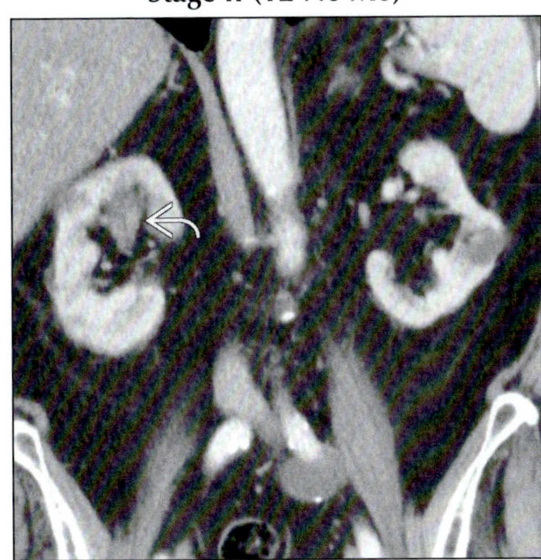

(Left) Axial CT IVP shows a mass → filling and distending the right upper calyx. Note the compressed renal sinus fat around the distended calyx →. Calcifications in the mass → are a common feature of TCC, which allow detection of tumors on a nonenhanced CT performed for evaluation of hematuria. (Right) Coronal CT IVP in the same patient shows a mass → filling the upper calyx (oncocalyx) without involvement of the renal sinus fat or renal parenchyma.

Stage II (T2 N0 M0)

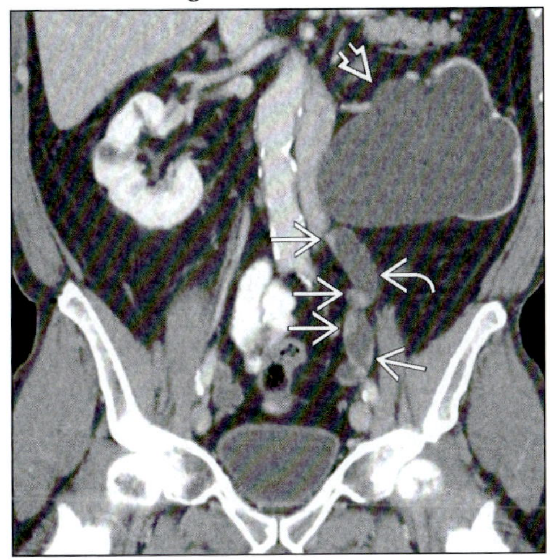

Stage II (T2 N0 M0)

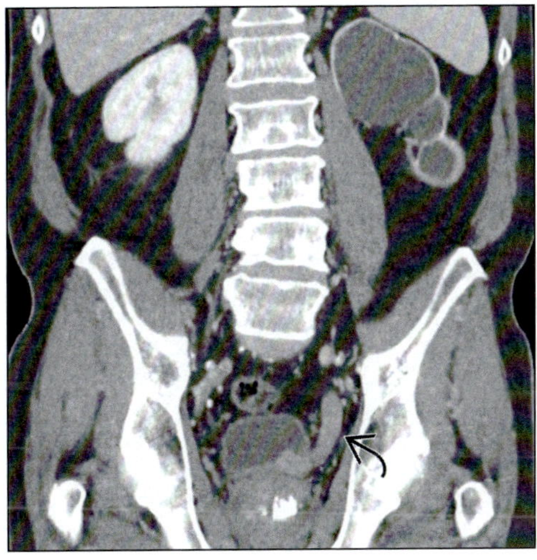

(Left) Coronal CECT shows severe hydronephrosis → and hydroureter →. Multiple ureteric masses are seen within the ureter →. It is difficult to show the extent of ureteric involvement on a single axial or coronal image. No contrast was seen in the renal pelvis or ureter, even an hour after contrast injection. (Right) Coronal CECT in the same patient shows that the distal ureter is filled with a large mass → extending to the ureterovesical junction.

Stage II (T2 N0 M0)

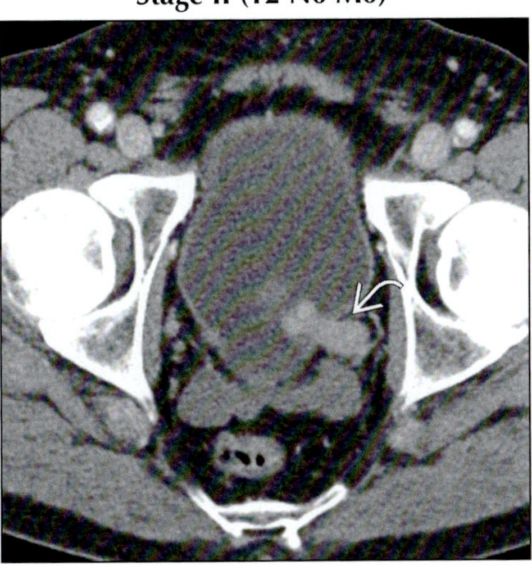

Stage II (T2 N0 M0)

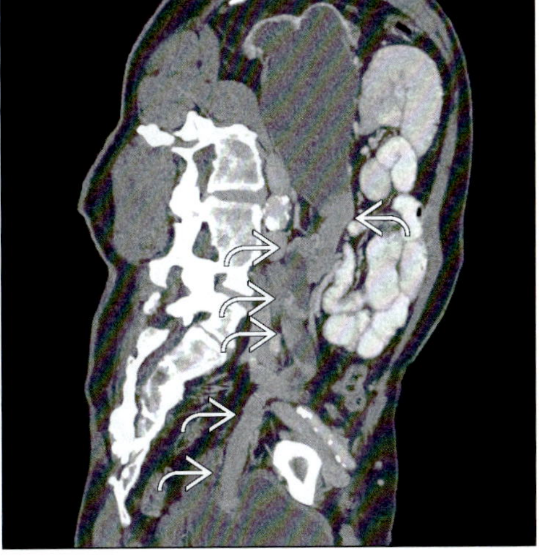

(Left) Axial CECT in the same patient shows the distal ureteric mass → protruding into the urinary bladder lumen. (Right) Curved multiplanar reformatting along the course of the ureter shows the extent of ureteric involvement with multiple masses →. The ureteric masses were all confined to the ureter without extraureteric extension. This case illustrates a common pathway of tumor spread through seeding along the ureter.

Stage II (T2 N0 M0)

Stage II (T2 N0 M0)

(Left) Axial CECT in a patient with horseshoe kidney shows a mass filling left posterior calyx ➡ without renal invasion. Note the clear fat plane ➡ around the distended calyx. *(Right)* Axial CECT in the same patient shows extension of the tumor to the renal pelvis ➡, again with preservation of peripelvic fat. The relative risk of TCC in a patient with horseshoe kidney is increased 3-4x.

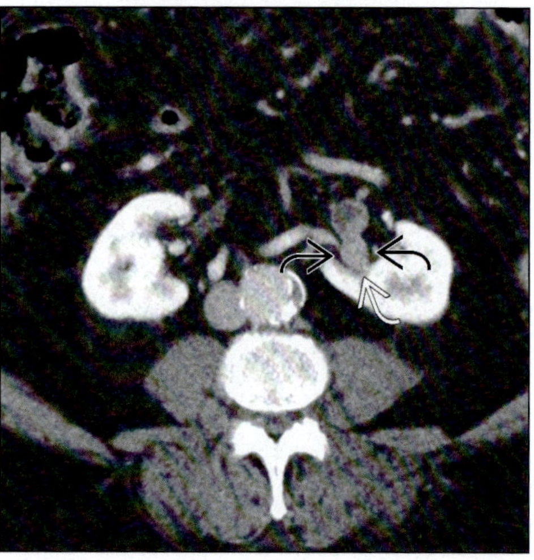

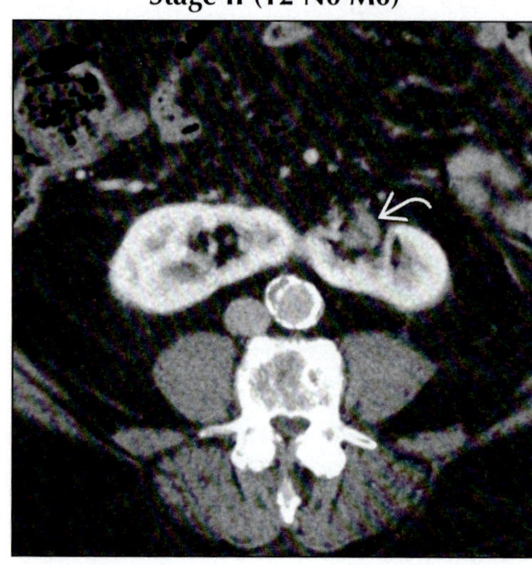

Stage II (T2 N0 M0)

Stage II (T2 N0 M0)

(Left) Coronal CECT shows an enlarged kidney with a staghorn stone in the renal pelvis ➡ and replacement of renal parenchyma by multiple low-density, fluid-filled areas ➡ surrounded by a thin rim of residual renal parenchyma, due to xanthogranulomatous pyelonephritis. Abnormal enhancing soft tissue fills the renal pelvis around the stone ➡. *(Right)* Axial CECT in the same patient shows tumor extending into the dilated calyces ➡. Biopsy specimen revealed squamous cell carcinoma.

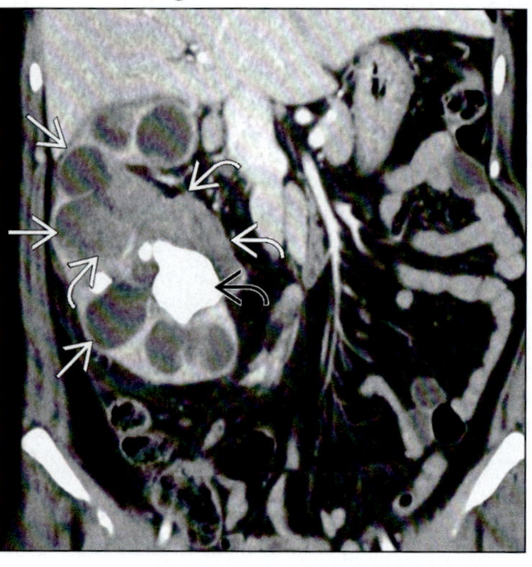

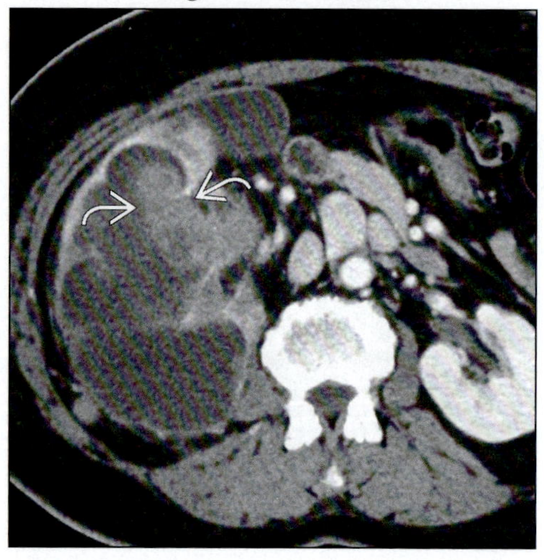

Stage II (T2 N0 M0)

Stage II (T2 N0 M0)

(Left) Axial T2WI MR shows a left renal pelvis mass ➡ with extension to the renal calyces ➡. There is no evidence of invasion into the peripelvic fat or into the renal parenchyma. *(Right)* Axial T1WI C+ FS MR shows a large mass ➡ filling the renal pelvis and calyces. The mass is hypoenhancing relative to the kidney. Although the mass is distending the renal pelvis, there is a complete circle of ureteric enhancement ➡, indicating that the peripelvic fat is not invaded by tumor.

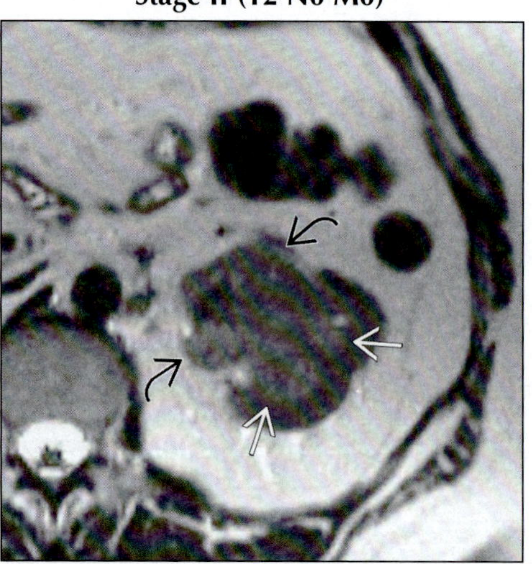

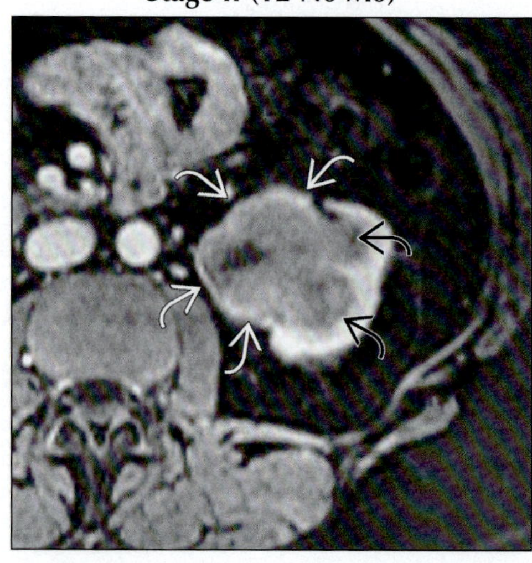

RENAL PELVIS AND URETERAL CARCINOMA

Stage II (T2 N0 M0)

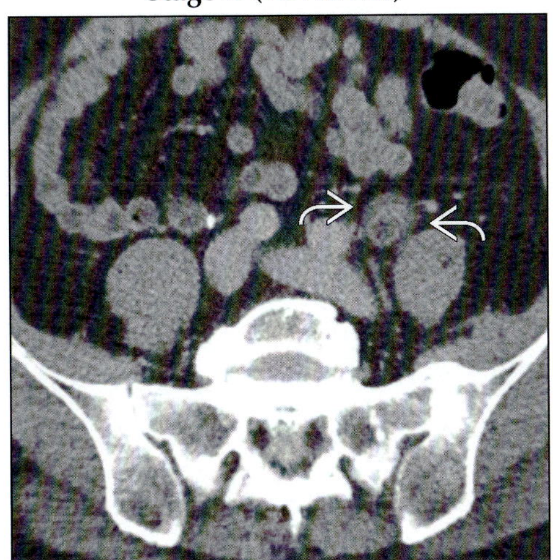

Stage II (T2 N0 M0)

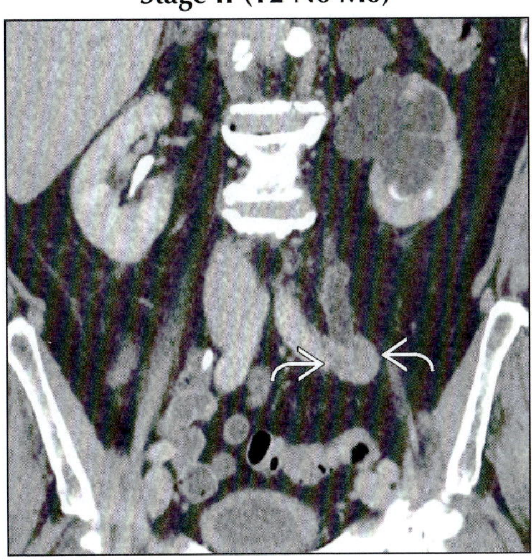

(Left) Axial CT IVP shows a mass ⇒ centered on the left ureter. Although the mass is large and appears to extend beyond the contour of the ureter, pathological evaluation of the resected specimen showed that the tumor invaded the muscularis and was surrounded by a concentric mass of fibrous tissue. *(Right)* Coronal CT IVP in the same patient shows the exophytic ureteral mass ⇒ causing hydronephrosis and dilatation of the proximal ureter.

Stage III (T3 N0 M0)

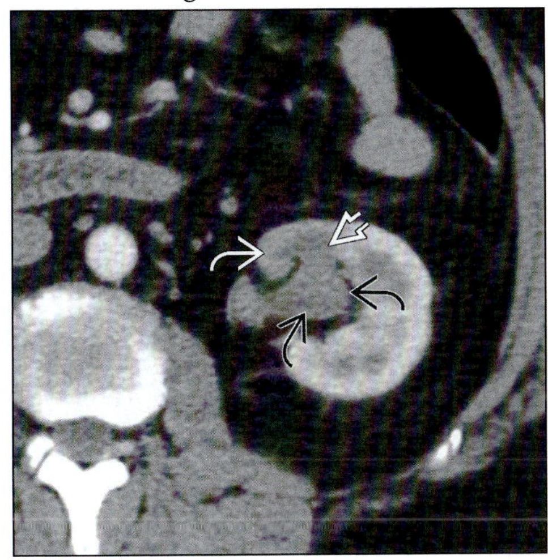

Stage III (T3 N0 M0)

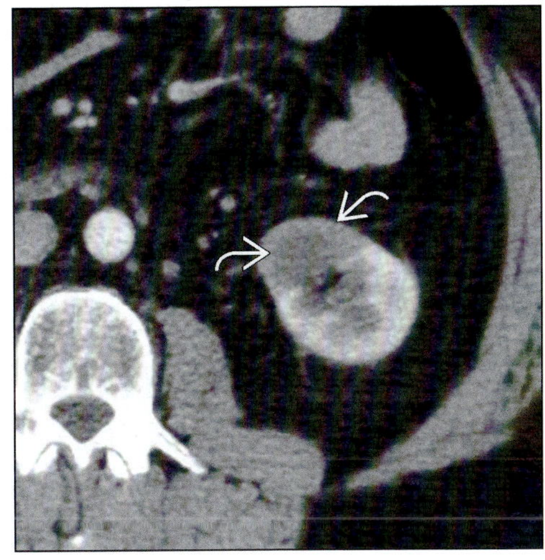

(Left) Axial CT IVP shows a soft tissue mass ⇒ distending the renal pelvis and extending into an anterior calyx ⇒. The mass also invades into the renal parenchyma ⇒; the tumor enhances less than the normal parenchyma. *(Right)* Axial CT IVP in the same patient shows renal parenchymal invasion ⇒. The involved kidney is hypoenhancing compared to the normal enhancing kidney. There is no evidence of perinephric fat involvement.

Stage IV (T4 N0 M0)

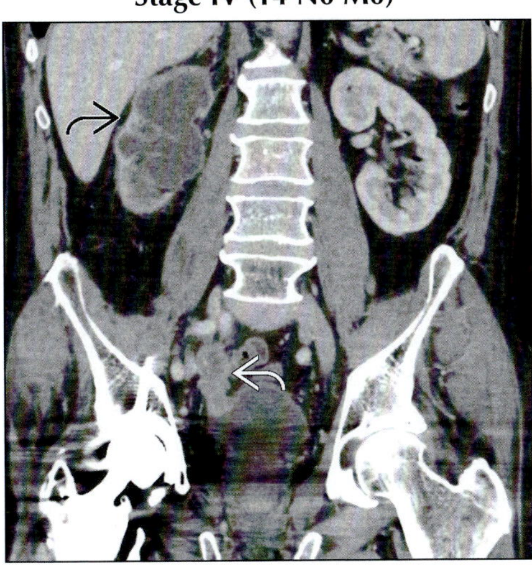

Stage IV (T4 N0 M0)

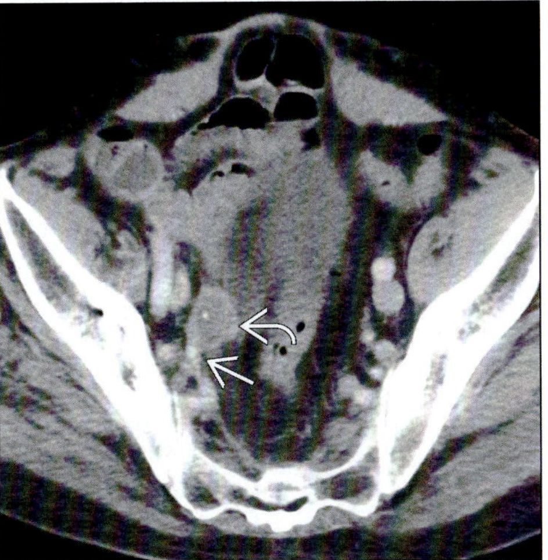

(Left) Coronal CECT shows right side hydronephrosis ⇒ and a right ureteric mass ⇒ involving the ureterovesical junction. *(Right)* Axial CECT in the same patient shows the right ureteric mass ⇒ invading into the periureteric fat to involve the right internal iliac artery ⇒.

RENAL PELVIS AND URETERAL CARCINOMA

Stage IV (T2 N1 M0)

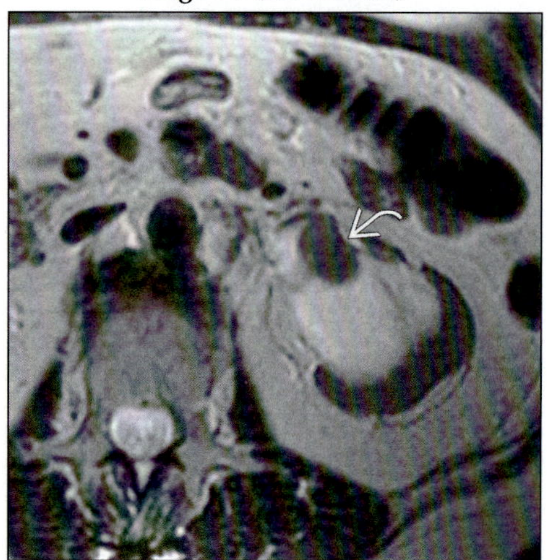

Stage IV (T2 N1 M0)

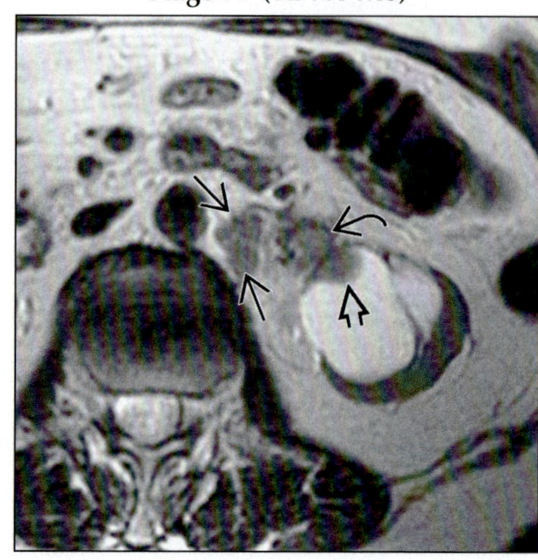

(Left) Axial T2WI MR shows a polypoid mass ⤷ of intermediate signal intensity within the left renal pelvis. The mass does not infiltrate into the renal sinus fat or the kidney. (Right) Axial T2WI MR in the same patient shows an intermediate signal intensity renal pelvis mass ⤷ infiltrating the upper ureter ⤷ and causing hydronephrosis. Multiple paraaortic lymph nodes ⤷, each less than 2 cm, are present.

Stage IV (T2 N1 M0)

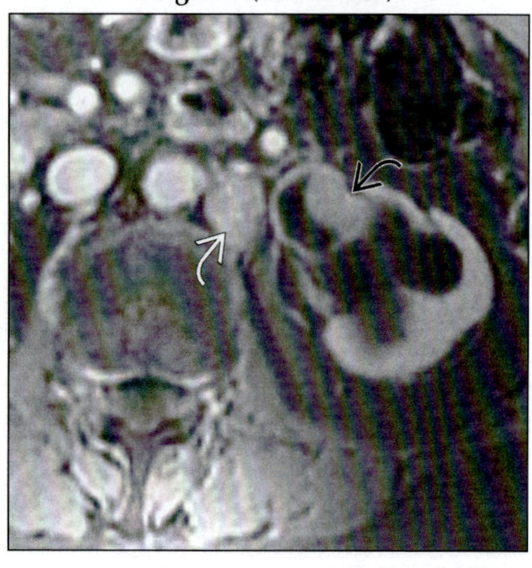

Stage IV (T2 N1 M0)

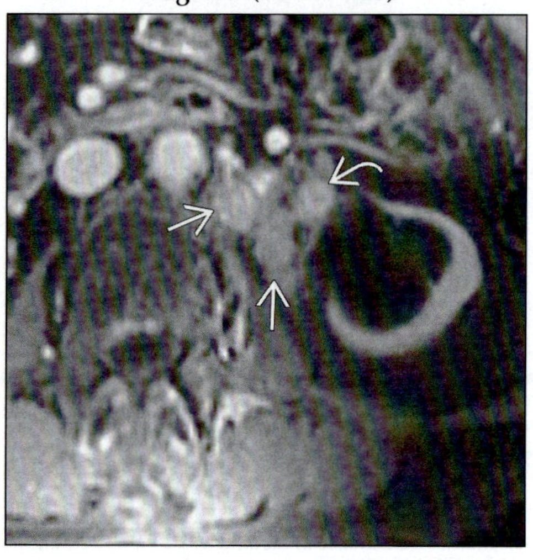

(Left) Axial T1WI C+ FS MR in the same patient shows an enhancing renal pelvis mass ⤷ with no evidence of invasion of renal parenchyma. There is an enhancing paraaortic lymph node ⤷ that measures just less than 2 cm. (Right) Axial T1 C+ FS MR in the same patient shows involvement of the upper ureter ⤷ and multiple paraaortic lymph nodes ⤷.

Stage IV (T2 N1 M0)

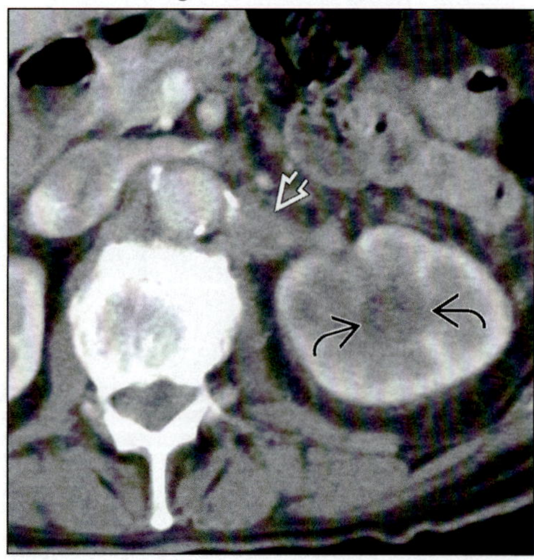

Stage IV (T2 N1 M0)

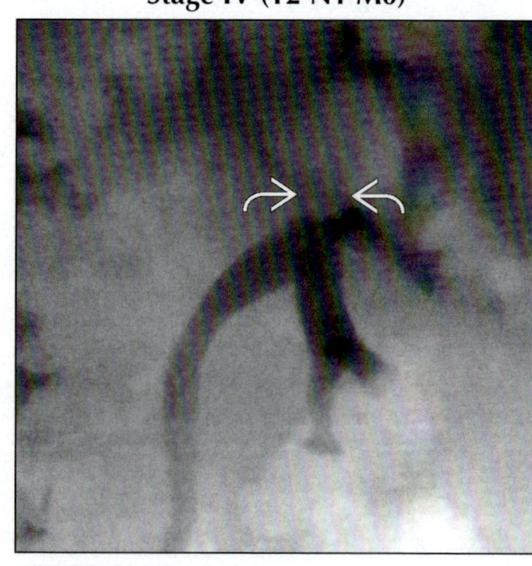

(Left) Axial CECT in a 76-year-old man who presented with hematuria shows an enhancing soft tissue mass ⤷ filling and expanding the left upper calyx (oncocalyx). An ill-defined, left, paraaortic, 1.8 cm lymph node ⤷ is also present. (Right) Retrograde pyelogram in the same patient shows amputation of the left upper calyx ⤷.

RENAL PELVIS AND URETERAL CARCINOMA

Stage IV (T3 N1 M0)

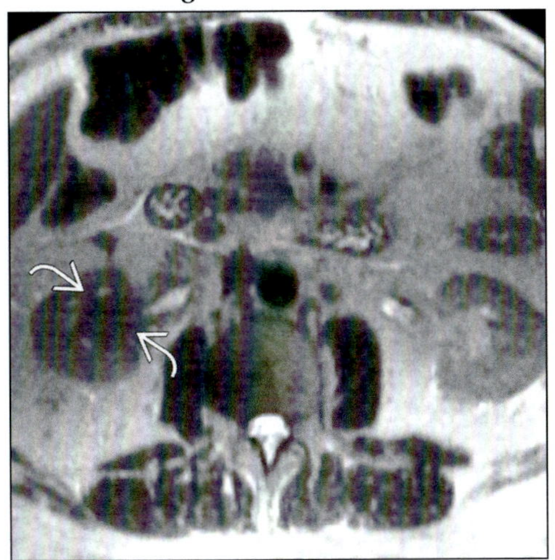

Stage IV (T3 N1 M0)

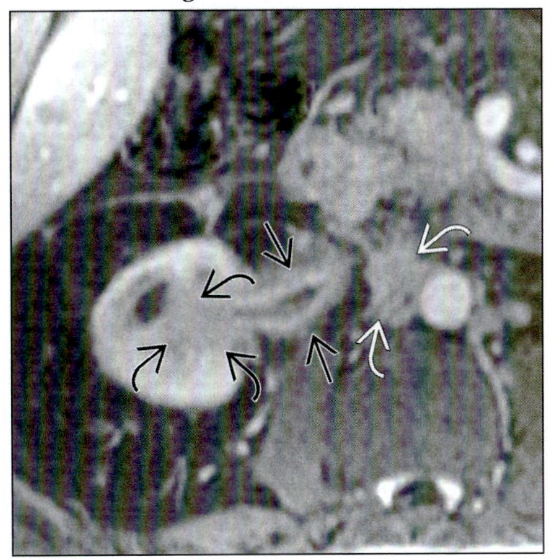

(Left) Axial T2WI MR shows a low signal intensity mass ➡ obliterating the right renal sinus fat. (Right) Axial T1 C+ FS MR shows an enhancing mass ➡ obliterating the renal sinus fat. Note thickening and mucosal enhancement of the renal pelvis ➡, which can be due to submucosal tumor spread or associated inflammatory changes. Also note the infiltrative enhancing nodal mass ➡ occluding the inferior vena cava.

Stage IV (T4 N1 M0)

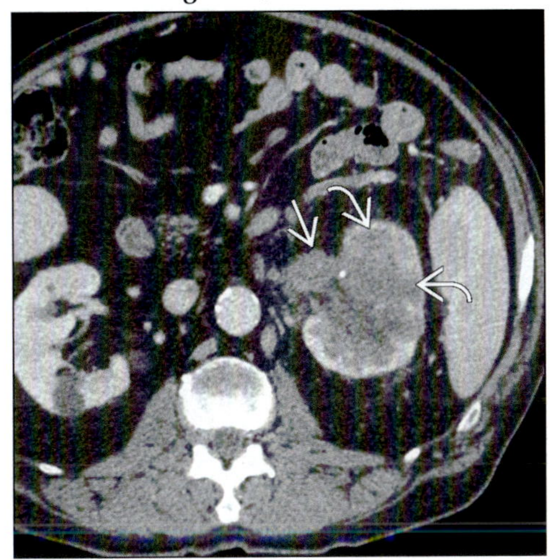

Stage IV (T4 N1 M0)

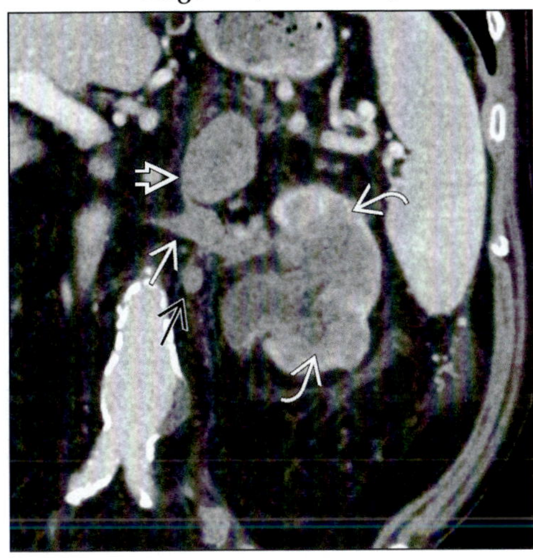

(Left) Axial CECT shows a mass filling the left renal pelvis and calyces, as well as invading the renal parenchyma ➡. The mass also infiltrates the renal vein ➡. (Right) Coronal CECT in the same patient shows the mass infiltrating most of the kidney ➡. There is involvement of the left renal vein ➡ and left adrenal vein, forming a mass ➡ that is separate from the adrenal gland. There is also a 2 cm enlarged lymph node ➡.

Stage IV (T4 N1 M0)

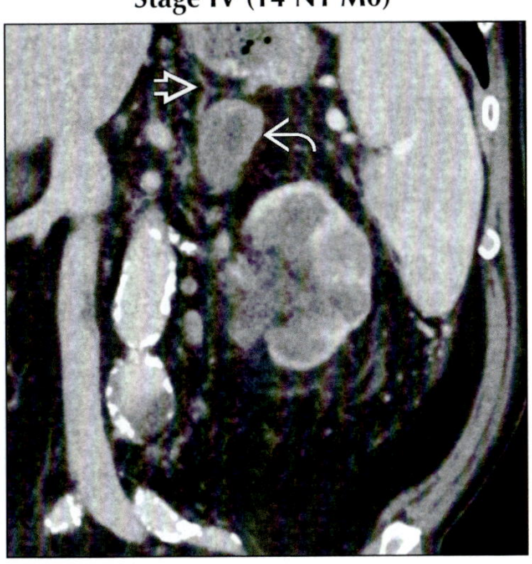

Stage IV (T4 N1 M0)

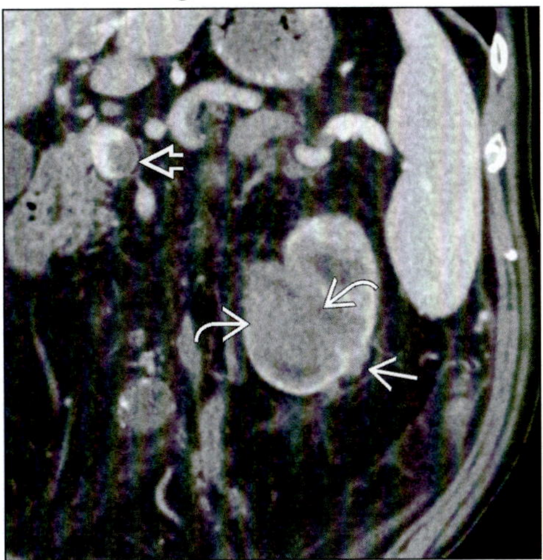

(Left) Coronal CECT in the same patient shows the mass involving the left adrenal vein ➡ separate from the normal adrenal gland ➡. (Right) Coronal CECT in the same patient shows the infiltrative mass ➡ involving almost the entire left kidney with violation of the renal capsule and extension into the perinephric fat ➡. An incidental finding was thrombosis of the portal vein ➡.

RENAL PELVIS AND URETERAL CARCINOMA

Stage IV (T2 N2 M0)

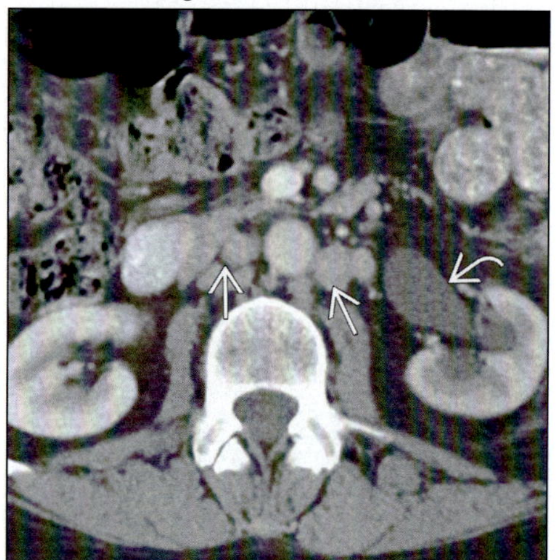

Stage IV (T2 N2 M0)

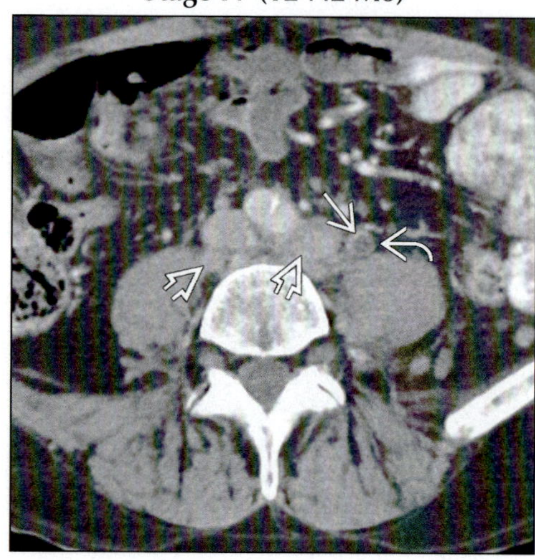

(Left) Axial CECT in a 56-year-old man who presented with hematuria shows left side hydronephrosis ➔ with delayed left renal contrast excretion. Multiple paraaortic lymph nodes ➔ are present. *(Right)* Axial CECT in the same patient shows left side hydroureter ➔ just above the level of obstruction with a rim of enhancing ureteral wall thickening ➔ due to tumor extension. Multiple paraaortic lymph nodes are present ➔.

Stage IV (T2 N2 M0)

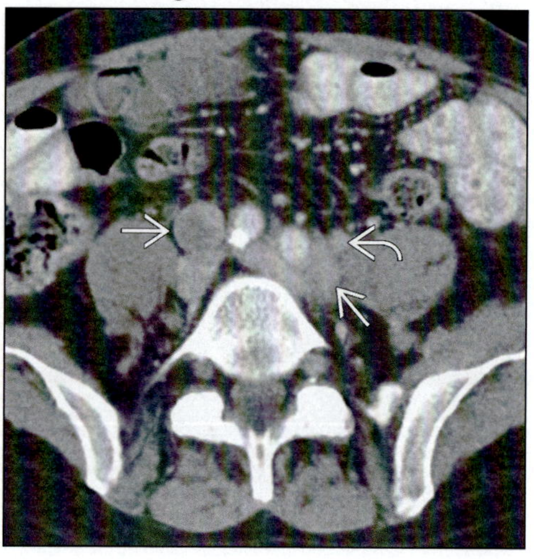

Stage IV (T2 N2 M0)

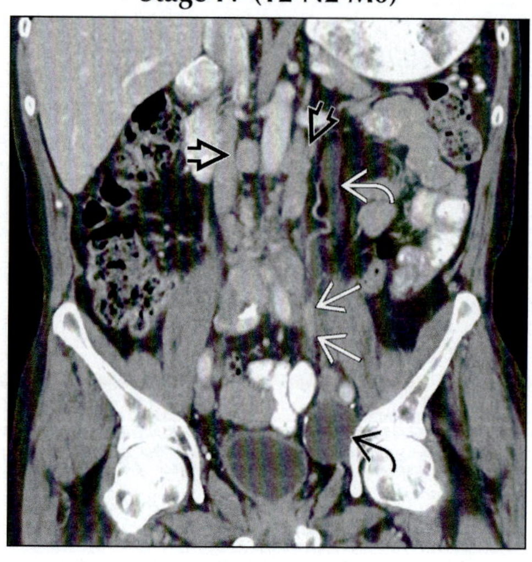

(Left) Axial CECT in the same patient shows an enhancing mass ➔ obstructing the ureter, as well as multiple retroperitoneal lymph nodes ➔. *(Right)* Coronal CECT in the same patient shows an enhancing ureteric soft tissue mass ➔ with dilatation of the proximal ureter ➔ and multiple paraaortic lymph nodes ➔. The cystic lesion in the left side of the pelvis ➔ is a lymphocele resulting from previous pelvic nodal dissection for prostate carcinoma.

Stage IV (T3 N2 M0)

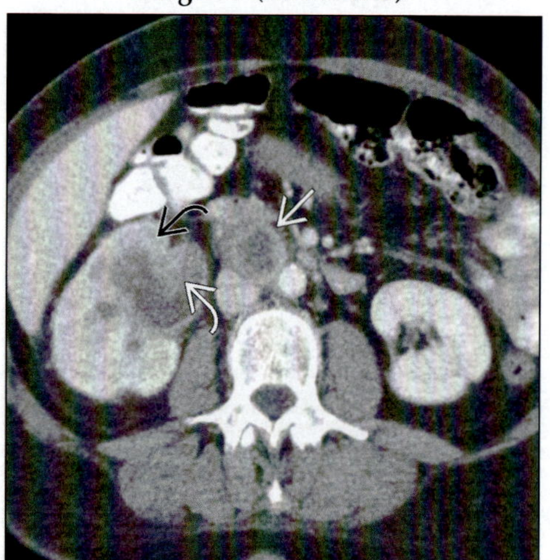

Stage IV (T3 N2 M0)

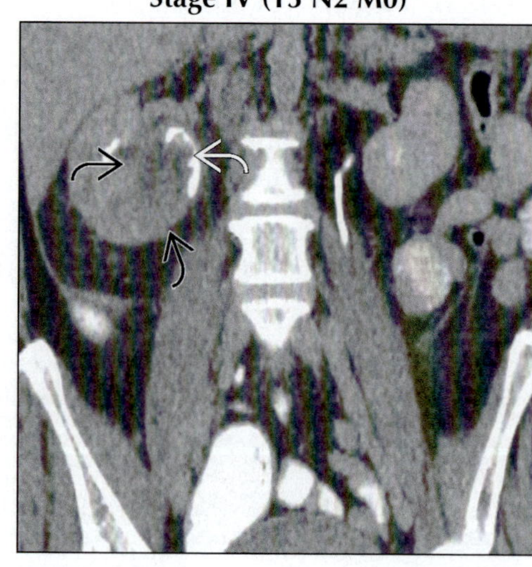

(Left) Axial CECT shows a right renal pelvis mass ➔ that invades into the renal parenchyma ➔ but not through the kidney into the perinephric fat. There is also a single enlarged necrotic aortocaval lymph node ➔ that measures 3 cm. *(Right)* Coronal CECT in the same patient shows the right renal pelvis mass ➔ invading into the renal parenchyma ➔. There is no invasion of the perinephric fat.

RENAL PELVIS AND URETERAL CARCINOMA

Stage IV (T3 N2 M1)

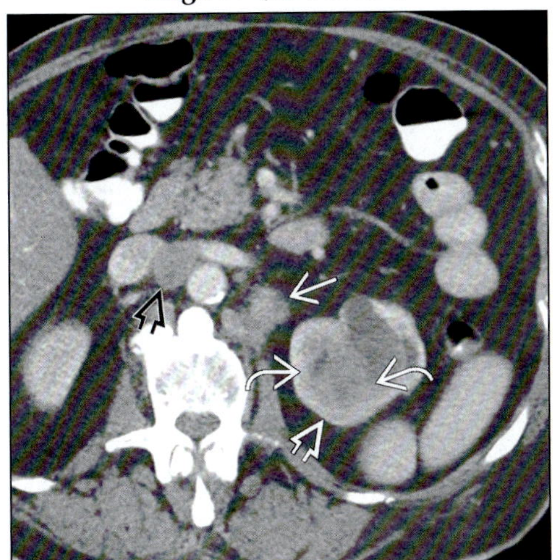

Stage IV (T3 N2 M1)

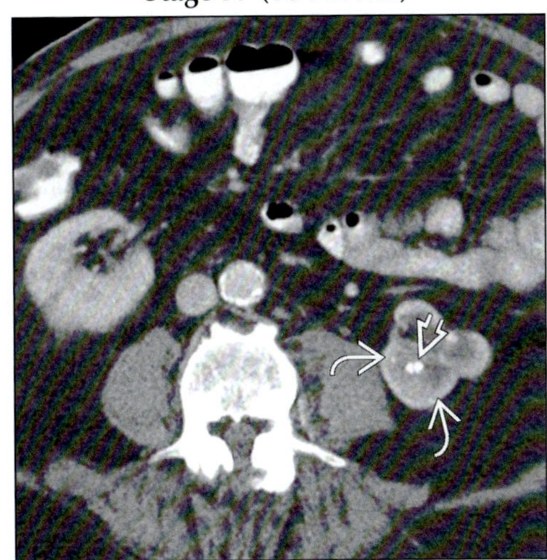

(Left) Axial CECT in a 77-year-old man who presented with gross hematuria shows an upper pole infiltrative renal mass ➡ that extends to, but not beyond, the renal capsule ➡. Multiple paraaortic ➡ and aortocaval ➡ lymph nodes are also present. (Right) Axial CECT in the same patient shows a lower pole renal mass ➡ that contains nodular calcifications ➡.

Stage IV (T3 N2 M1)

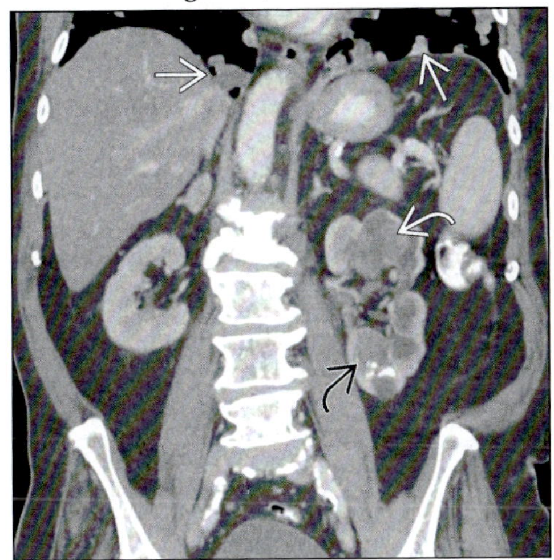

Stage IV (T3 N2 M1)

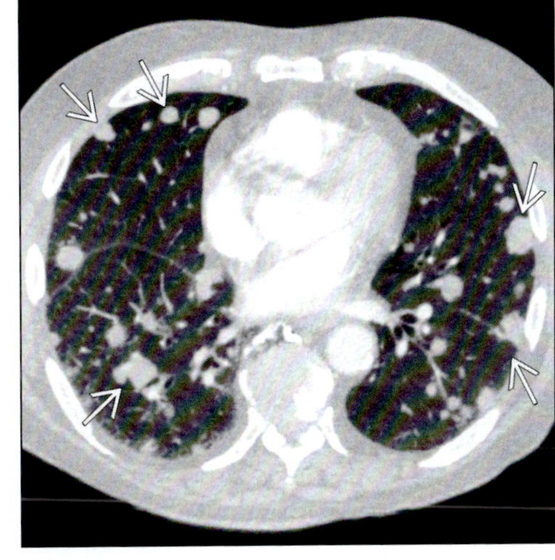

(Left) Coronal CECT in the same patient shows 2 renal masses, 1 in the upper pole ➡ and 1 in the lower pole ➡. It is difficult to determine whether these masses are renal cell carcinomas or transitional cell carcinomas arising from the collecting system. Note also numerous pulmonary metastases ➡. (Right) Axial CECT in the same patient shows numerous pulmonary nodules ➡ due to parenchymal pulmonary metastases.

Stage IV (T3 N2 M1)

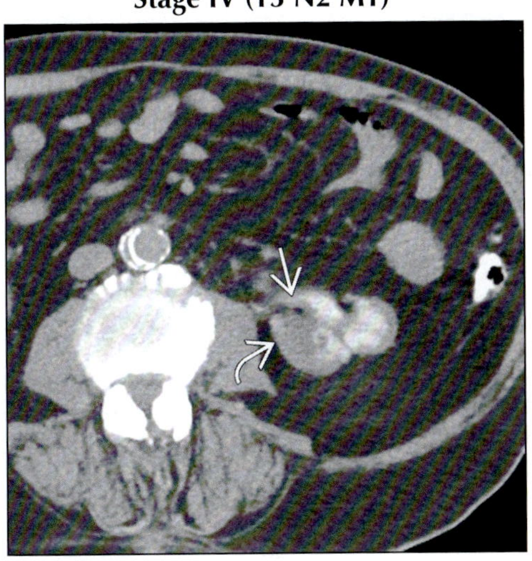

Stage IV (T3 N2 M1)

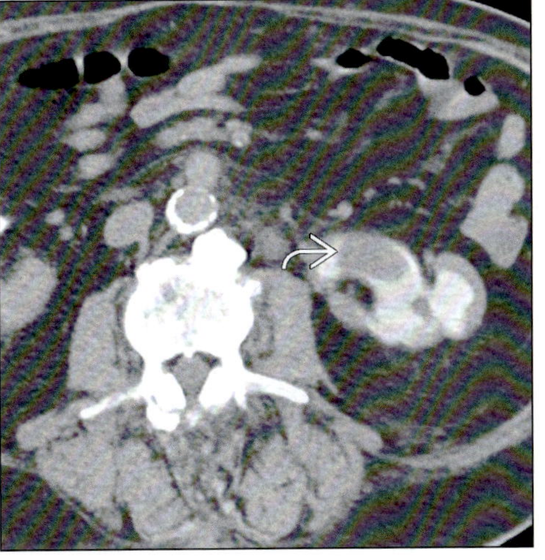

(Left) Axial CECT in the same patient 1 day later shows high-density contrast within the collecting system. The lower pole mass ➡ extends to involve the adjacent part of the renal pelvis ➡. (Right) Axial CECT in the same patient shows a large filling defect ➡ that changed position after the patient assumed a prone position, behavior consistent with a floating blood clot.

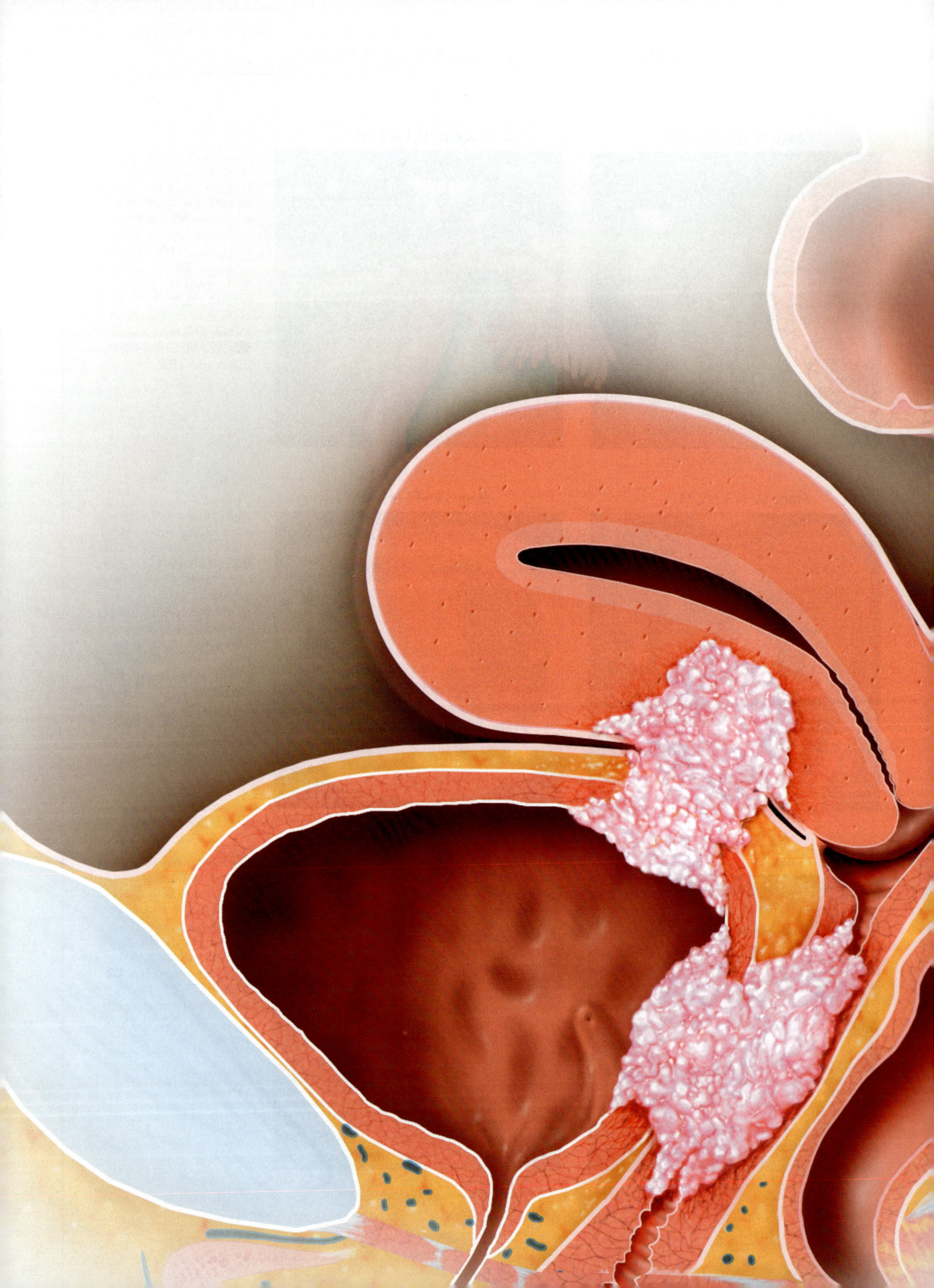

Urinary Bladder Carcinoma

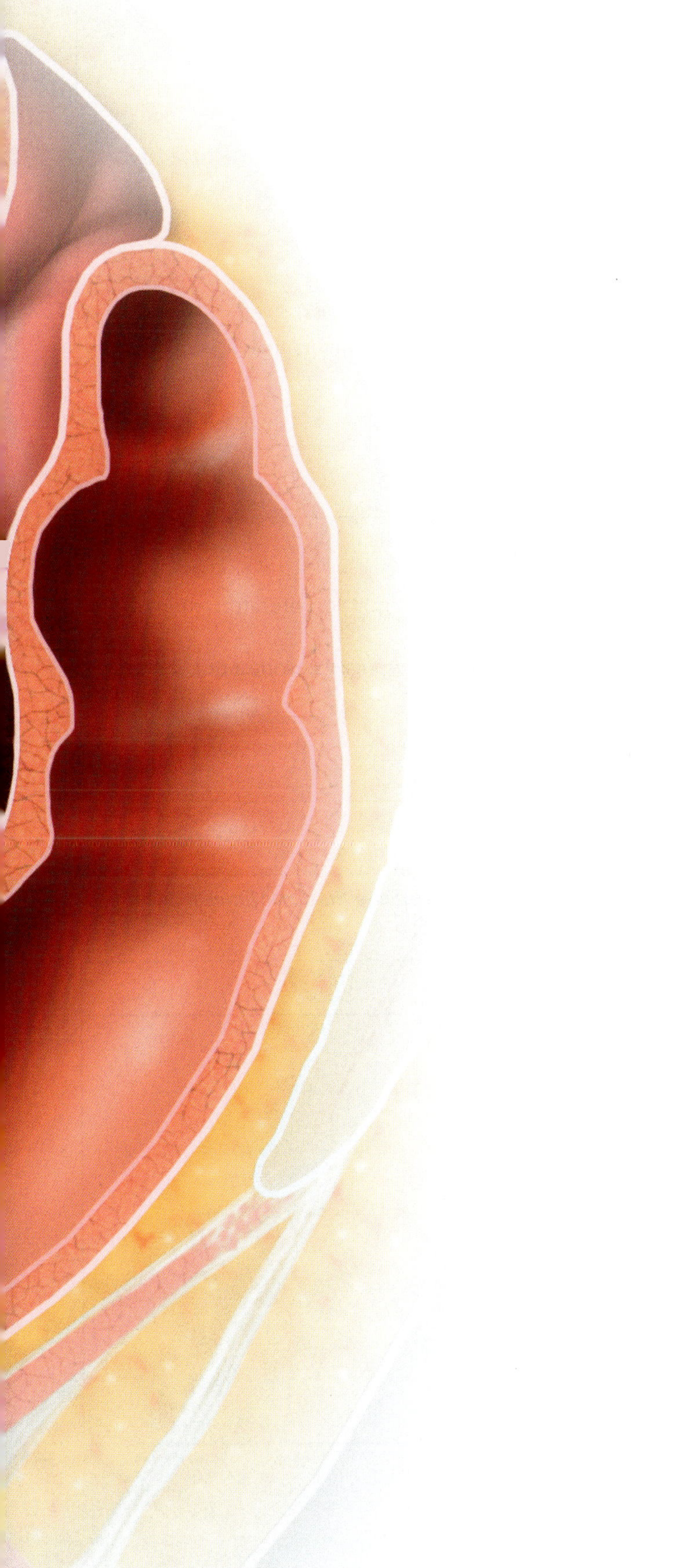

URINARY BLADDER CARCINOMA

(T) Primary Tumor

Adapted from 7th edition AJCC Staging Forms.

TNM	Definitions
TX	Primary tumor cannot be assessed
T0	No evidence of primary tumor
Ta	Noninvasive papillary carcinoma
Tis	Carcinoma in situ: "Flat tumor"
T1	Tumor invades subepithelial connective tissue
T2	Tumor invades muscularis propria
pT2a	Tumor invades superficial muscularis propria (inner half)
pT2b	Tumor invades deep muscularis propria (outer half)
T3	Tumor invades perivesical tissue
pT3a	Tumor invades perivesical tissue microscopically
pT3b	Tumor invades perivesical tissue macroscopically (extravesical mass)
T4	Tumor invades any of the following: Prostatic stroma, uterus, vagina, pelvic wall, abdominal wall
T4a	Tumor invades prostatic stroma, uterus, vagina
T4b	Tumor invades pelvic wall, abdominal wall

(N) Regional Lymph Nodes

NX	Regional lymph nodes cannot be assessed
N0	No regional lymph node metastasis
N1	Single regional lymph node metastasis in true pelvis (hypogastric, obturator, external iliac, or presacral lymph node)
N2	Multiple regional lymph node metastases in true pelvis (hypogastric, obturator, external iliac, or presacral lymph node)
N3	Lymph node metastasis to common iliac lymph nodes

(M) Distant Metastasis

M0	No distant metastasis
M1	Distant metastasis

Regional lymph nodes include both primary and secondary drainage regions. All other nodes above the aortic bifurcation are considered distant lymph nodes.

AJCC Stages/Prognostic Groups

Adapted from 7th edition AJCC Staging Forms.

Stage	T	N	M
0a	Ta	N0	M0
0is	Tis	N0	M0
I	T1	N0	M0
II	T2a	N0	M0
	T2b	N0	M0
III	T3a	N0	M0
	T3b	N0	M0
	T4a	N0	M0
IV	T4b	N0	M0
	Any T	N1-3	M0
	Any T	Any N	M1

T Staging of Urinary Bladder Carcinoma

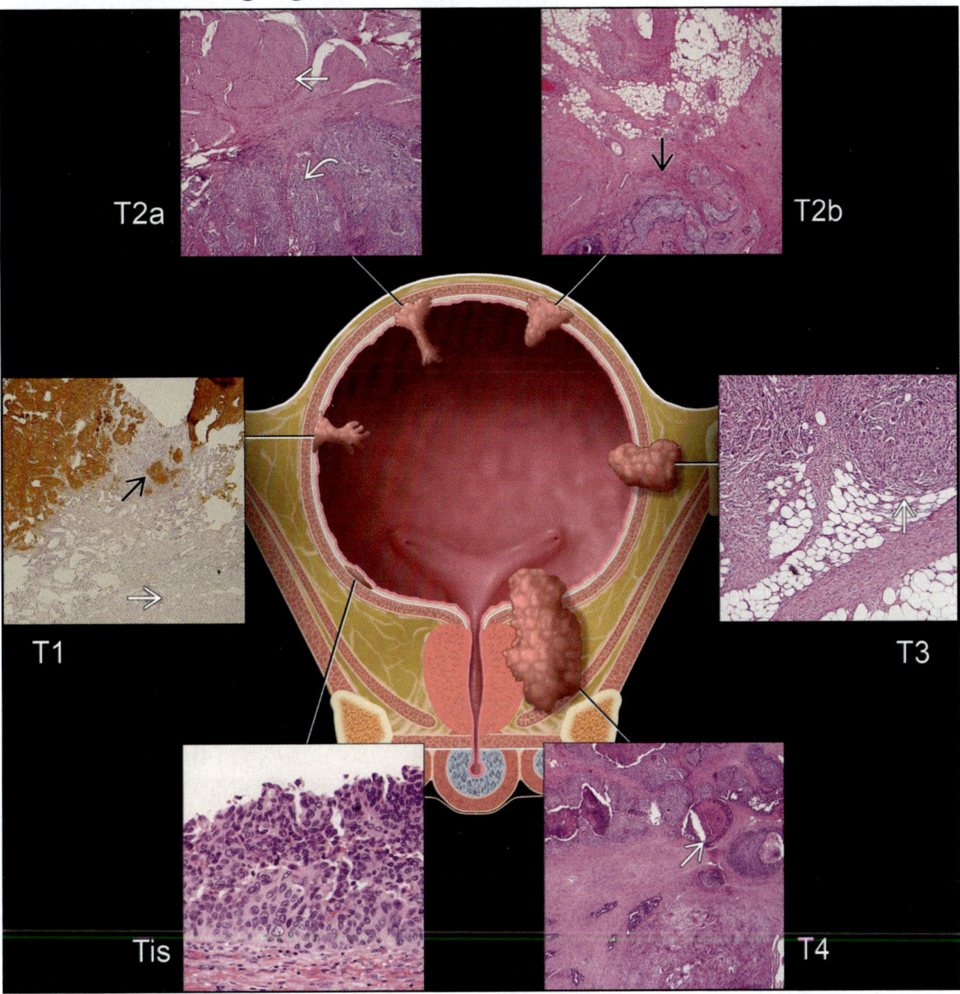

Graphics show the T stages of urinary bladder carcinoma with histologic correlation. **Tis** or carcinoma in situ refers to a nonpapillary (flat) mucosa in which the normal urothelium has been replaced by cancer cells that have not invaded through the basement membrane. The carcinoma in situ is a high-grade lesion and essentially recognized because of cytologic abnormalities similar to those noted in high-grade papillary tumors. The neoplastic cells are pleomorphic, hyperchromatic, and occupy a portion of the thickness of the urothelium. They lack polarity in relation to the basement membrane. (Original magnification 400x.) **T1** describes urothelial tumor invasion through the basement membrane into the subepithelial connective tissue. In this photomicrograph, cytokeratin immunohistochemical stain is used to highlight tumor ➥ invading into the subepithelial connective tissue but not to the muscularis propria ➥. (Original magnification 200x.) **T2** designates tumor that invades the muscularis propria. **T2a**: H&E stain shows tumor cell invading superficial/inner half of the muscularis propria ➥. Note that the outer half of the muscularis propria is not involved ➥. (Original magnification 100x.) **T2b**: H&E stain shows tumor cells ➥ invading the outer half of the muscularis propria. (Original magnification 100x.) **T3** is tumor invading perivesical tissue. H&E stain shows tumor cells ➥ invading perivesical fat tissue. (Original magnification 200x.) Tumor is considered T3a if perivesical fat involvement is microscopic (not evident by imaging) and T3b if macroscopic (potentially detected by imaging). **T4** is tumor invading any of the following: Prostate, uterus, vagina, pelvic wall, or abdominal wall. It is T4a when tumor invades the prostate, uterus, and vagina; the tumor is T4b when it invades the pelvic wall and abdominal wall. H&E stain demonstrates neoplastic transitional cell carcinoma cells ➥ invading the prostate. (Original magnification 100x.)

URINARY BLADDER CARCINOMA

T4a: Male

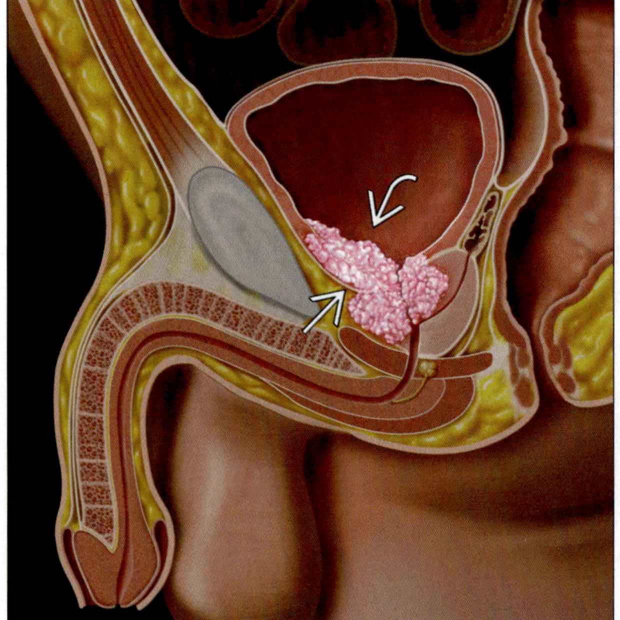

Graphic shows a bladder neck tumor ➡ in a male patient; the tumor invades the prostate ➡, constituting stage T4a. To be considered T4a disease, the tumor should have prostatic stromal invasion directly from the bladder tumor. Subepithelial invasion of prostatic urethra will not constitute T4 staging status.

T4a: Female

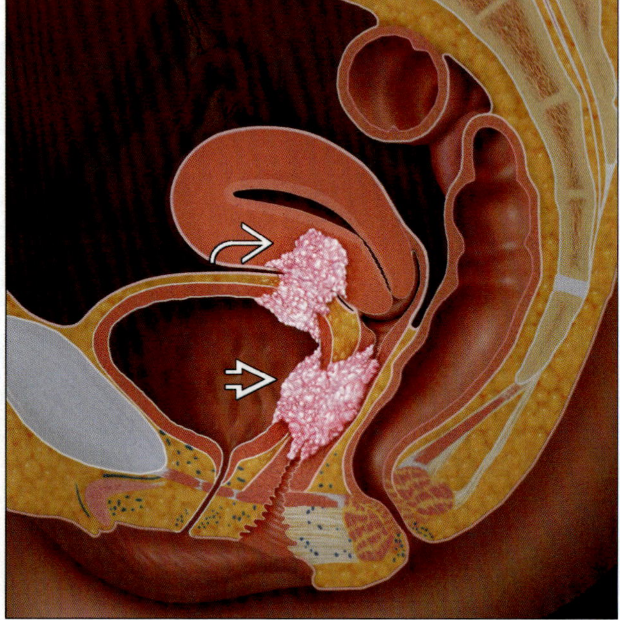

Graphic shows posterior wall bladder tumors in a female patient invading the uterus ➡ and vagina ➡. Invasion of the uterus &/or vagina constitutes stage T4a.

T4b: Male

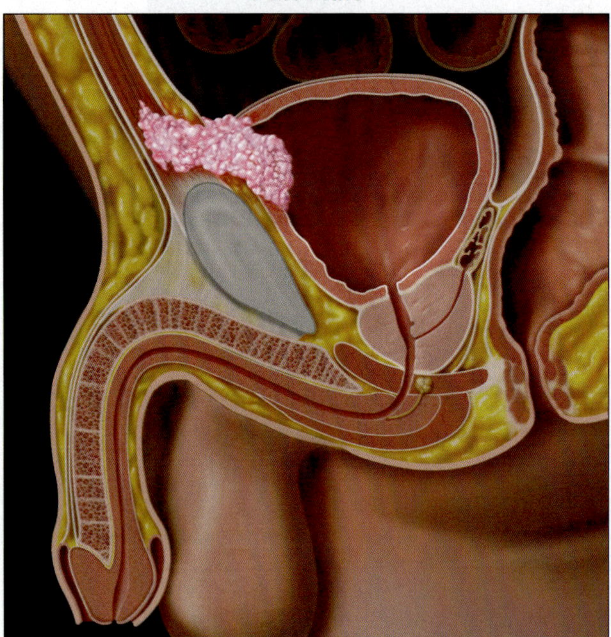

Graphic shows a tumor of the anterior wall of the urinary bladder that invades into the extraperitoneal prevesical fat (space of Retzius) and eventually the muscles of the anterior abdominal wall, constituting stage T4b.

T4b: Female

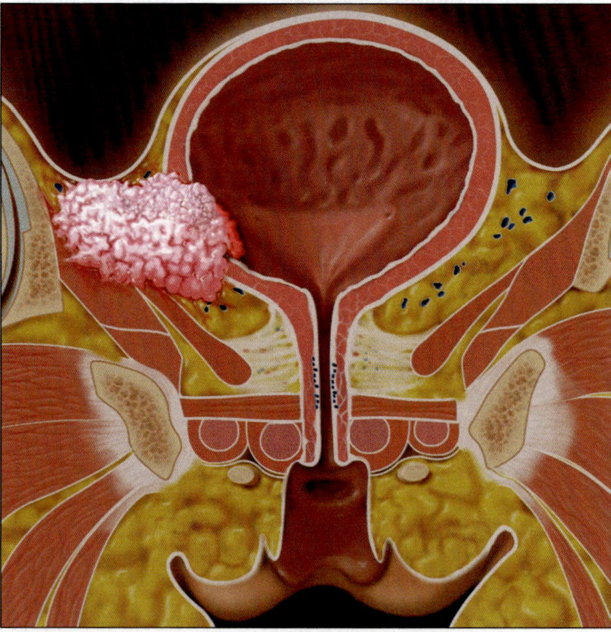

Graphic shows a lateral wall bladder tumor invading the muscles of the lateral pelvic wall, constituting stage T4b.

URINARY BLADDER CARCINOMA

N1 and N2

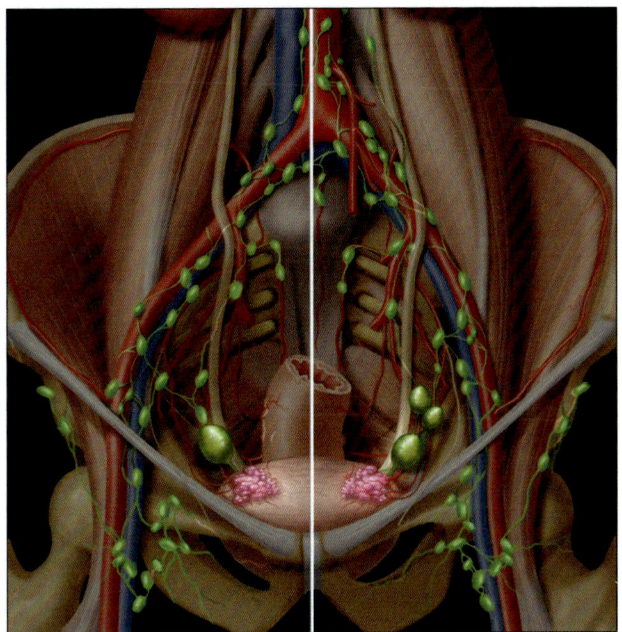

N3 and Distant Nodal Metastases

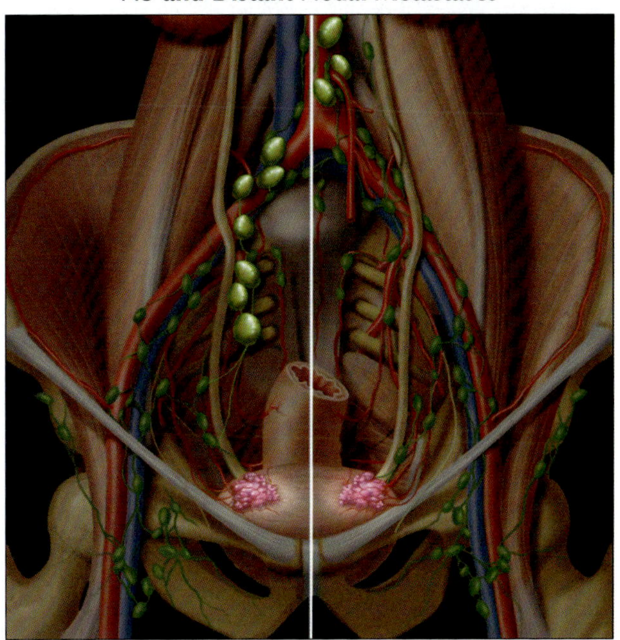

Graphics show N1 and N2 disease in urinary bladder carcinoma. Both classifications describe nodal metastases confined to the true pelvis. N1 (left) is a single metastatic pelvic lymph node, whereas N2 (right) is defined as multiple metastatic pelvic lymph nodes.

The graphic on the left shows N3 disease, which describes involvement of the common iliac lymph nodes. The graphic on the right shows involvement of paraaortic lymph nodes, which constitute distant metastases and M1 staging in the 7th edition of the AJCC Cancer Staging Manual.

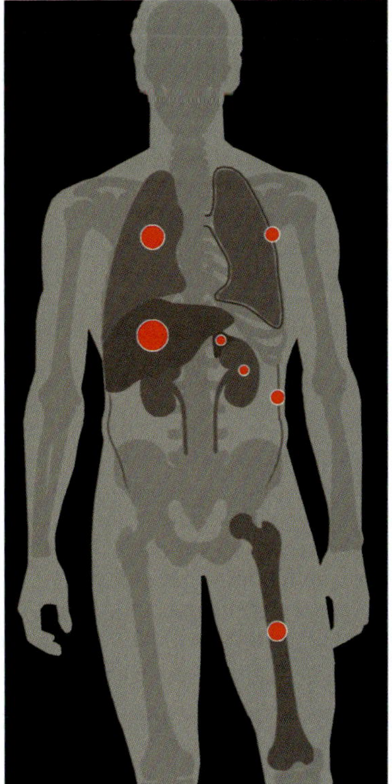

METASTASES, ORGAN FREQUENCY

Liver	47%
Lung	45%
Bone	32%
Peritoneum	19%
Pleura	16%
Kidney	14%
Adrenal	14%

Adapted from Wallmeroth A et al: Patterns of metastasis in muscle-invasive bladder cancer (pT2-4): an autopsy study on 367 patients. Urol Int. 62:69-75, 1999.

URINARY BLADDER CARCINOMA

OVERVIEW

General Comments
- Most common urinary tract malignancy

Classification
- Uroepithelial (95%)
  - Transitional cell carcinoma (TCC) (90%)
  - Squamous cell carcinoma (6-8%)
  - Adenocarcinoma (2%)
    - Urachal origin
    - Nonurachal origin (usually chronic irritation)
  - Neuroendocrinal (1%)
  - Mixed
- Mesenchymal (5%) includes
  - Neurofibrosarcoma
  - Pheochromocytoma
  - Lymphoma
  - Angiosarcoma
  - Leiomyosarcoma
  - Rhabdomyosarcoma
  - Liposarcoma
  - Chondrosarcoma
  - Osteosarcoma
  - Plasmacytoma

PATHOLOGY

Routes of Spread
- Local spread
  - Extension through layers of bladder wall into perivesical fat
  - Invasion of local pelvic organs
    - Seminal vesicles
    - Prostate
    - Uterus
    - Ovaries
    - Rectum
    - Perineum
  - Later spread to pelvic side wall or anterior abdominal wall
- Lymphatic spread
  - Depends on depth of invasion of bladder wall
    - Superficial tumors (< T2b): Rarely spread to local nodes
    - Deep muscle invasion (T2b): 30% risk of nodal metastases
    - Perivesical extension (T3): 50-60% risk of nodal metastases
  - Initially to perivesical, presacral, and sacral nodes
  - Later to internal iliac, obturator, and external iliac nodes, and eventually to common iliac and paraaortic nodes
  - Regional lymph node metastases are those confined to true pelvis (hypogastric, obturator, external iliac, or presacral lymph node)
    - N1: Single regional lymph node
    - N2: Multiple regional lymph nodes
  - Common iliac nodes are defined as N3 disease
  - All other nodes above aortic bifurcation are considered distant metastases (M1 disease)
- Hematogenous spread
  - Occurs late and with recurrent disease
    - Common sites are bones, lung, brain, and liver
      - Bone metastases occur mainly to pelvic bones and spine (perivesical venous plexus → Batson paravertebral plexus → vertebral bodies)
      - Direct extension to pelvic bones is also common

General Features
- Etiology
  - Direct prolonged contact with excreted carcinogens
    - Smoking is most important risk factor
      - Smokers' risk is 2x that of nonsmokers
    - Industrial carcinogens (aniline, benzidine, arylamine)
    - High level of arsenic in drinking water
  - Recurrent urinary tract infections and stone disease
    - Squamous cell carcinoma
  - *Schistosoma hematobium* infection
    - Squamous cell carcinoma
- Epidemiology & cancer incidence
  - Most common tumor of urinary system
    - 4th most common cancer in men
    - 10th most common cancer in women
  - Median age at diagnosis is 73 years
  - Incidence differs by sex and race
    - 4x more common in men than women
    - 2x more common in whites than in African-Americans
  - Age-adjusted incidence of 21.2/100,000
    - Estimated 70,980 new cases in USA in 2009
  - Age-adjusted death rate of 4.3/100,000
    - Estimated 14,330 deaths in USA in 2009
- Associated diseases, abnormalities
  - Metaplastic changes can involve extensive areas of bladder epithelium
  - 30% present with multifocal urinary bladder disease
    - Often widespread bladder squamous metaplasia and carcinoma in situ
  - 50% of patients presenting with upper urinary tract carcinoma will develop metachronous tumors in urinary bladder
  - 5% of patients presenting with urinary bladder carcinoma will develop metachronous tumors in upper urinary tract
    - More likely in patients with multiple bladder lesions

Gross Pathology & Surgical Features
- Urothelial neoplasms of urinary bladder may be subdivided into
  - Papillary
    - Papillomas
    - Low malignant potential papillary tumors
    - Papillary carcinoma
  - Nonpapillary
    - Urothelial carcinoma in situ
    - Invasive carcinoma
      - Invasive urothelial carcinoma may present as polypoid, sessile, ulcerated, or infiltrative lesion

Microscopic Pathology
- H&E
  - Carcinoma in situ (CIS)
    - Malignant urothelial cells within nonpapillary urothelial lining

URINARY BLADDER CARCINOMA

- Characterized by extensive (often full thickness) replacement of urothelium by cells demonstrating severe cytologic atypia
  - ○ Papillary lesions
    - Microscopic appearance
      - Contain well-defined fibrovascular cores
      - Lining urothelium may vary from indistinguishable from normal (papilloma) to markedly anaplastic (high-grade urothelial carcinoma)
    - Papillary urothelial neoplasia of low malignant potential (PUNLMP)
      - Papillary tumor characterized by cytologically bland, yet thickened, epithelium when compared to papilloma
      - Lower rate of recurrence than low-grade urothelial carcinoma
    - Papillary lesions with cytological atypia
      - Low-grade papillary urothelial carcinoma (LGPUC)
      - High-grade papillary urothelial carcinoma (HGPUC)
  - ○ Invasive carcinoma
    - Neoplastic cells invade bladder wall as nests, cords, trabeculae, small clusters, or single cells that are usually separated by desmoplastic stroma

IMAGING FINDINGS

Detection

- **Cystoscopy** is considered gold standard for detection of bladder cancer
- **Intravenous urography (IVP)**
  - ○ Traditionally modality of choice in evaluating hematuria
  - ○ Largely replaced by CT IVP
  - ○ Used primarily to access upper urinary tract + cystoscopy
  - ○ Only 60% of bladder cancers are detected by IVP
    - Small tumors may be obscured in contrast-filled urinary bladder
  - ○ Tumors appear as sessile or pedunculated filling defects
- **Ultrasound**
  - ○ Bladder tumors may be found incidentally or during work-up for hematuria
  - ○ Sonographic features include
    - Focal hypoechoic or mixed echogenicity nonmobile mass projecting into bladder lumen
    - No posterior shadowing
    - Focal bladder wall thickening
    - Color Doppler shows ↑ vascularity (differentiate bladder masses from blood clots)
  - ○ Sonographic detection of bladder tumors depends on size and location
    - Difficult to detect tumors < 5 mm in size and tumors located in neck or dome of bladder
  - ○ Transrectal US can be useful in differentiating bladder neck from prostatic tumor
- **NECT**
  - ○ Modality of choice in patients presenting with painful hematuria to assess for stones

- ○ Polypoid bladder tumors, isodense to bladder wall, may be seen against background of fluid density urine
  - Changing window sittings can make it easier to detect bladder tumors
- ○ Factors that can make tumor easier to detect against isodense urine
  - Presence of tumor calcifications
    - Tumoral calcifications in approximately 5% of cases of transitional cell carcinoma
    - Calcification typically encrusts tumor surface
  - Presence of high-density hemorrhage in bladder lumen
- **CT IVP**
  - ○ Modality of choice in evaluating patients presenting with painless hematuria
  - ○ Evaluation of upper urinary tract for synchronous tumors in patients with known or suspected carcinoma
  - ○ Consistent performance in detection of bladder tumors
    - Sensitivity (79%)
    - Specificity (94%)
    - Accuracy (91%)
    - Positive predictive value (75%)
    - Negative predictive value (95%)
  - ○ Imaging features
    - Tumors appear as polypoid or flat lesions of similar attenuation compared to bladder wall
    - Larger tumors tend to be more heterogeneous with areas of low density due to necrosis
    - Urachal carcinoma
      - Midline mass anterosuperior to bladder dome
      - Low-attenuation components, which represent pools of mucin at pathologic examination
      - Peripheral calcifications in masses of soft tissue attenuation occur in 50–70% of cases (pathognomonic for urachal adenocarcinoma)
- **MR**
  - ○ Not used routinely for tumor detection
    - Tumors may be detected during pelvic imaging for other indications
  - ○ As good as CT IVP for detection of bladder tumors
    - Sensitivity and positive predictive value > 90%
  - ○ Imaging features
    - T1WI
      - Intermediate signal intensity, isointense to bladder wall, higher than urine and lower than perivesical fat
    - T2WI
      - Slightly hyperintense to bladder wall and hypointense to urine
    - Dynamic gadolinium-enhanced T1WI
      - Earlier and more pronounced enhancement than bladder wall
    - Diffusion-weighted imaging (DWI) under free breathing is very promising in detection of urinary bladder carcinoma
      - ADC values of urinary bladder carcinoma are lower compared to urine, normal bladder wall, prostate, and seminal vesicles
      - Sensitivity (98.1%); specificity (92.3%); positive predictive value (100%); negative predictive value (92.3%); and accuracy (97.0%)

URINARY BLADDER CARCINOMA

- Dynamic contrast-enhanced MR parameters: Peak time enhancement in 1st minute (E(max/1)) after contrast administration and steepest slope
  - E(max/1) and steepest slope correlate with histologic grade

Staging

- Determined by depth of invasion of bladder wall during cystoscopic examination, which includes
  - Deep biopsy, encompassing all layers of bladder wall
  - Examination under anesthesia to assess
    - Size and mobility of palpable masses
    - Degree of induration of bladder wall
    - Presence of extravesical extension or invasion of adjacent organs
- Unfortunately, clinical staging is not perfect
  - Errors reported in 25–50% of cases
- Patients shown to have muscle-invasive disease following cystoscopy are referred for imaging, usually CT or MR, for complete staging
- **Imaging techniques for local staging**
  - **MR** is imaging modality of choice in local staging of urinary bladder carcinoma
    - Sensitivity and positive predictive value > 90% and overall diagnostic accuracy of 62-75%
    - Inherent high soft tissue contrast
    - Multiplanar capabilities
    - Nonnephrotoxic contrast
    - Superior to CT in assessing depth of muscular invasion
    - Diffusion-weighted MR improves specificity for detection of invasive urinary bladder tumors
  - **CT** is useful to distinguish tumors confined to bladder wall from those spreading into perivesical fat
    - Cannot determine depth of wall invasion to differentiate T2a from T2b disease
  - **Transabdominal US** is not useful for staging
  - **Transurethral US** can be used for staging
    - Can distinguish between T2 and T3 disease
    - Invasive
    - Does not provide more staging information than CT or MR
  - **FDG PET** has limited role in local staging
    - Increased tumor uptake may be obscured by radioisotope excretion into bladder
    - Early results suggest promising role of tracer 11C-choline in evaluation of bladder cancer because of its minimal urinary excretion
- **Local staging**
  - Urinary bladder carcinoma stages
    - Not possible to differentiate Ta from T1 by imaging
    - T1: Intraluminal filling defect with normal underlying wall
    - T2: Localized wall thickening and retraction indicate muscle involvement
    - T3a: Microscopic perivesical invasion cannot be resolved with CT or MR
    - T3b: Loss of clear interface between bladder wall and perivesical fat → perivesical fat stranding and nodularity
    - T4: Tumor invading adjacent organs, abdominal or pelvic wall, and perineum → distortion and irregularity between tumor and adjacent organs

- T4 disease includes prostatic stromal invasion; subepithelial invasion of prostatic urethra does not constitute T4 disease
  - Presence of ureteral obstruction strongly suggests muscle invasion
  - MR imaging tends to overestimate local extent of tumor
    - Improved detection of perivesical fat stranding, which may be reactive or inflammatory rather than metastatic
  - MR is particularly helpful to differentiate muscle-invasive from noninvasive disease
    - T2WI
      - Interrupted low signal intensity muscle layer → muscle invasion (T2 disease)
    - Dynamic gadolinium-enhanced T1WI
      - Can differentiate T2a from T2b by showing depth of muscle invasion
    - Improved accuracy of T stage diagnosis from 67% for T2WI alone to 88% for T2WI + DW images
  - Staging CT or MR should be delayed > 7 days after transurethral resection (TUR) because focal wall thickening and perivesical fat stranding can be seen following TUR → overstaging
  - Tumors arising in bladder diverticula are challenging from staging point of view
    - Tend to invade perivesical fat early due to absence of muscle layer in diverticular wall
    - Thinner wall makes accurate staging difficult
    - Omission of T2 has been suggested
      - Tumor either confined to diverticulum (T1) or extradiverticular tumor (T3)
- **Nodal metastases**
  - Nodal size and morphology criteria
    - Nodal metastases in oval nodes > 10 mm and round nodes > 8 mm
  - CT and routine MR have similar accuracy for detection of nodal disease
    - Reported accuracy (73-92%)
    - Sensitivity (83%) and specificity (98%)
  - Improved detection of nodal metastases using ultrasmall superparamagnetic iron oxide (ferumoxtran-10) particles
    - Can detect metastases in normal-sized nodes and exclude metastases in enlarged reactive nodes
    - Normal nodal tissue shows contrast material uptake → ↓ signal intensity on T2- or T2*-weighted images
    - Nodal metastases lack ferumoxtran-10 uptake and retain high signal intensity on ferumoxtran-10–enhanced images
  - PET can be used for detection of nodal metastases
- **Distant metastases**
  - Lung metastases are common and can present as
    - Solitary nodule
    - Multiple nodules
    - Cavitary nodules
    - Diffuse multinodular opacities
  - Bony metastases are usually lytic, although sclerotic and mixed lesions are also common
    - Bone scan may be used if there is suspicion of bone metastases
    - T1WI MR is useful to assess pelvic bone marrow involvement

URINARY BLADDER CARCINOMA

○ Brain metastases
  ■ Rare manifestation of metastatic bladder carcinoma
  ■ Usually occurs with advanced metastatic disease
  ■ May present as single or multiple enhancing parenchymal masses
  ■ Can rarely present as leptomeningeal carcinomatosis
○ PET can be used for detection of distant metastases

Restaging

• Routine imaging follow-up is **not** indicated for patients with superficial TCC and no additional risk factors
  ○ Cystoscopy every 3 months for 2 years, then every 6 months for 2 years, and then yearly thereafter
• Patients with invasive TCC, especially those with risk factors, should have CT IVP every 1-2 years
• Patients requiring cystectomy for invasive bladder cancer should have
  ○ Abdominal and pelvic CT (or MR) at 6, 12, and 24 months
    ■ Local recurrence can present as
      - Pelvic lymphadenopathy
      - Well-defined or poorly defined pelvic soft tissue masses
      - Tumor invading adjacent structures, such as vagina, urethra, pelvic sidewall, anterior abdominal wall, seminal vesicle, and spermatic cord
  ○ Chest x-ray at 6, 12, 18, 24, 36, 48, and 60 months postoperatively

CLINICAL ISSUES

Presentation

• Macroscopic painless hematuria
  ○ 80% of cases of bladder carcinoma present with painless hematuria
  ○ Bladder carcinoma is detected in up to 13-28% of patients presenting with macroscopic hematuria
• Urinary frequency, urgency, and dysuria
• Urinary tract infections
• Urinary obstruction
• Urinary bladder rupture is rare; can result
  ○ Spontaneously
  ○ Following biopsy
  ○ From endovesical chemotherapy with mitomycin C
  ○ As long-term complication of radiotherapy

Cancer Natural History & Prognosis

• Approximately 70% of newly diagnosed cases of bladder cancer represent superficial disease
  ○ High risk of local recurrence
  ○ Rarely progress to invasive or metastatic disease
• Risk of disease relapse following radical cystectomy may be as high as 70%
• As many as 50% of patients who have muscle-invasive tumors will have occult metastases that will present within 5 years of diagnosis
• 78% of patients who developed metastases did so within 1 year of cystectomy
  ○ Suggests that metastases must be present at time of cystectomy

• Presence of ≥ 1 of the following risk factors ↑ likelihood of recurrent or metastatic disease in TCC
  ○ Extent of bladder wall invasion
  ○ Tumor size
    ■ Tumors > 3 cm have up to 35% chance of progression
  ○ Pathological tumor grade (i.e., degree of differentiation)
    ■ 5-year survival of patients with grade I tumors is 94% and only 40% for patients with grade III tumors
    ■ < 10% of grade I tumors, 50% of grade II tumors, and > 80% of grade III tumors are invasive at time of initial diagnosis
  ○ Adjacent or remote bladder mucosal changes
    ■ Carcinoma in situ (CIS) in patients with low-grade, low-stage lesions may be associated with progression to muscle invasion (> 80% within 4 years of diagnosis)
  ○ Multiplicity of foci
    ■ Recurrence rate is almost 1/3 higher in patients with multiple lesions than in patients with single lesions
  ○ Upper tract obstruction
    ■ 5-year survival of 31% for patients with bilateral hydronephrosis
    ■ 5-year survival of 45% for patients with unilateral hydronephrosis
    ■ 5-year survival of 63% for patients with no hydronephrosis
  ○ Lymphatic invasion in lamina propria
    ■ Very poor prognostic sign
    ■ Most patients die within 6 years
  ○ Involvement of prostate
    ■ Increased risk of urethral recurrence
• 70-80% present with superficial bladder tumors (i.e., stage Ta, Tis, or T1)
  ○ Complete cure is expected
• 5 year survival rate for bladder cancer by stage
  ○ Stage 0 (95%)
  ○ Stage I (85%)
  ○ Stage II (55%)
  ○ Stage III (38%)
  ○ Stage IV (16%)

Treatment Options

• Treatment options by stage
  ○ **Stage 0 and I**
    ■ Transurethral resection (TUR) and fulguration
    ■ TUR with fulguration followed by intravesical bacille Calmette-Guérin (BCG)
    ■ TUR with fulguration followed by intravesical chemotherapy
    ■ Segmental cystectomy (rarely indicated)
    ■ Radical cystectomy in selected patients with extensive or refractory superficial tumor
    ■ Interstitial implantation of radioisotopes with or without external beam radiation therapy (EBRT)
  ○ **Stage II and III**
    ■ Radical cystectomy ± pelvic lymph node dissection
    ■ Urinary diversion becomes necessary and can be accomplished through
      - Cutaneous ureterostomy
      - Ileal conduit with ureteroileocutaneostomy

- – Ureterosigmoidostomy
- – Orthotopic neobladder reconstruction with ileal or ileocecal segments
- ■ Neoadjuvant platinum-based combination chemotherapy followed by radical cystectomy
- ■ EBRT ± concurrent chemotherapy
- ■ Interstitial implantation of radioisotopes before or after EBRT
- ■ TUR with fulguration (in selected patients)
- ■ Segmental cystectomy (in selected patients)
- ○ Locally advanced stage IV
  - ■ Radical cystectomy + pelvic lymph node dissection
  - ■ EBRT
  - ■ Urinary diversion or cystectomy for palliation
  - ■ Chemotherapy as an adjunct to local treatment
- ○ Stage IV with distant metastases
  - ■ Chemotherapy ± adjunct to local treatment
  - ■ EBRT for palliation
  - ■ Urinary diversion or cystectomy for palliation

REPORTING CHECKLIST

T Staging

- Depth of bladder wall invasion
  - ○ MR to evaluate muscle layer invasion
  - ○ Ureteric orifice involvement strongly suggests muscle invasion
  - ○ Focal retraction of outer bladder contour suggests muscle invasion
- Perivesical fat invasion
  - ○ Microscopic perivesical fat invasion cannot be resolved by imaging
- Invasion of surrounding pelvic organs
- Tumors arising in diverticula and involving wall are at least T3 disease

N Staging

- N1: Single lymph node metastasis confined to true pelvis
- N2: Multiple lymph nodes metastases confined to true pelvis
- N3: Lymph node metastases confined to common iliac lymph nodes

M Staging

- Common sites include bones, lungs, and liver
  - ○ Bone metastases can be lytic, mixed, or sclerotic
- Nodal metastases above aortic bifurcation are classified as M1 disease

SELECTED REFERENCES

1. American Joint Committee on Cancer: AJCC Cancer Staging Manual. 7th ed. New York: Springer, 2010
2. Abou-El-Ghar ME et al: Bladder cancer: diagnosis with diffusion-weighted MR imaging in patients with gross hematuria. Radiology. 251(2):415-21, 2009
3. Koster IM et al: Best cases from the AFIP: urachal carcinoma. Radiographics. 29(3):939-42, 2009
4. Takeuchi M et al: Urinary bladder cancer: diffusion-weighted MR imaging--accuracy for diagnosing T stage and estimating histologic grade. Radiology. 251(1):112-21, 2009
5. Tuncbilek N et al: Value of dynamic contrast-enhanced MRI and correlation with tumor angiogenesis in bladder cancer. AJR Am J Roentgenol. 192(4):949-55, 2009
6. Watanabe H et al: Preoperative T staging of urinary bladder cancer: does diffusion-weighted MRI have supplementary value? AJR Am J Roentgenol. 192(5):1361-6, 2009
7. Canter D et al: Hydronephrosis is an independent predictor of poor clinical outcome in patients treated for muscle-invasive transitional cell carcinoma with radical cystectomy. Urology. 72(2):379-83, 2008
8. Sadow CA et al: Bladder cancer detection with CT urography in an Academic Medical Center. Radiology. 249(1):195-202, 2008
9. Matsuki M et al: Diffusion-weighted MR imaging for urinary bladder carcinoma: initial results. Eur Radiol. 17(1):201-4, 2007
10. Zhang J et al: Imaging of bladder cancer. Radiol Clin North Am. 45(1):183-205, 2007
11. Wong-You-Cheong JJ et al: From the Archives of the AFIP: neoplasms of the urinary bladder: radiologic-pathologic correlation. Radiographics. 26(2):553-80, 2006
12. Tekes A et al: Dynamic MRI of bladder cancer: evaluation of staging accuracy. AJR Am J Roentgenol. 184(1):121-7, 2005
13. Tekes A et al: MR imaging features of transitional cell carcinoma of the urinary bladder. AJR Am J Roentgenol. 180(3):771-7, 2003
14. Wallmeroth A et al: Patterns of metastasis in muscle-invasive bladder cancer (pT2-4): An autopsy study on 367 patients. Urol Int. 62(2):69-75, 1999

URINARY BLADDER CARCINOMA

Stage 0a (Ta N0 M0)

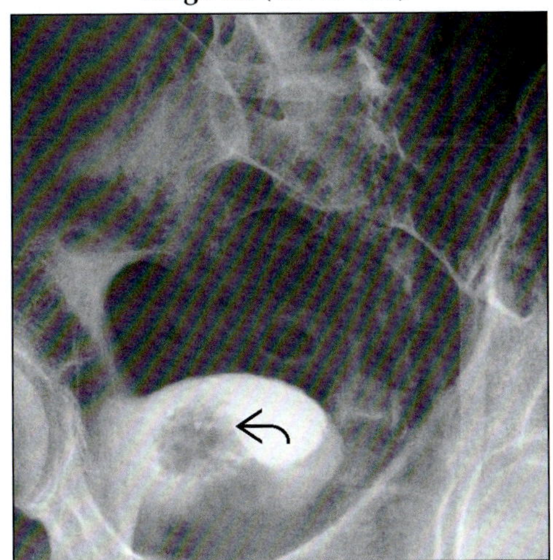

Stage 0a (Ta N0 M0)

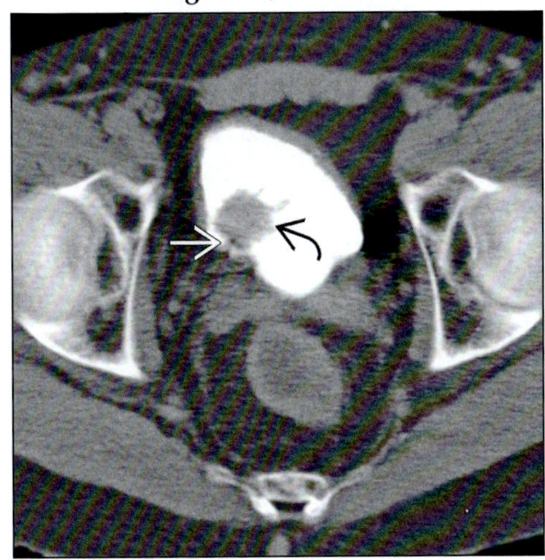

(Left) Right posterior oblique intravenous pyelography in a patient who presented with gross hematuria shows a papillary mass ➔ projecting into the contrast-filled lumen of the urinary bladder. *(Right)* Axial CECT in the same patient shows a pedunculated papillary mass ➔ with a narrow stalk ➔ attached to the right posterolateral aspect of the urinary bladder. The tumor was found to be noninvasive papillary carcinoma.

Stage I (T1 N0 M0)

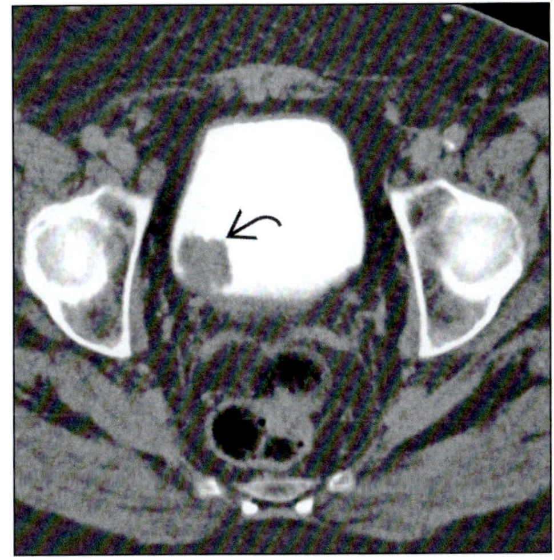

Stage I (T1 N0 M0)

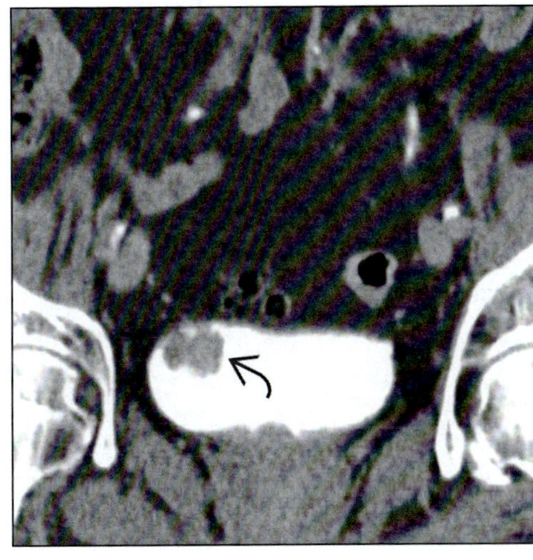

(Left) Axial CECT shows a polypoid mass ➔ involving the right side of the posterior wall of the bladder lateral to the ureteric orifice. The tumor was found to invade into the subepithelial connective tissue without extension into the muscle layer. *(Right)* Coronal CECT in the same patient shows the polypoid tumor ➔ attached to the superior aspect of the right posterior bladder wall.

Stage II (T2a N0 M0)

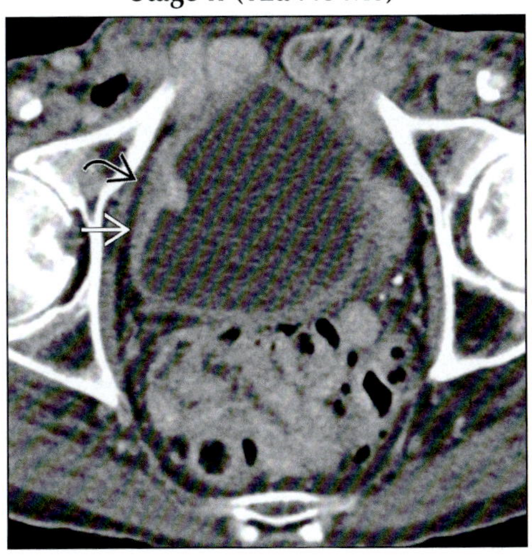

Stage II (T2a N0 M0)

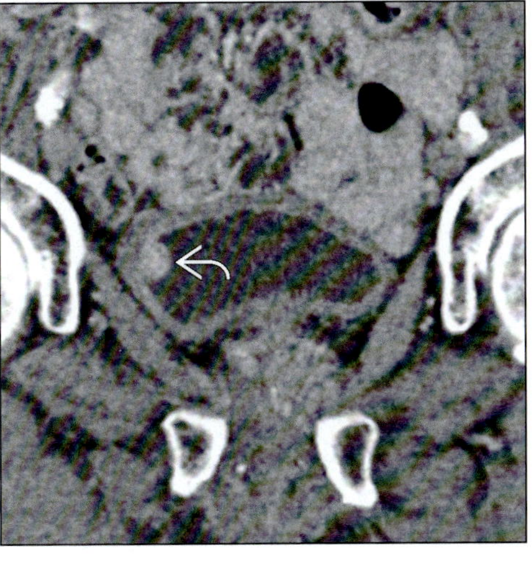

(Left) Axial CECT shows an enhancing polypoid mass arising from the right lateral wall of the urinary bladder ➔. There is associated thickening of the adjacent bladder wall ➔. *(Right)* Coronal CECT in the same patient shows the enhancing urinary bladder mass ➔. Enhancement is limited to the mass without involvement of the underlying wall, suggesting the absence of muscle invasion, although CT is not adequate to definitely make this distinction. This was found to be a T2a tumor.

URINARY BLADDER CARCINOMA

Stage II (T2a N0 M0)

Stage II (T2a N0 M0)

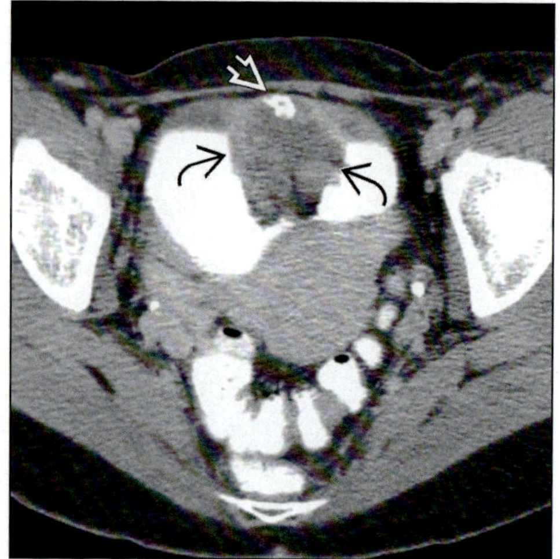

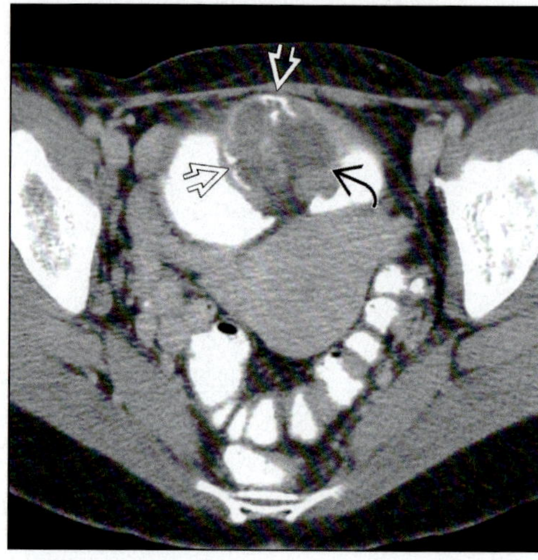

(Left) Axial CECT in a 38-year-old woman who presented with repeated urinary tract infection and gross hematuria shows a heterogeneous mass ➡ in the anterior aspect of the dome of the urinary bladder with focal calcifications ⇨. There is no evidence of extravesical extension. *(Right)* Axial CECT in the same patient shows the bladder dome mass ➡ with peripheral curvilinear calcifications ⇨, which is pathognomonic for urachal adenocarcinoma.

Stage II (T2b N0 M0)

Stage II (T2b N0 M0)

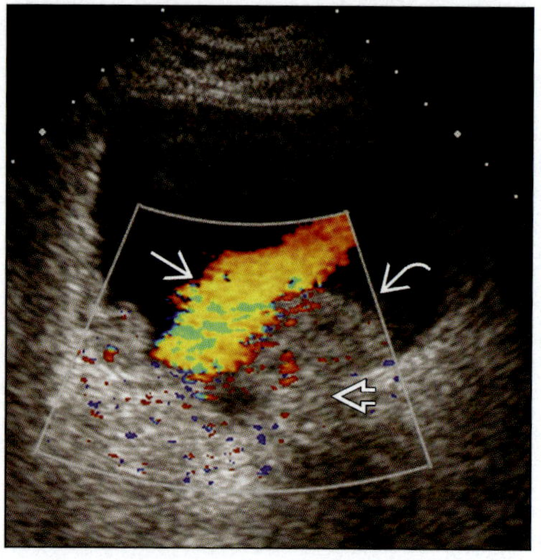

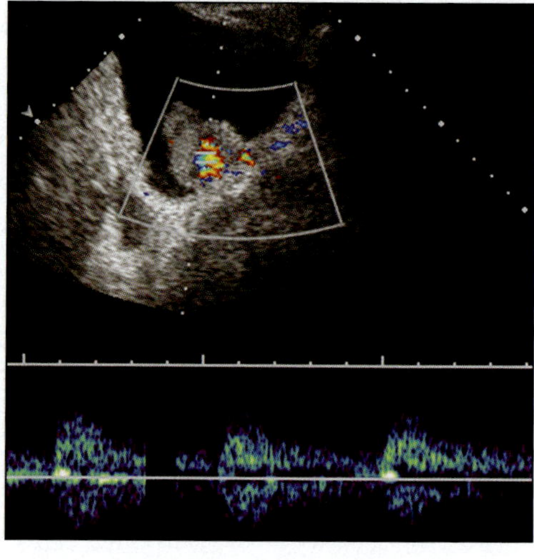

(Left) Transverse ultrasound image of the urinary bladder shows an echogenic mass ➡ centered on and obstructing the left ureteric orifice ⇨. Note the normal right side ureteric jet ➡. Ultrasound is not useful for staging bladder carcinoma but can help in tumor detection and evaluation of ureteric orifice. *(Right)* Longitudinal duplex Doppler ultrasound in the same patient shows blood flow in the mass, which helps differentiate a solid mass from blood clot.

Stage II (T2b N0 M0)

Stage II (T2b N0 M0)

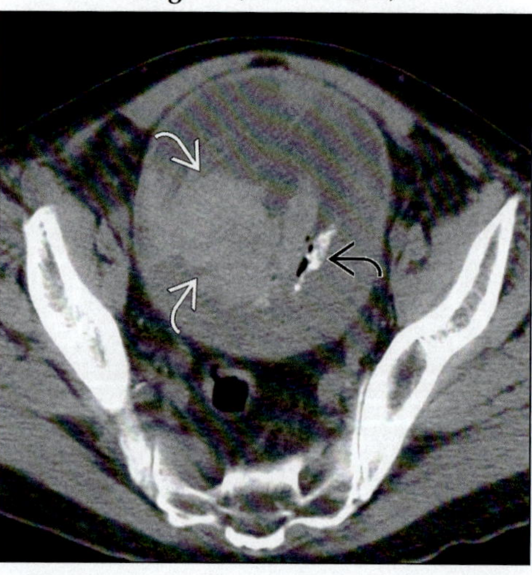

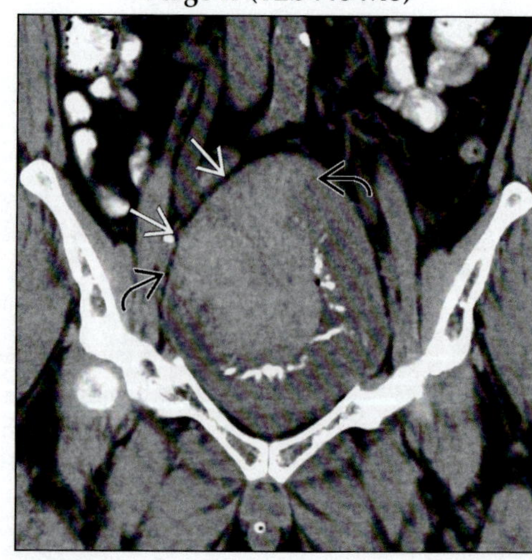

(Left) Axial CECT shows a large mass filling the bladder ➡ without evidence of perivesical infiltration. Calcifications ➡ are seen on the surface of the mass. *(Right)* Coronal CECT in the same patient shows that the mass ➡ is attached to the superior wall of the bladder. Note the smooth outer contour of the bladder at the site of tumor attachment ➡, indicating the absence of perivesical infiltration despite the large tumor size.

URINARY BLADDER CARCINOMA

Stage II (T2b N0 M0)

Stage II (T2b N0 M0)

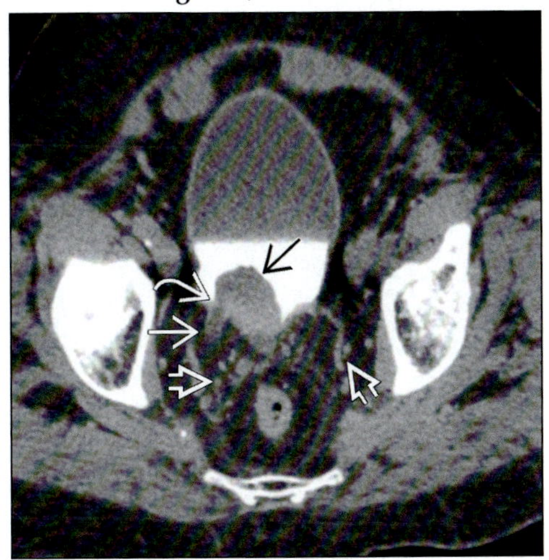

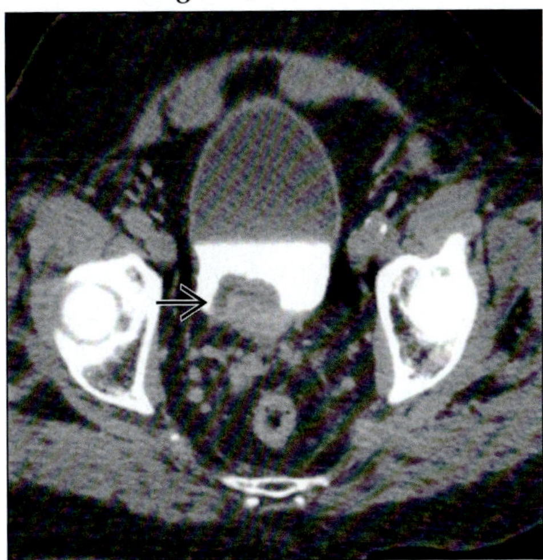

(Left) Axial CECT in a patient who presented with hematuria shows a posterior wall bladder mass ⇨ that involves the ureteric orifice ⇨. The right ureter is slightly dilated ⇨. No regional adenopathy is present. Small nodular densities in the perivesical fat represent dilated veins ⇨. *(Right)* Axial CECT in the same patient shows involvement of the right ureteric orifice ⇨. Ureteric involvement is a strong indication of muscle-invasive (T2) disease.

Stage II (T2b N0 M0)

Stage III (T3b N0 M0)

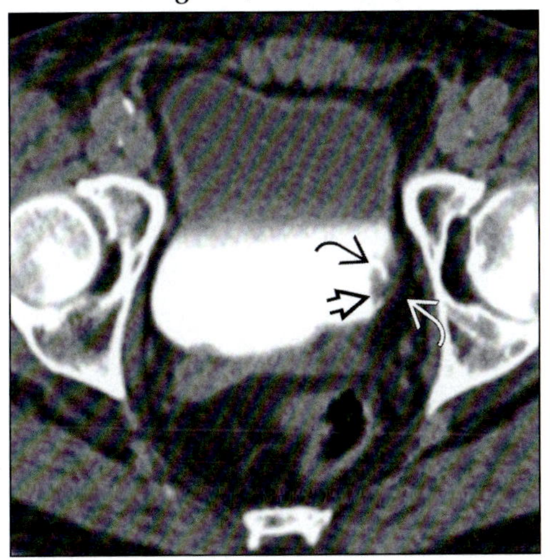

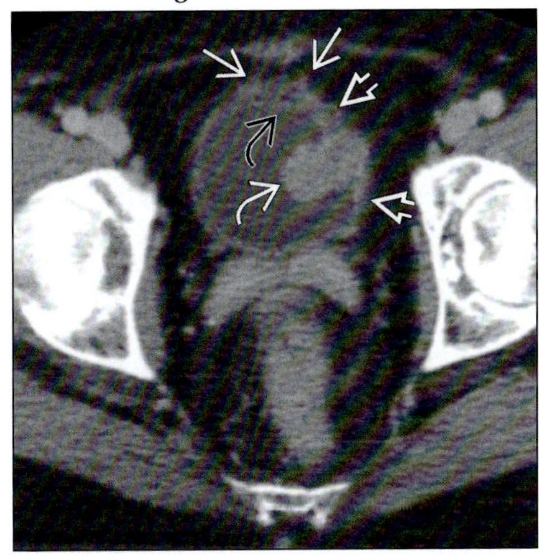

(Left) Axial CECT shows a polypoid lesion arising from the left lateral wall of the urinary bladder ⇨. Contrast is extending into a superficial ulcer ⇨. There is no perivesical tumor extension ⇨. *(Right)* Axial CECT shows thickening of the anterior ⇨ and left lateral wall of the urinary bladder ⇨ with a large polypoid mass projecting into the bladder lumen ⇨. There is stranding of the perivesical fat almost reaching to the anterior abdominal wall ⇨.

Stage III (T3b N0 M0)

Stage III (T3b N0 M0)

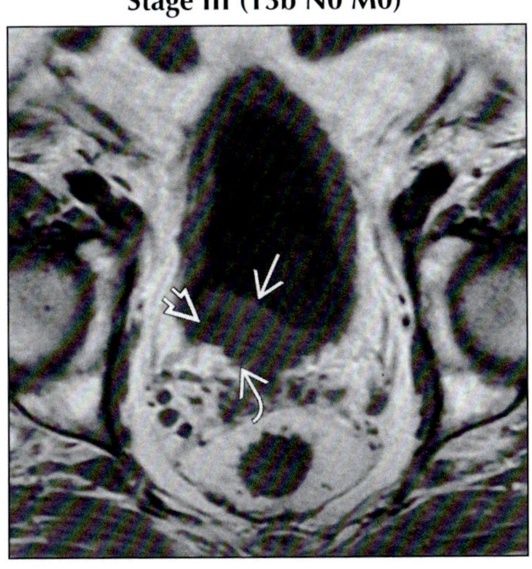

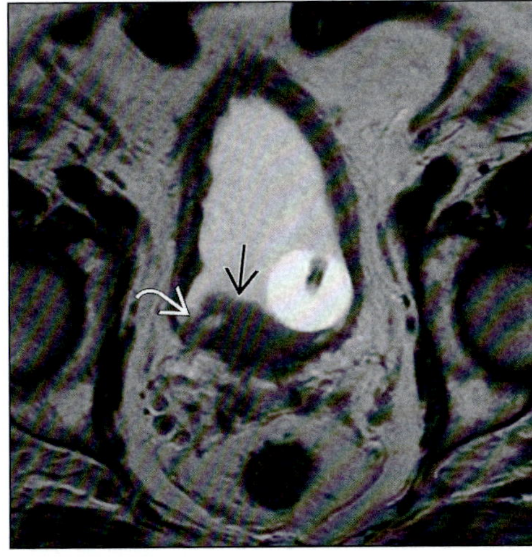

(Left) Axial T1WI MR shows an intermediate signal intensity posterior wall bladder mass ⇨ that is hyperintense to urine, hypointense to fat, and isointense to muscle. Tumor nodules extend into high signal perivesical fat ⇨. The ureteric orifice is embedded in the mass ⇨. *(Right)* Axial T2WI MR in the same patient shows an intermediate signal bladder mass ⇨ that is hypointense to the urine and perivesical fat. Note also involvement of the ureteric orifice ⇨.

URINARY BLADDER CARCINOMA

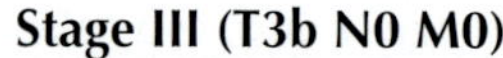

Stage III (T3b N0 M0)

Stage III (T3b N0 M0)

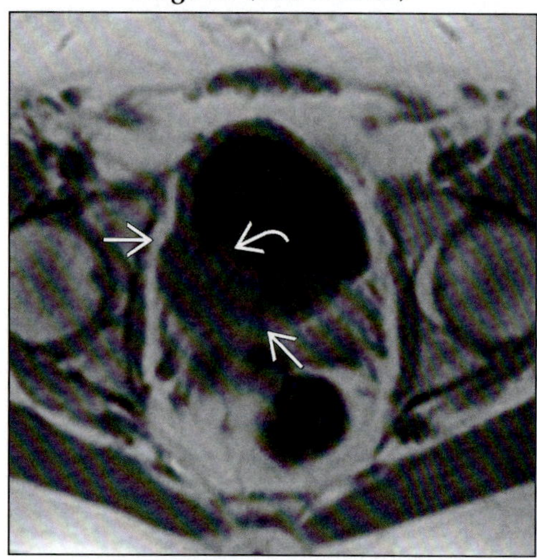

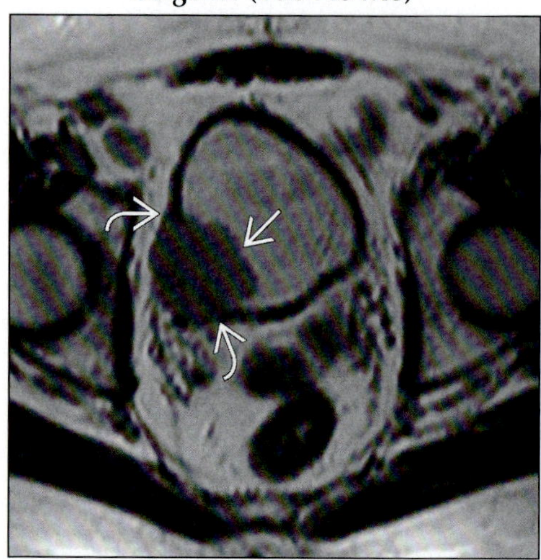

(Left) Axial T1WI MR shows a right posterolateral urinary bladder mass → that has a large extravesical component →. The mass is isointense to the bladder wall on T1WI MR. (Right) Axial T2WI MR shows a bladder mass → that is hyperintense relative to the dark urinary bladder wall and hypointense relative to urine and perivesical fat. Note the interruption of the dark urinary bladder wall signal where the mass extends into the perivesical fat →.

Stage III (T3b N0 M0)

Stage III (T3b N0 M0)

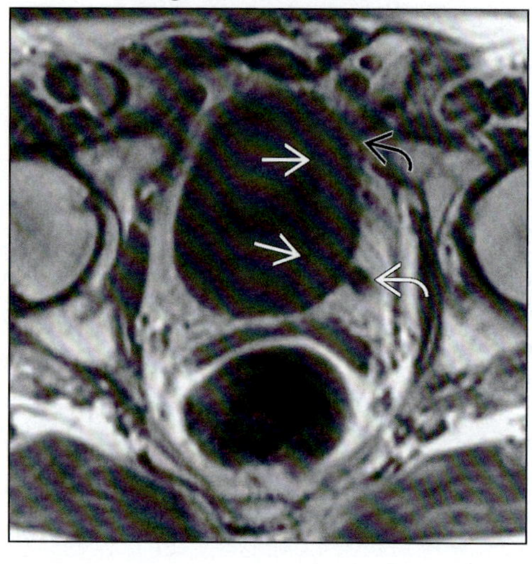

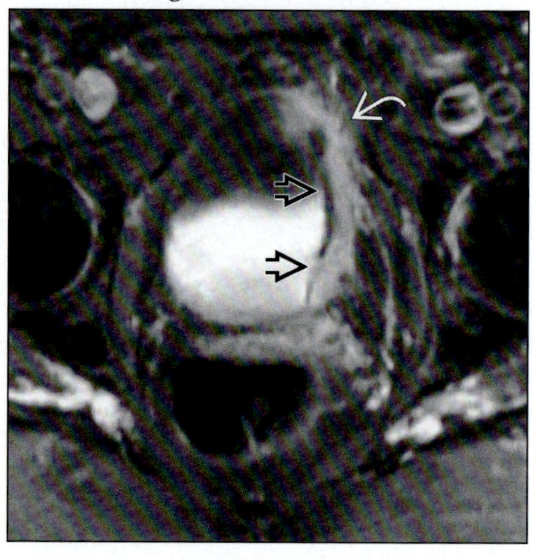

(Left) Axial T1WI MR shows diffuse thickening of the left lateral urinary bladder wall →. Note focal disruption of the smooth outer contour of the bladder → and tumor extension into the high signal perivesical fat. The left ureter → is dilated, which suggests muscle-invasive disease. (Right) Axial T1WI C+ FS MR in the same patient shows tumor enhancement → and confirms the extension of enhancing tumor tissue into the low signal perivesical fat →.

Stage III (T4a N0 M0)

Stage III (T4a N0 M0)

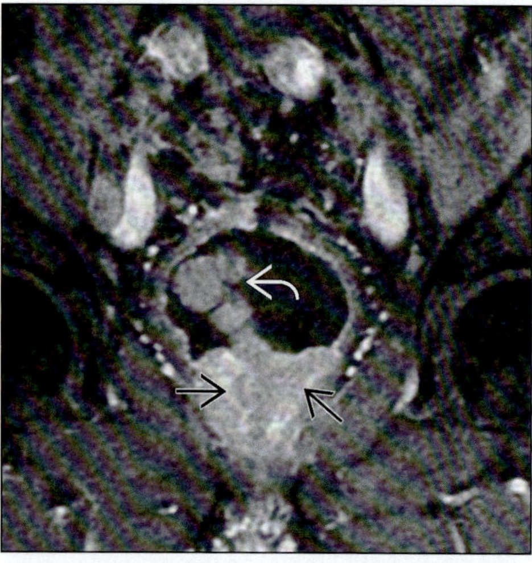

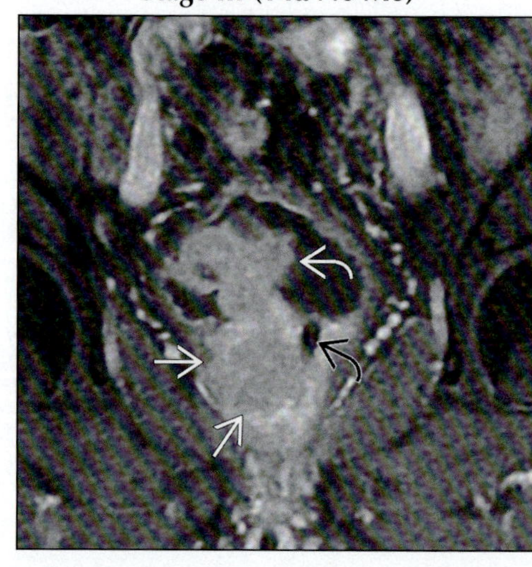

(Left) Coronal T1WI C+ FS MR in the same patient shows a polypoid bladder mass → that infiltrates into the prostate →. (Right) Coronal T1WI C+ FS MR in the same patient again shows the bladder mass → invading into the prostate → and displacing the Foley catheter → toward the left side. It can be difficult to differentiate primary bladder masses invading the prostate from prostate carcinoma invading the neck of the urinary bladder.

URINARY BLADDER CARCINOMA

Stage III (T4a N0 M0)

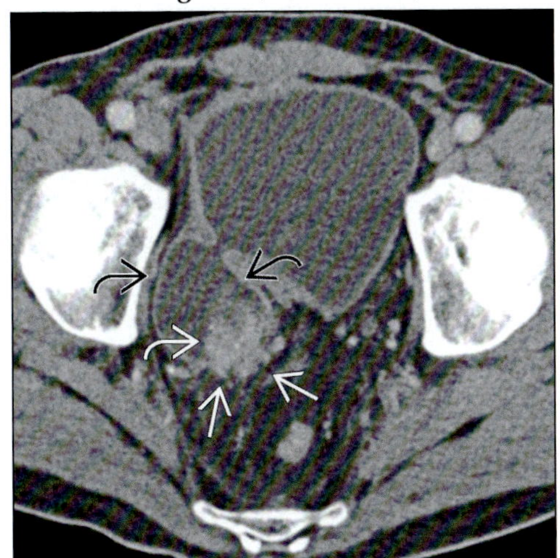

Stage III (T4a N0 M0)

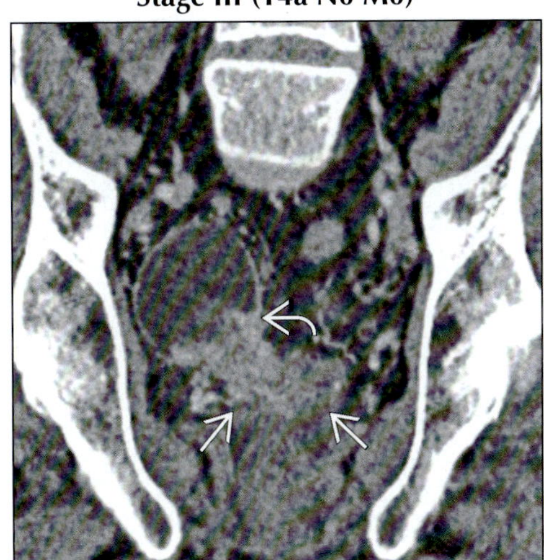

*(Left) Axial CECT shows a right posterolateral bladder diverticulum ⟹ with a polypoid mass ⟹ arising within the diverticulum and infiltrating into the perivesical fat ⟹. Pathology confirmed the diagnosis of squamous cell carcinoma. **(Right)** Coronal CECT in the same patient shows that the mass ⟹ within the diverticulum invades into the prostate ⟹. Because bladder diverticula lack a muscle layer, tumors arising within a diverticulum and invading the wall are at least T3.*

Stage III (T4a N0 M0)

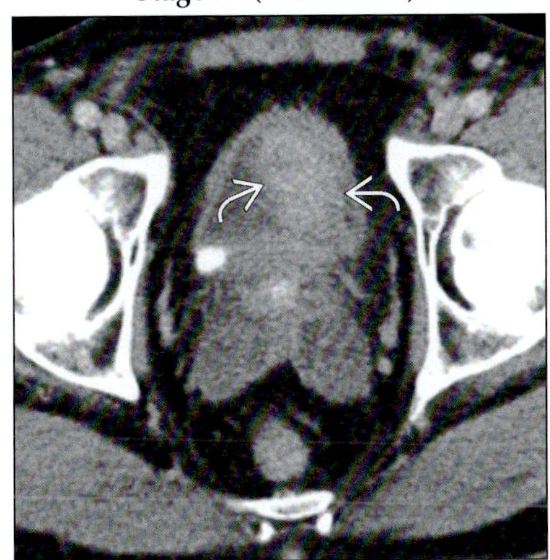

Stage III (T4a N0 M0)

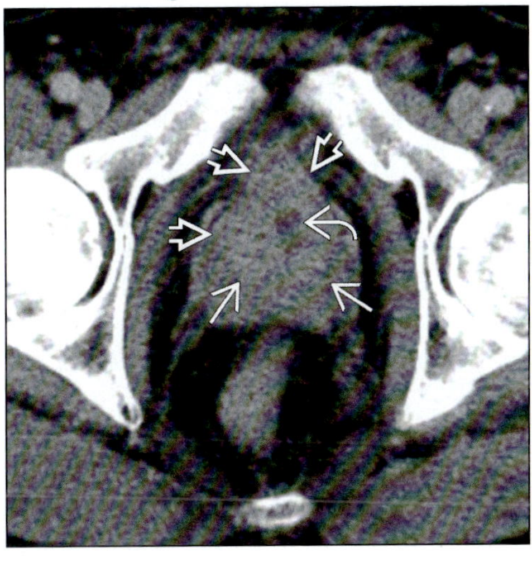

*(Left) Axial CECT shows an enhancing mass in the region of the neck of the urinary bladder ⟹. **(Right)** Axial CECT in the same patient at the level of the prostate shows tumor ⟹ surrounding the urethra ⟹ and invading into the prostate ⟹. It can be difficult to differentiate prostatic tumor invading the bladder neck from bladder tumors invading the prostate. The presence of prostate invasion makes this T4a disease.*

Stage IV (T4b N0 M0)

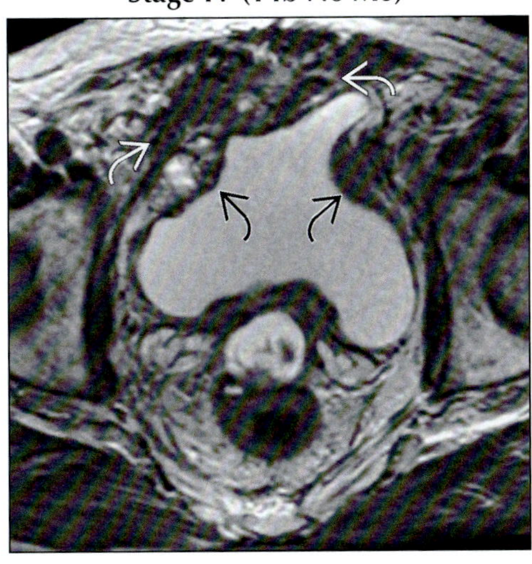

Stage IV (T4b N0 M0)

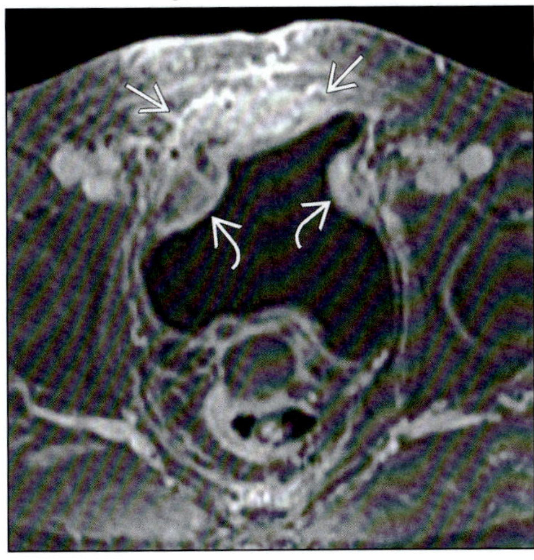

*(Left) Axial T2WI MR shows extensive infiltrative tumor ⟹ involving mainly the anterior bladder wall with focal invasion of the rectus abdominus muscle ⟹. The tumor shows heterogeneous T2 signal intensity. **(Right)** Axial T1WI C+ FS MR in the same patient shows heterogeneously enhancing tumor of the anterior wall of the bladder ⟹. Enhancing tumor fills the prevesical space and invades the rectus muscles ⟹.*

URINARY BLADDER CARCINOMA

Stage IV (T4b N0 M0)

Stage IV (T4b N0 M0)

(Left) Sagittal T2WI MR in the same patient shows marked circumferential thickening of the wall of the urinary bladder ➡, as well as invasion of the rectus muscles anteriorly ➡. *(Right)* Sagittal T1WI C+ FS MR in the same patient shows diffuse enhancement of the bladder wall with tumor extension into the wall of the rectum ➡ and the anterior abdominal wall muscles ➡.

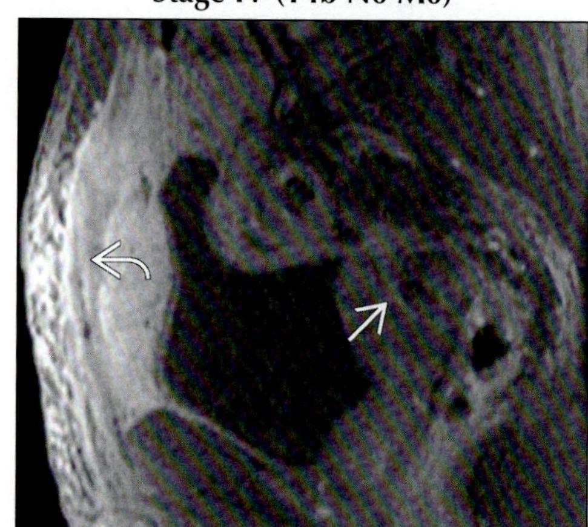

Stage IV (T4b N0 M0)

Stage IV (T4b N0 M0)

(Left) Axial CECT shows a large dumbbell-shaped polypoid mass that has a large intraluminal component ➡ and a large extraluminal component ➡. The extraluminal component invades into the anterior abdominal wall ➡. *(Right)* Coronal CECT in the same patient shows the intraluminal ➡ and large extraluminal ➡ components. This lesion was initially thought to be a mesenchymal mural tumor but was found at surgery to be transitional cell carcinoma.

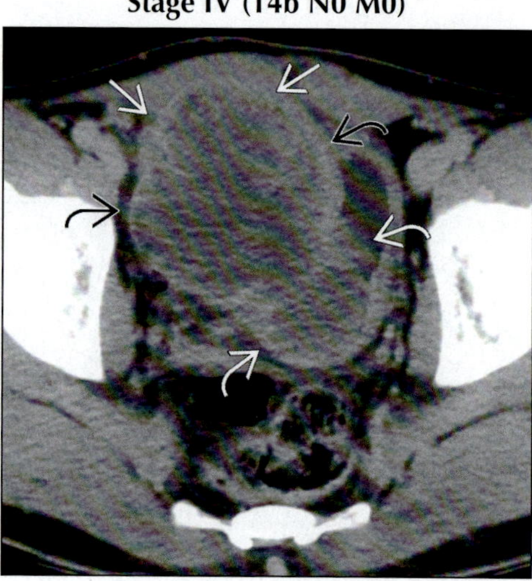

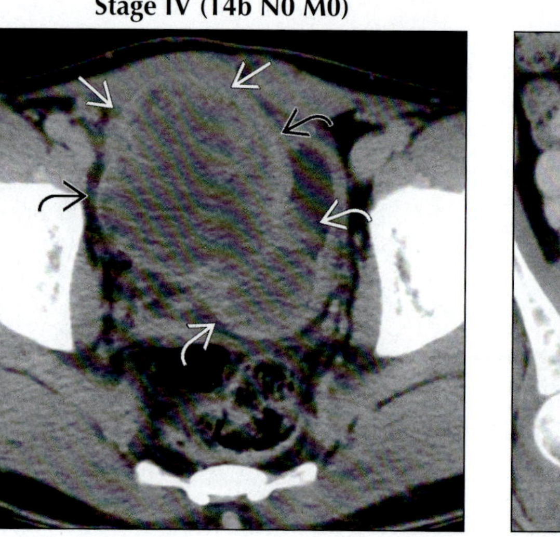

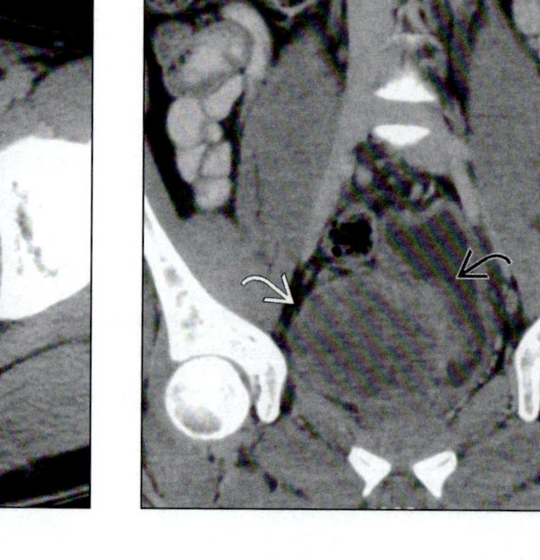

Stage IV (T2b N1 M0)

Stage IV (T2b N1 M0)

(Left) Axial T2WI MR shows 2 urinary bladder masses. The 1st mass ➡ is superficial and does not invade through the muscle layer (uniform low signal intensity muscle layer at the base of the lesion ➡). The 2nd lesion invades and interrupts the muscle layer ➡. A perivesical lymph node is present ➡. *(Right)* Axial T1WI C+ FS MR in the same patient shows enhancement of both lesions ➡, as well as similar enhancement of the perivesical lymph node ➡.

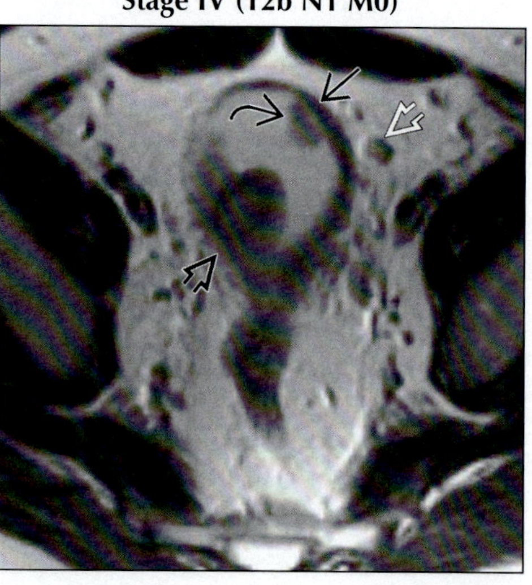

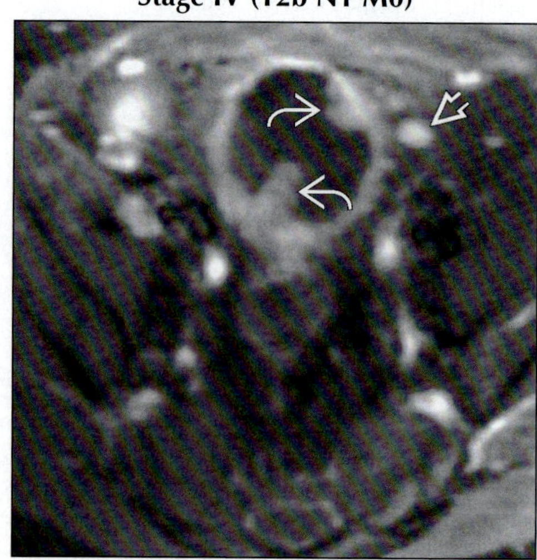

URINARY BLADDER CARCINOMA

Stage IV (T2b N1 M0)

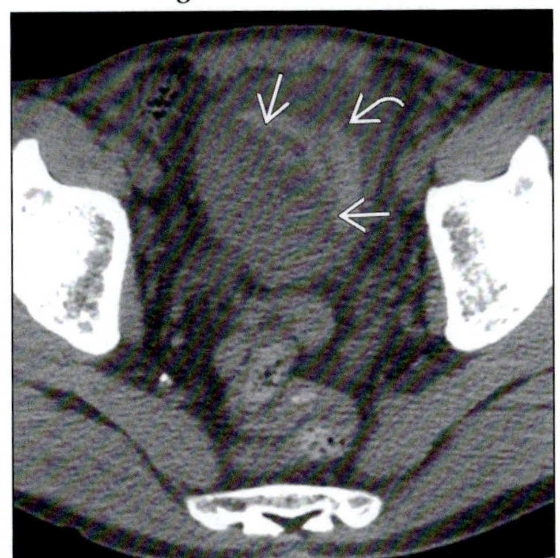

Stage IV (T2b N1 M0)

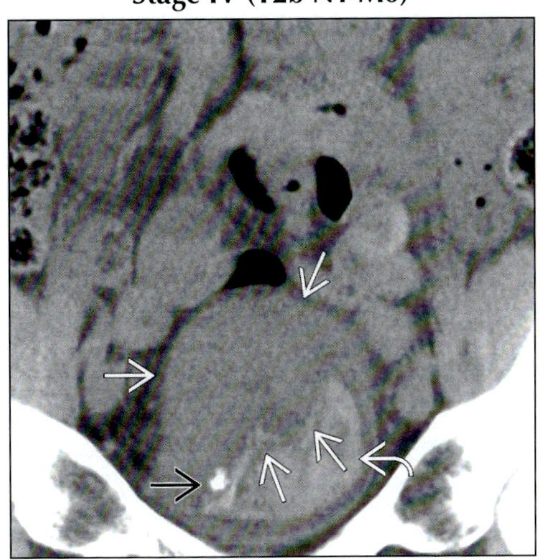

(Left) Axial NECT in a patient who presented with gross hematuria shows high-density blood within the urinary bladder ➡. The intraluminal blood outlines a large urinary bladder tumor ➡ that is otherwise isodense to urine. (Right) Coronal NECT in the same patient shows intravesical blood ➡ outlining the bladder tumor ➡. There are focal tumoral calcifications ➡. The bladder has a smooth outer contour, indicating the absence of perivesical invasion.

Stage IV (T2b N1 M0)

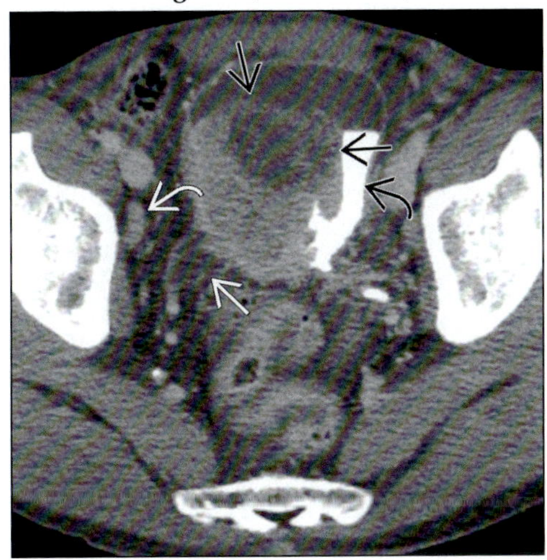

Stage IV (T2b N1 M0)

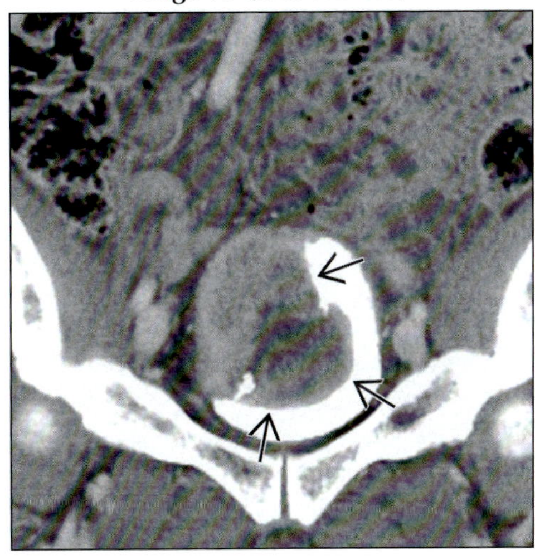

(Left) Axial CECT in the same patient shows contrast material ➡ within the urinary bladder outlining the large necrotic bladder mass ➡. Note involvement of the ureteric orifice and mild ureteric dilatation ➡. There is a single obturator lymph node ➡, which constitutes N1 disease (stage IV). (Right) Coronal CECT in the same patient shows the tumor outlined by intravesical contrast ➡.

Stage IV (T2b N2 M0)

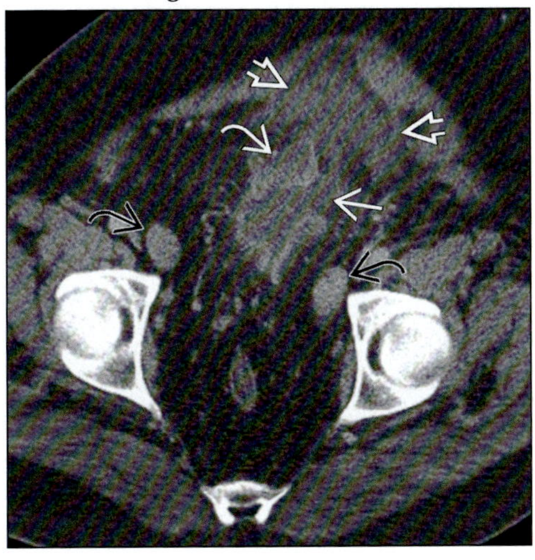

Stage IV (T2b N2 M0)

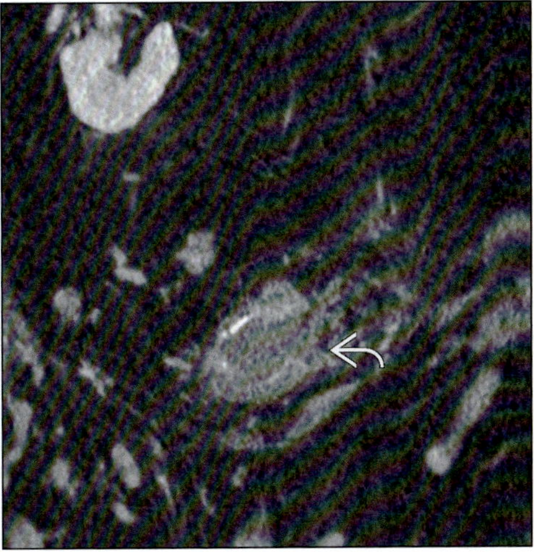

(Left) Axial CECT in a morbidly obese patient with pathologically proven T2b disease, who presented with severe lower abdominal pain, shows focal thickening of the anterior wall of the urinary bladder ➡ with a large defect of the bladder wall ➡ and fluid collection in the prevesical space ➡ due to bladder rupture. Bilateral enlarged external iliac nodes are seen ➡. (Right) Coronal CECT in the same patient shows the bladder defect ➡.

URINARY BLADDER CARCINOMA

Stage IV (T3b N2 M0)

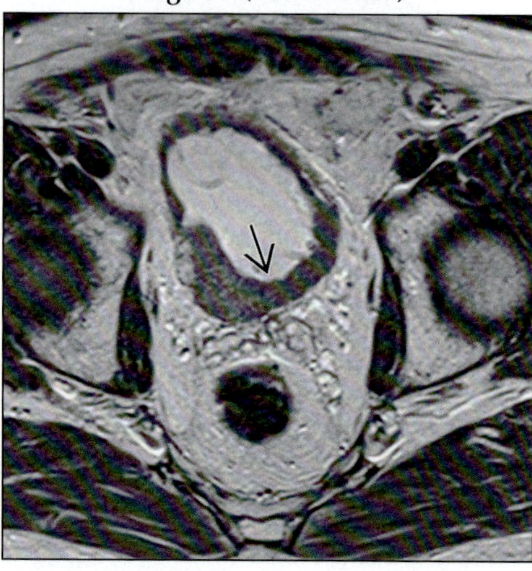

Stage IV (T3b N2 M0)

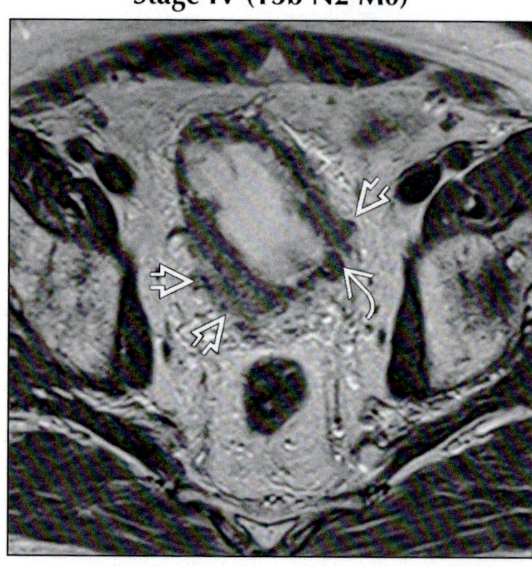

(Left) Axial T2WI MR in a 72-year-old man who presented with painless hematuria shows posterior urinary bladder wall thickening ➡ with loss of the low signal bladder wall indicating muscle invasion. *(Right)* Axial T2WI MR in the same patient shows thickening of the wall of the distal left ureter due to tumor invasion ➡ and irregular outer contour of the urinary bladder ➡ due to gross invasion of the perivesical fat, constituting T3b disease.

Stage IV (T3b N2 M0)

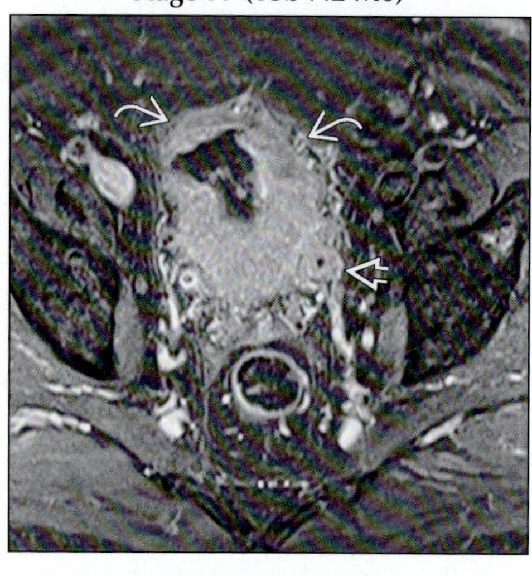

Stage IV (T3b N2 M0)

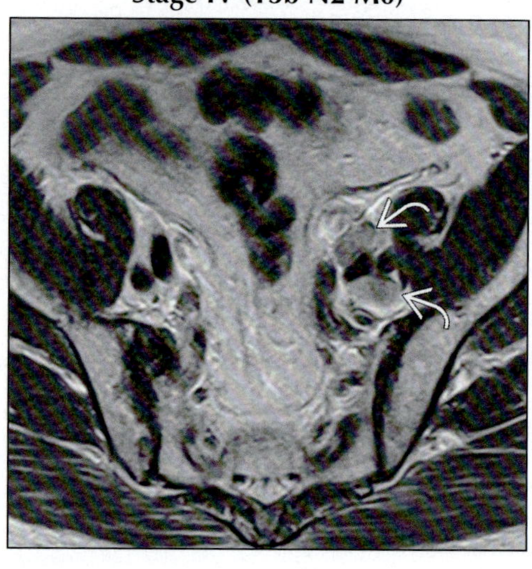

(Left) Axial T1WI C+ FS MR obtained at a higher level in the same patient shows diffuse enhancing wall thickening ➡ involving the dome of the urinary bladder with circumferential thickening of the distal left ureter ➡ due to tumor invasion. *(Right)* Axial T2WI MR in the same patient shows 2 enlarged left external iliac lymph nodes ➡. The presence of multiple lymph nodes metastases within the true pelvis constitutes N2 disease.

Stage IV (T4a N2 M0)

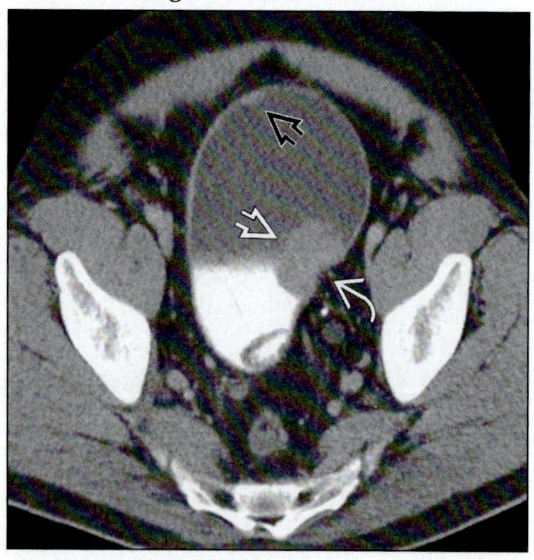

Stage IV (T4a N2 M0)

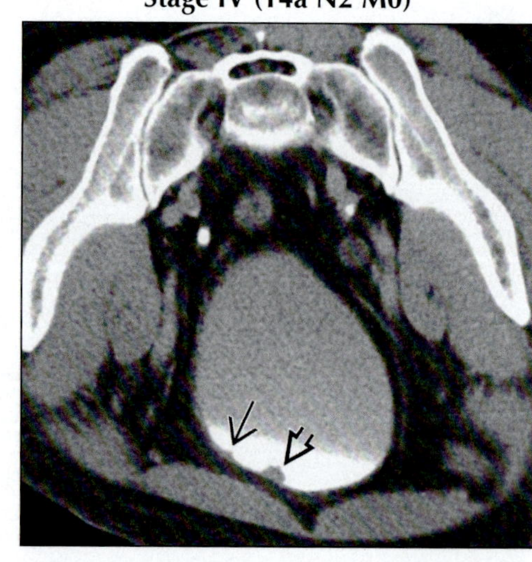

(Left) Axial CECT in a 54-year-old man shows a large polypoid lesion ➡ with indentation of the urinary bladder wall ➡ at the site of tumor attachment indicating muscle invasion. Note the subtle nodular lesion ➡ of the anterior bladder wall. *(Right)* Axial CECT in the same patient obtained in the prone position confirms the presence of the anterior wall polypoid lesion ➡ and shows another subtle flat lesion ➡, which was pathologically proven to be carcinoma in situ.

URINARY BLADDER CARCINOMA

Stage IV (T4a N2 M0)

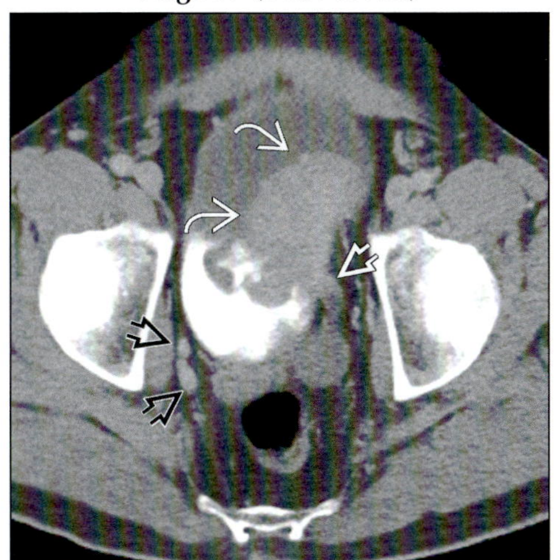

Stage IV (T4a N2 M0)

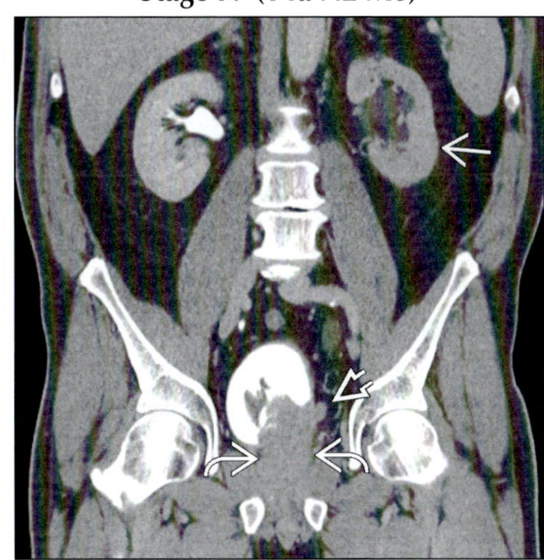

(Left) Axial CECT in the same patient shows the large polypoid mass ⮞ invading the left ureter ⮞. Two metastatic obturator lymph nodes ⮞ are present. The presence of multiple metastatic lymph nodes within the true pelvis constitute N2 disease. (Right) Coronal CECT in the same patient shows invasion of the prostate ⮞ and the left ureteric orifice ⮞. The left kidney ⮞ shows delayed nephrogram due to left ureteric obstruction.

Stage IV (T2b N0 M1)

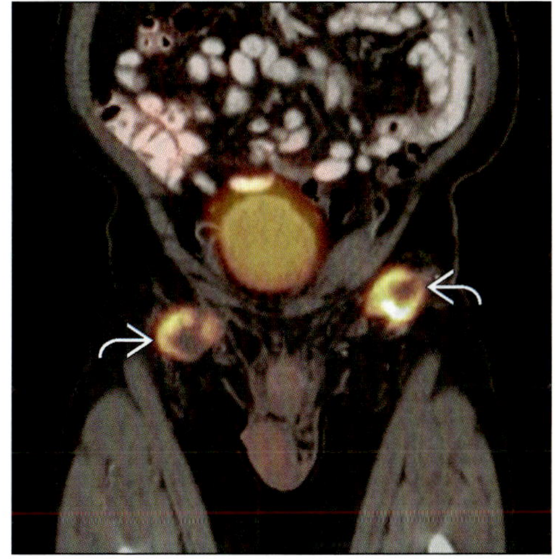

Stage IV (T2b N0 M1)

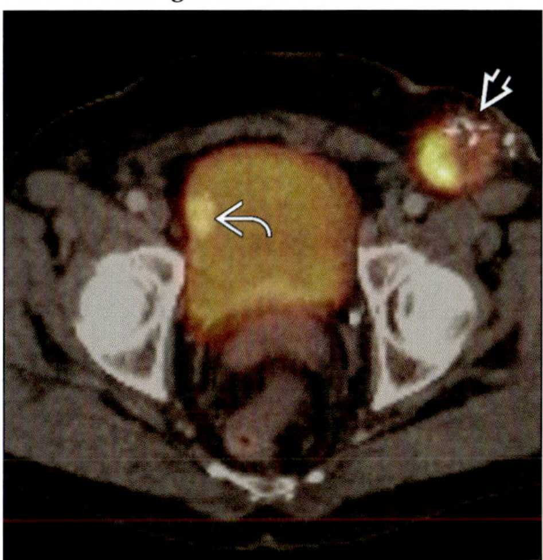

(Left) Coronal PET/CT was obtained after forced diuresis in a patient who presented with bilateral inguinal lymphadenopathy that was pathologically proven to be metastatic transitional cell carcinoma. Bilateral FDG-avid inguinal lymph nodes ⮞ are seen. (Right) Axial PET/CT in the same patient shows inguinal lymphadenopathy ⮞. A polypoid bladder mass is seen ⮞, representing the primary tumor that was found to be T2b tumor at surgery.

Stage IV (T3b N0 M1)

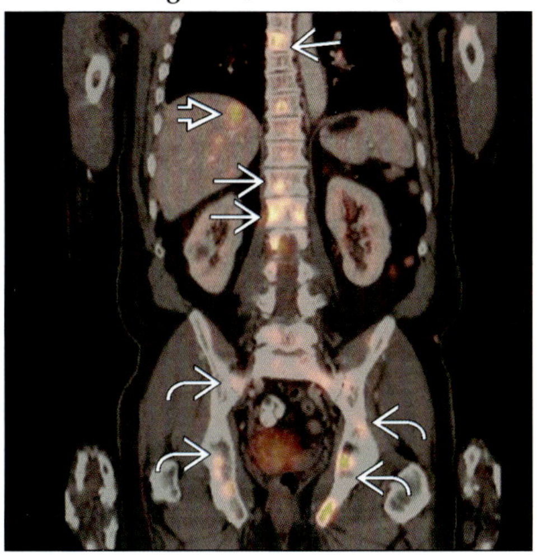

Stage IV (T3b N0 M1)

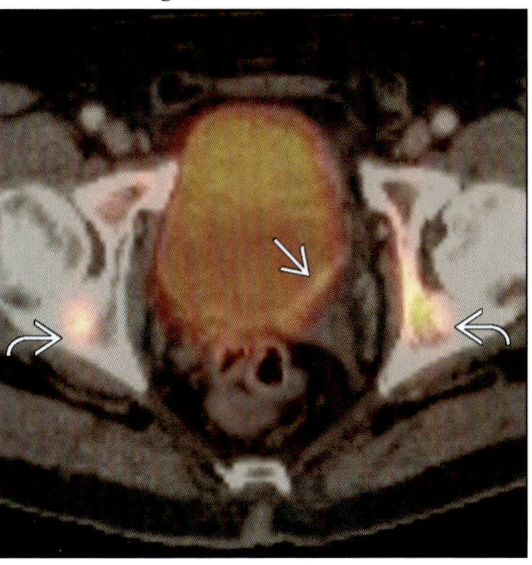

(Left) Coronal PET/CT shows liver metastases ⮞, multiple spine metastases ⮞, as well as multiple pelvic bony metastases ⮞. Spine and bony pelvic metastases are common due to tumor spread through the Batson venous plexus. (Right) Axial PET/CT in the same patient shows uptake ⮞ along the left posterolateral wall of the urinary bladder following resection of a muscle-invasive tumor and bilateral acetabular uptake ⮞ due to pelvic bony metastases.

URINARY BLADDER CARCINOMA

Stage IV (T3b N2 M1)

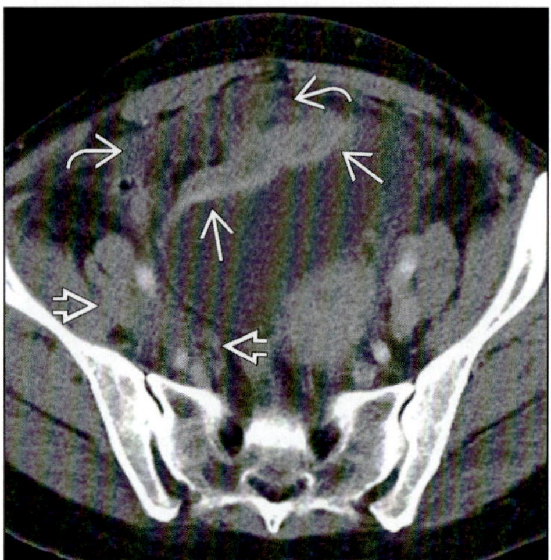

Stage IV (T3b N2 M1)

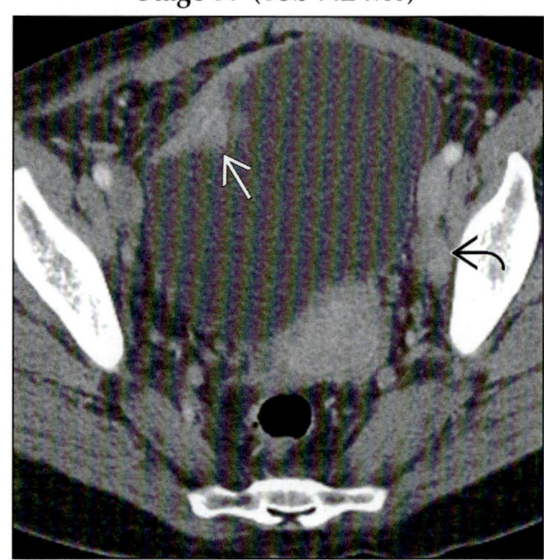

(Left) Axial CECT in a patient who presented with hematuria shows a large anterior bladder wall mass ➡ with stranding of the fat anterior to the bladder ➡. Visible involvement of the perivesical fat constitutes T3b disease. Right iliac adenopathy ➡ is present. (Right) Axial CECT in the same patient shows the anterior wall bladder mass ➡. There is an enlarged left obturator lymph node ➡.

Stage IV (T3b N2 M1)

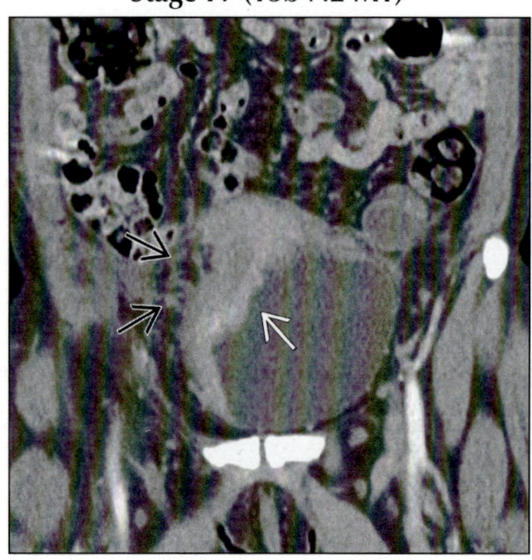

Stage IV (T3b N2 M1)

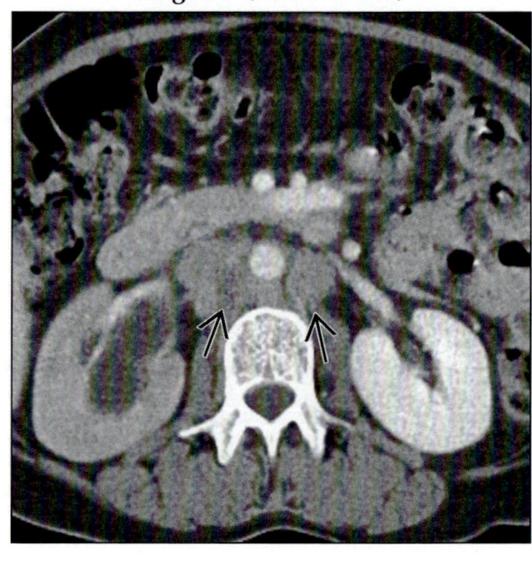

(Left) Coronal CECT in the same patient shows the bladder mass ➡, as well as soft tissue nodules and streaks within the perivesical fat ➡. (Right) Axial CECT in the same patient shows multiple periaortic enlarged lymph nodes ➡. The presence of metastatic nodes above the level of aortic bifurcation constitutes M1 disease. There is right hydronephrosis and delayed contrast excretion due to ureteric compression by the periaortic nodes.

Stage IV (T3 N3 M1)

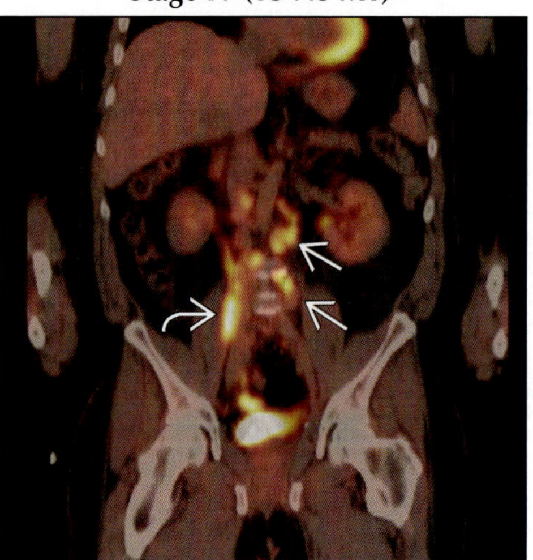

Stage IV (M1)

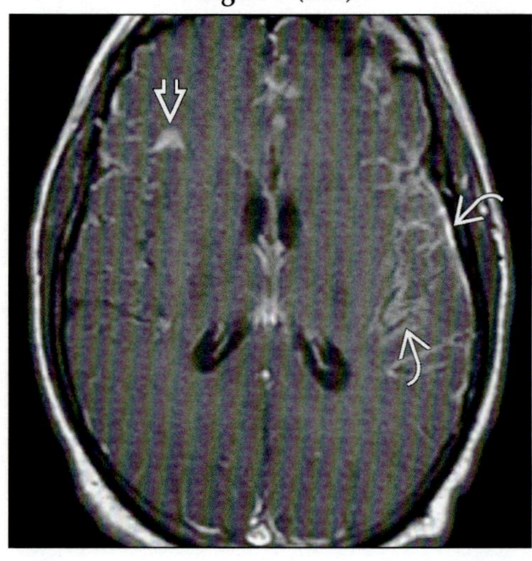

(Left) Coronal PET/CT in a patient with muscle-invasive disease shows hypermetabolic right common iliac ➡ and paraaortic lymph nodes ➡. Common iliac lymph nodes metastases are classified as N3, but nodal metastases above the level of aortic bifurcation are classified as distant metastases (M1 disease). (Right) Axial T1WI C+ FS MR of the brain in a patient with muscle-invasive TCC shows parenchymal ➡ and extensive leptomeningeal enhancement ➡ due to metastatic disease.

URINARY BLADDER CARCINOMA

Recurrent Locally Advanced Urinary Bladder Carcinoma

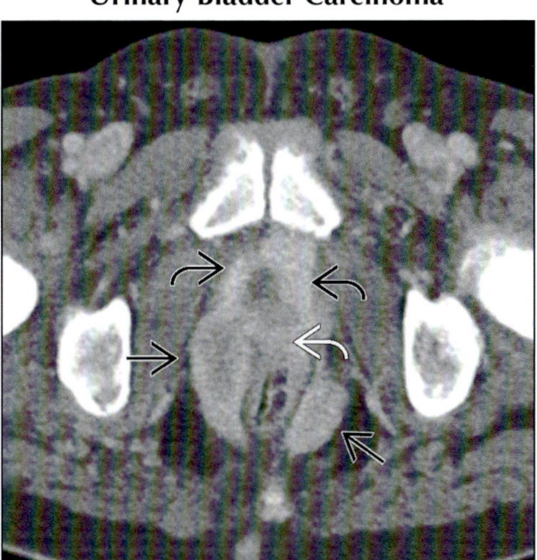

Recurrent Locally Advanced Urinary Bladder Carcinoma

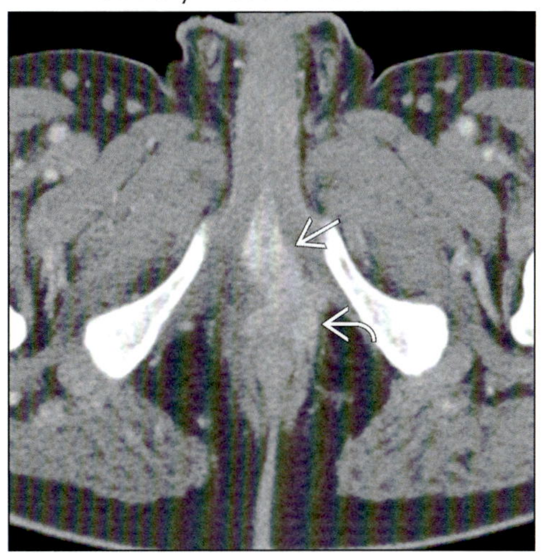

(Left) Axial CECT in a 68-year-old man following cystectomy for stage III (T3b N0 M0) bladder transitional cell carcinoma shows an enhancing soft tissue mass ⮕ in the cystectomy bed with posterior extension into the ischiorectal fossae ⮕. The tumor also invades the anterior wall of the rectum ⮕. *(Right)* Axial CECT in the same patient shows tumor invading the levator ani muscle ⮕ and extending anteriorly to invade the root of the penis ⮕.

Recurrent Locally Advanced Urinary Bladder Carcinoma

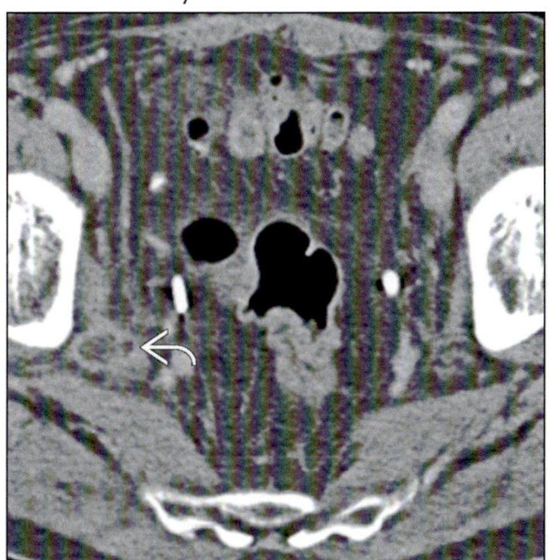

Recurrent Locally Advanced Urinary Bladder Carcinoma

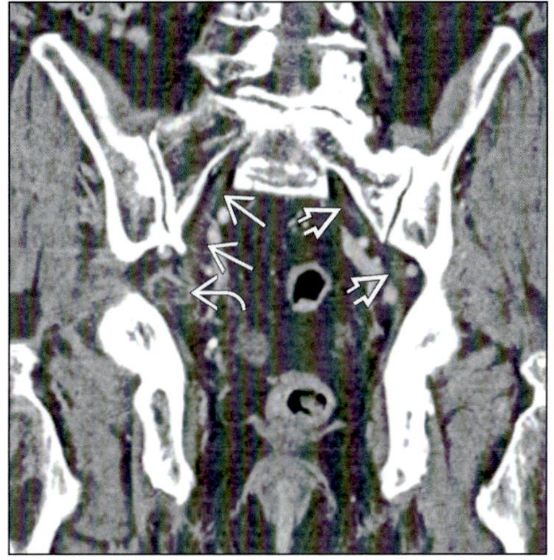

(Left) Axial CECT in a patient with advanced metastatic urinary bladder carcinoma shows a peripherally enhancing mass ⮕ involving the right sciatic nerve, an unusual site for metastatic disease. *(Right)* Coronal CECT in the same patient shows the peripherally enhancing mass ⮕ involving the right sciatic nerve. Note the normal appearance of the nerve proximal to the mass ⮕ and the normal appearance of the left sciatic nerve ⮕.

Recurrent Metastatic Urinary Bladder Carcinoma

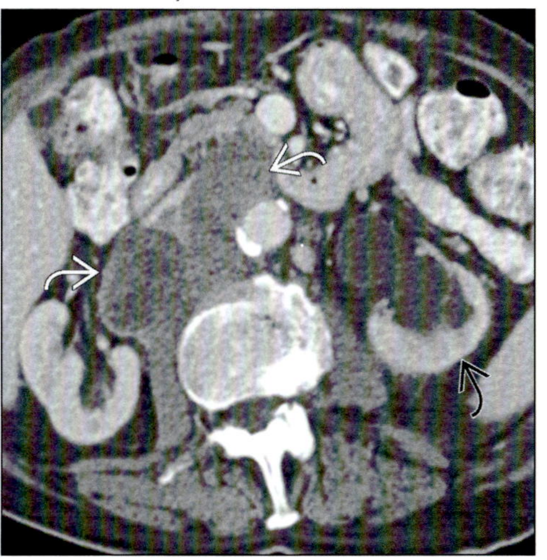

Recurrent Metastatic Urinary Bladder Carcinoma

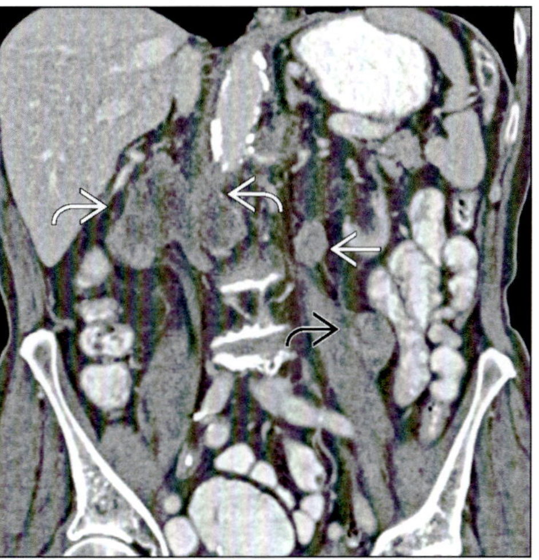

(Left) Axial CECT in a patient with recurrent metastatic bladder carcinoma after cystectomy shows multiple large paraaortic lymph nodes ⮕. Note left hydronephrosis and delayed contrast excretion by the left kidney ⮕. *(Right)* Coronal CECT in the same patient shows paraaortic lymph nodes ⮕ and retroperitoneal metastatic masses; the higher mass ⮕ involves the left ureter and causes hydronephrosis, while the lower invades into the psoas muscle ⮕.

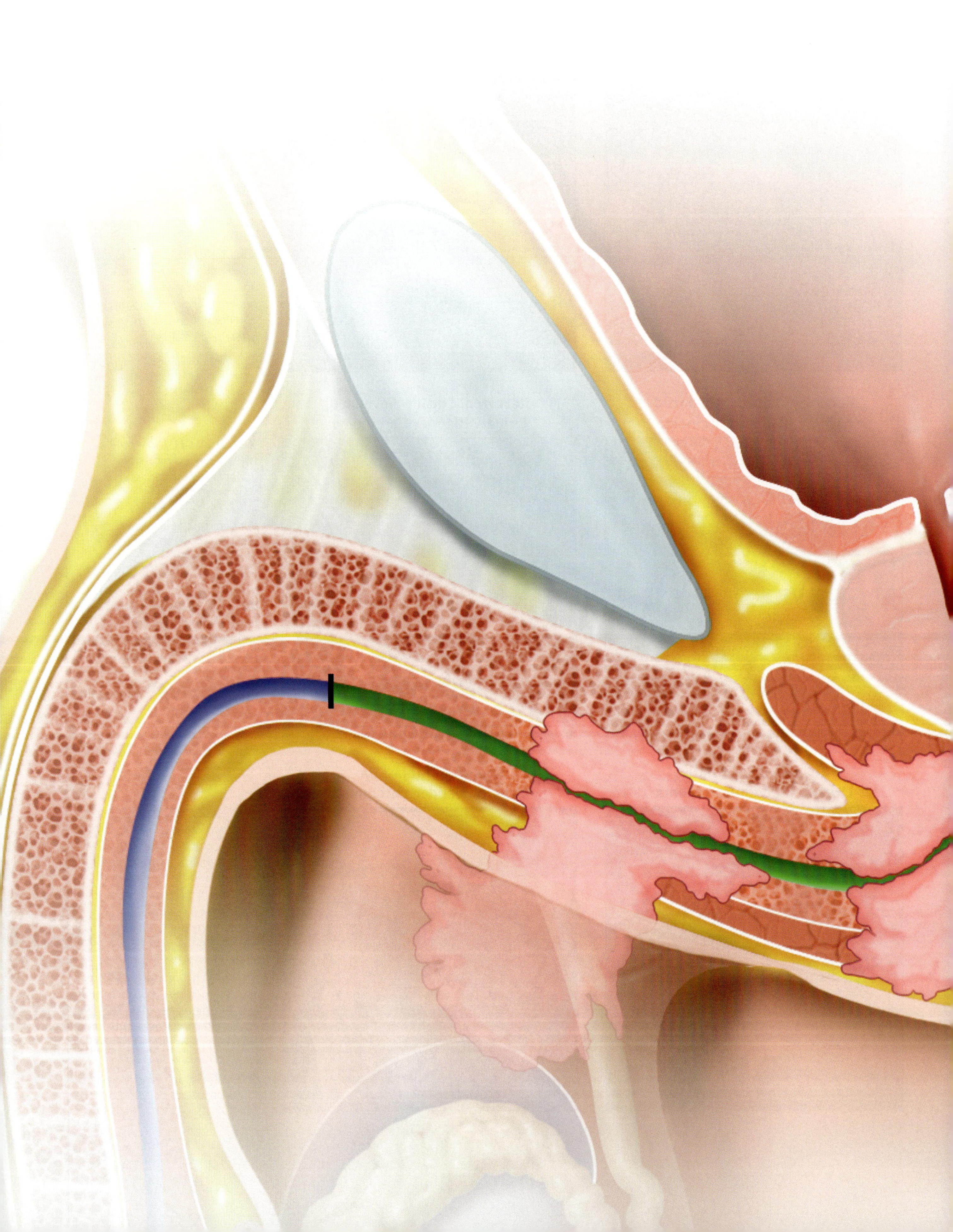

Urethral Carcinoma

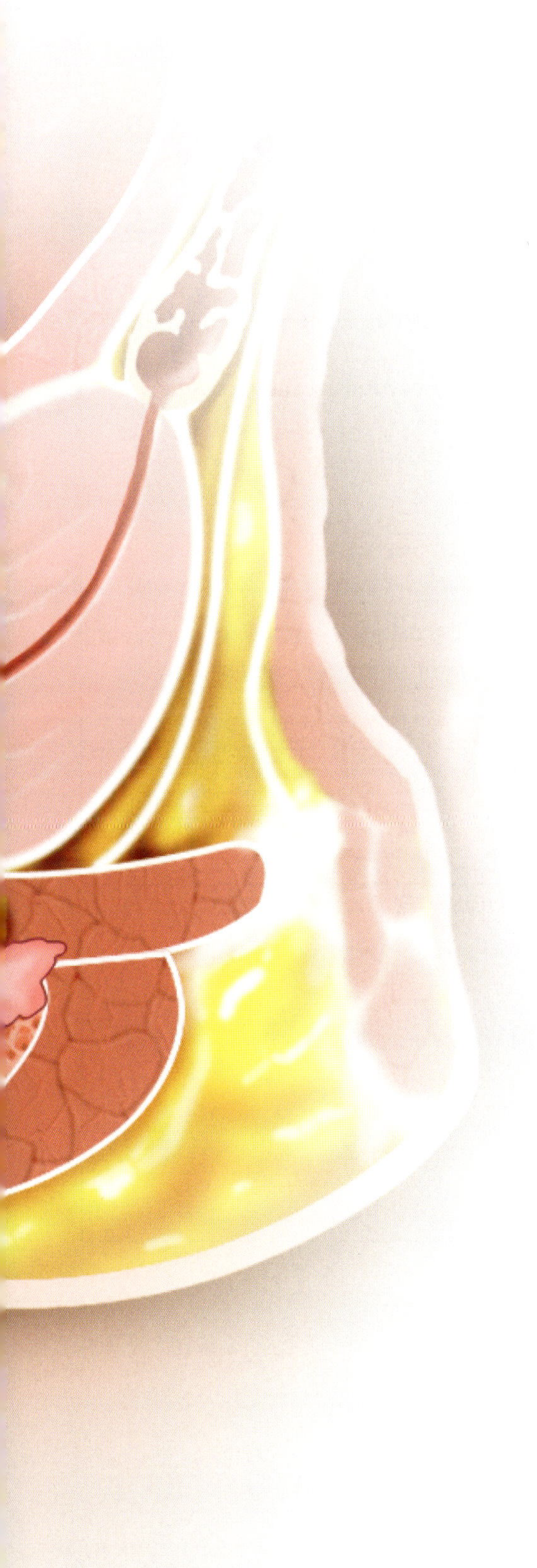

URETHRAL CARCINOMA

(T) Primary Tumor

Adapted from 7th edition AJCC Staging Forms.

TNM	Definitions
TX	Primary tumor cannot be assessed
T0	No evidence of primary tumor
Ta	Noninvasive papillary, polyoid, or verrucous carcinoma
Tis	Carcinoma in situ
T1	Tumor invades subepithelial connective tissue
T2	Tumor invades any of the following: Corpus spongiosum, prostate, periurethral muscle
T3	Tumor invades any of the following: Corpus cavernosum, beyond prostatic capsule, anterior vagina, bladder neck
T4	Tumor invades other adjacent organs

Urothelial (Transitional Cell) Carcinoma of the Prostate

Tis pu	Carcinoma in situ, involvement of the prostatic urethra
Tis pd	Carcinoma in situ, involvement of the prostatic ducts
T1	Tumor invades urethral subepithelial connective tissue
T2	Tumor invades any of the following: Prostatic stroma, corpus spongiosum, periurethral muscle
T3	Tumor invades any of the following: Corpus cavernosum, beyond prostatic capsule, bladder neck (extraprostatic extension)
T4	Tumor invades other adjacent organs (invasion of the bladder)

(N) Regional Lymph Nodes

NX	Regional lymph nodes cannot be assessed
N0	No regional lymph node metastasis
N1	Metastasis in a single lymph node ≤ 2 cm in greatest dimension
N2	Metastasis in a single node > 2 cm in greatest dimension or in multiple nodes

(M) Distant Metastasis

M0	No distant metastasis
M1	Distant metastasis

(G) Histologic Grade

World Health Organization/International Society of Urologic Pathology (WHO/ISUP) Grading System

LG	Low grade
HG	High grade

General Histologic Grading System

GX	Grade cannot be assessed
G1	Well differentiated
G2	Moderately differentiated
G3	Poorly differentiated
G4	Undifferentiated

URETHRAL CARCINOMA

AJCC Stages/Prognostic Groups

Adapted from 7th edition AJCC Staging Forms.

Stage	T	N	M
0a	Ta	N0	M0
0is	Tis	N0	M0
	Tis pu	N0	M0
	Tis pd	N0	M0
I	T1	N0	M0
II	T2	N0	M0
III	T1	N1	M0
	T2	N1	M0
	T3	N0	M0
	T3	N1	M0
IV	T4	N0	M0
	T4	N1	M0
	Any T	N2	M0
	Any T	Any N	M1

Incidence of Primary Urethral Carcinoma

Histologic Subtype	Incidence in Males	Incidence in Females
Transitional cell carcinoma	70.2%	33.9%
Squamous cell carcinoma	18.4%	31.1%
Adenocarcinoma	11.4%	35.0%

Data from Swartz MA et al: Incidence of primary urethral carcinoma in the United States. Urology. 68(6):1164-8, 2006. The data were calculated from the U.S. SEER database, 1973-2002.

Observed and Overall 1- and 5-Year Survival Rates

Stage	1-Year Survival	5-Year Survival
0a	97%	79%
0is	93%	62%
I	90%	59%
II	82%	51%
III	79%	28%
IV	59%	22%

Data from American Joint Committee on Cancer: AJCC Cancer Staging Manual. 7th ed. New York: Springer, 2010.

URETHRAL CARCINOMA

T1: Female

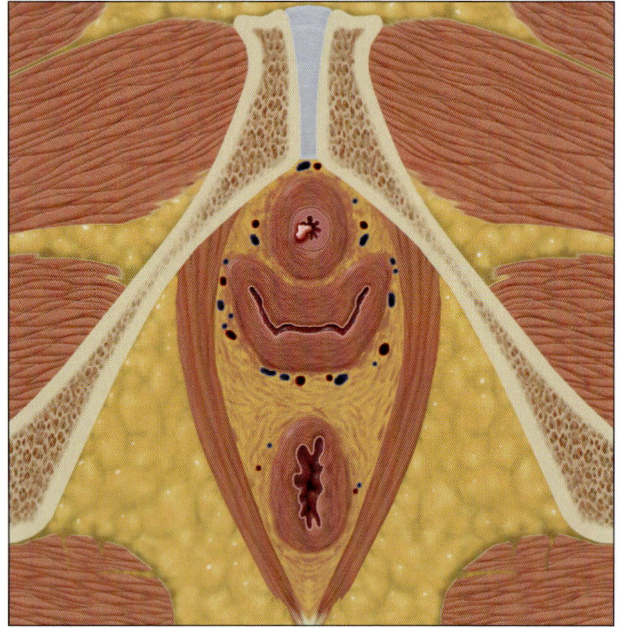

Axial illustration demonstrates T1 disease, which is limited to focal tumor with submucosal invasion. Periurethral tissue is not involved. It is unlikely that this minimal disease burden would be visible on imaging.

T2: Female

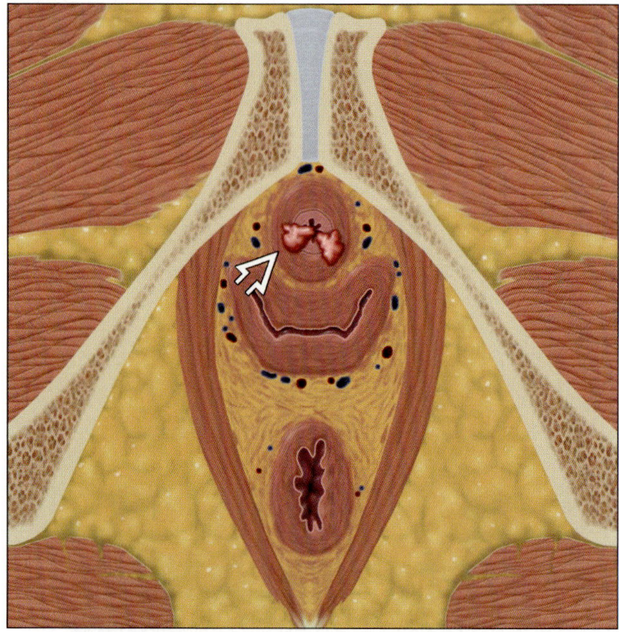

Axial illustration demonstrates T2 disease, which is centered in the urethra, extending through the subepithelial tissue into the periurethral muscle ➡ layer.

T3: Female

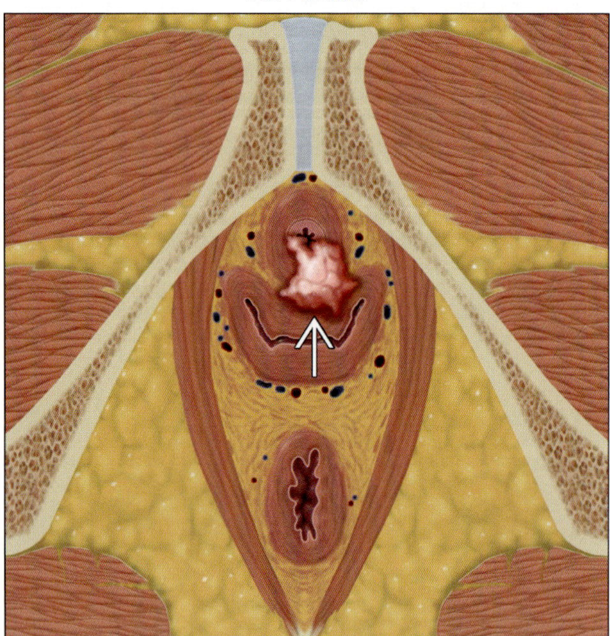

Axial illustration demonstrates T3 disease, which extends through the periurethral muscle into the adjacent anterior vagina ➡.

T4: Female

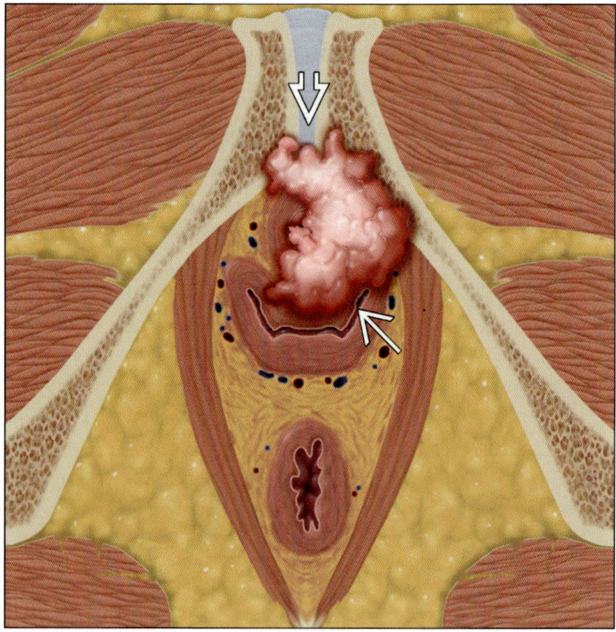

Axial illustration demonstrates T4 disease, which is locally advanced, involving both the anterior vagina ➡ and the pubic symphysis ➡.

T1 and T2: Female

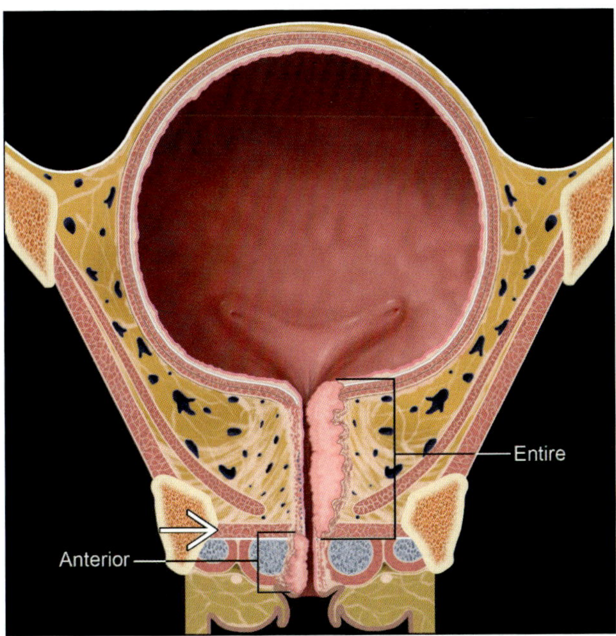

Coronal illustration through the bladder demonstrates primary urethral cancer. The distribution of disease is divided into anterior and entire urethra. Anterior urethral cancer is limited to the distal 1/3 of the urethra, external to the urogenital diaphragm ➡. Entire urethral cancer is usually high grade and locally advanced.

T3 and T4: Female

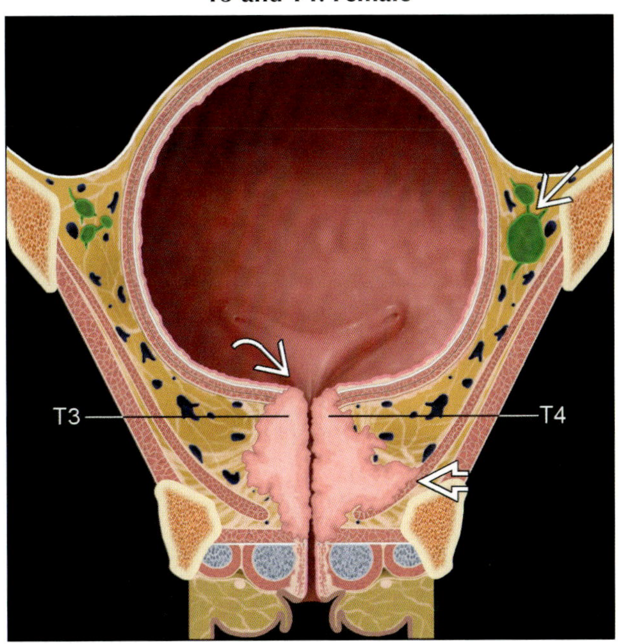

Coronal illustration through the bladder shows T3 disease on the left. This extends into the periurethral soft tissues and may involve the bladder neck ➡. T4 disease, shown on the right, involves the entire urethra and periurethral muscles ➡. N1 disease is illustrated by the enlarged regional lymph node ➡, which measures < 2 cm.

Tis and T1: Male

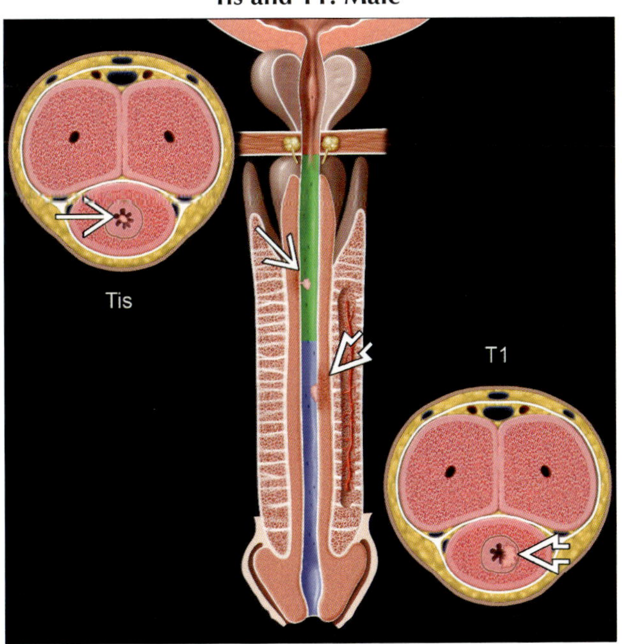

Primary urethral cancer in a male is divided into anterior (penile urethra in blue) and posterior (bulbomembranous urethra in green) distributions. On the left, Tis disease ➡ is papillary and localized, without submucosal invasion. On the right, T1 disease ➡ extends into the submucosal layer.

T2 and T3: Male

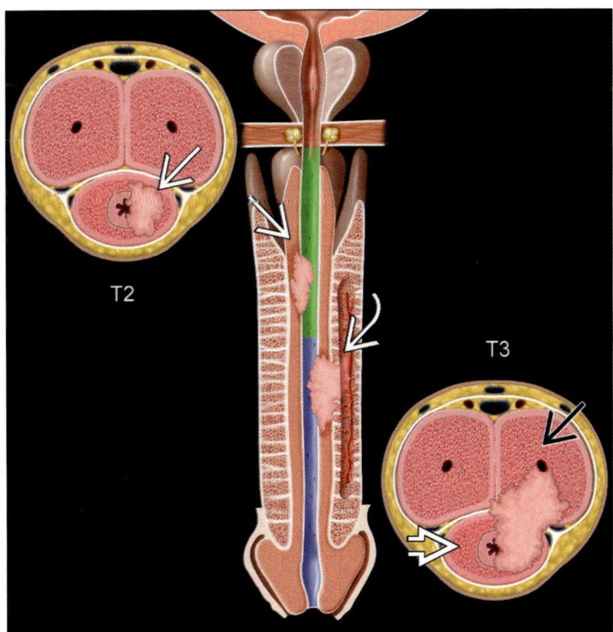

On the left, T2 disease extends into the corpus spongiosum ➡. On the right, T3 disease ➡ extends beyond the corpus spongiosum ➡ into the corpus cavernosum ➡. If prostatic urethra is involved, the etiology is more often prostatic or bladder cancer extending into prostatic urethra.

URETHRAL CARCINOMA

T2: Male

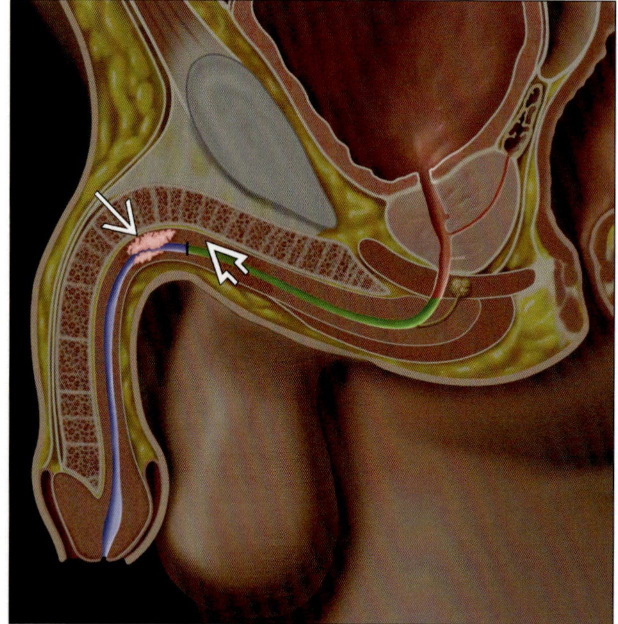

Sagittal illustration through the bladder and penis demonstrates anterior disease ➡ in the penile urethra (blue). Disease extends into the corpus spongiosum ➡, making this at least T2/stage II disease.

T2: Male

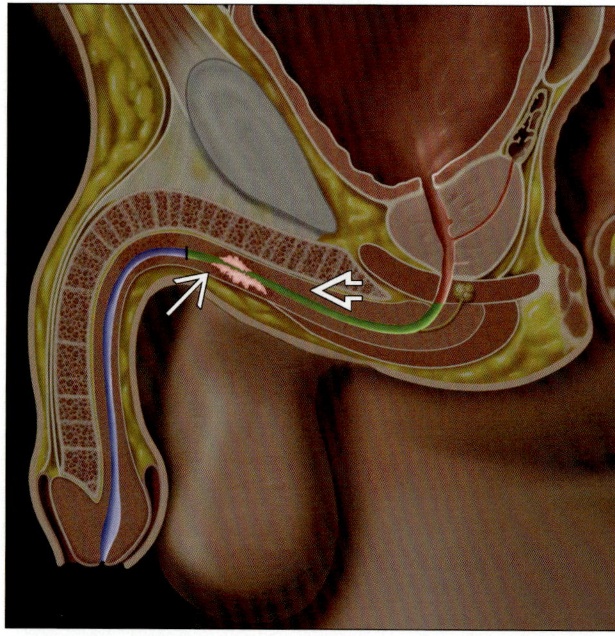

Sagittal illustration through the bladder and penis demonstrates posterior disease ➡ centered in the bulbous urethra (green). Again demonstrated is disease extending into the corpus spongiosum ➡, resulting in at least T2/stage II classification.

T3: Male

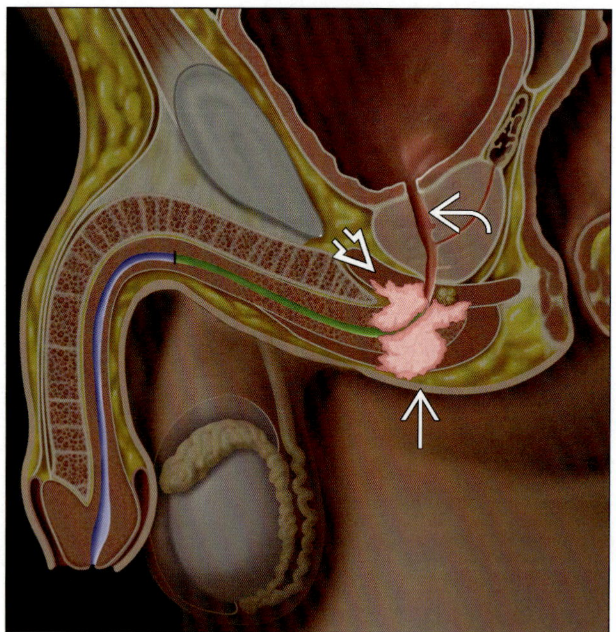

Locally advanced disease in the bulbomembranous urethra (green) is demonstrated. The tumor invades periurethral muscle, urogenital diaphragm ➡, and perineal tissues ➡. Note the normal prostatic urethra ➡, which is consistent with the tumor arising primarily from the urethra rather than from the bladder or prostate.

T4: Male

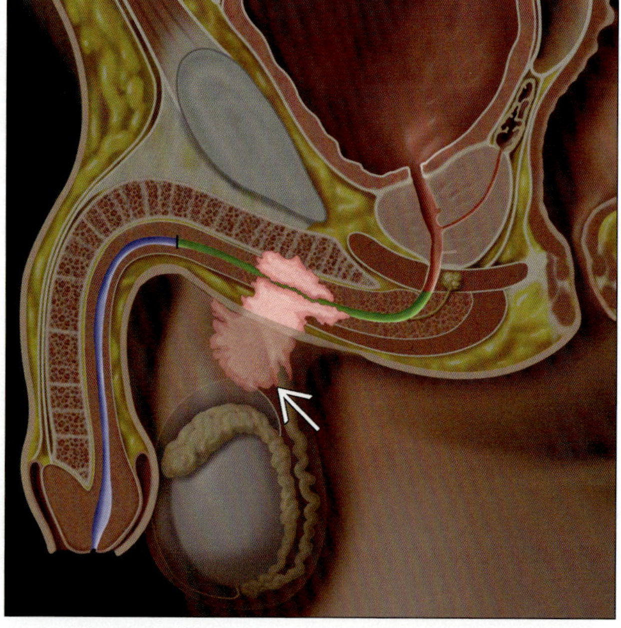

Sagittal illustration through the bladder and perineum demonstrates locally advanced posterior disease in the bulbomembranous urethra (green). This lesion extends beyond the corpus spongiosum to the scrotum ➡. Patient may present with a nonhealing scrotal ulcer in such cases.

URETHRAL CARCINOMA

N1

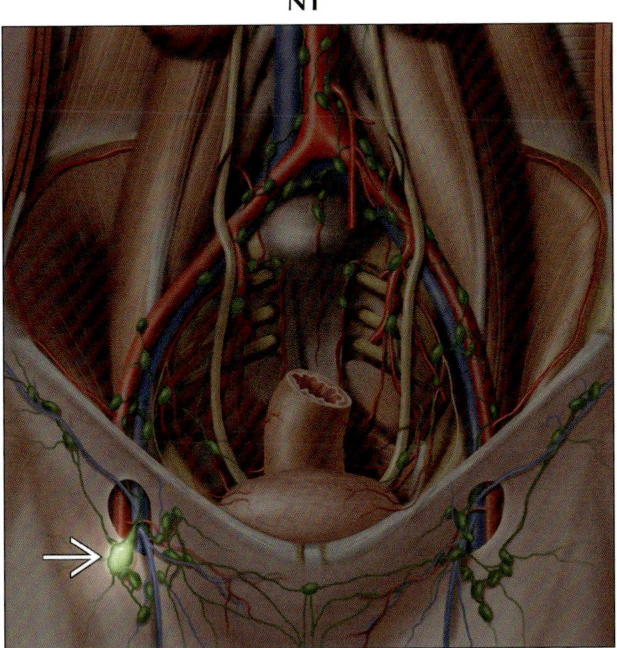

A single enlarged superficial inguinal node ➡ is present, which measures less than or equal to 2 cm. The presence of N1 disease upgrades disease severity to stage III.

N2

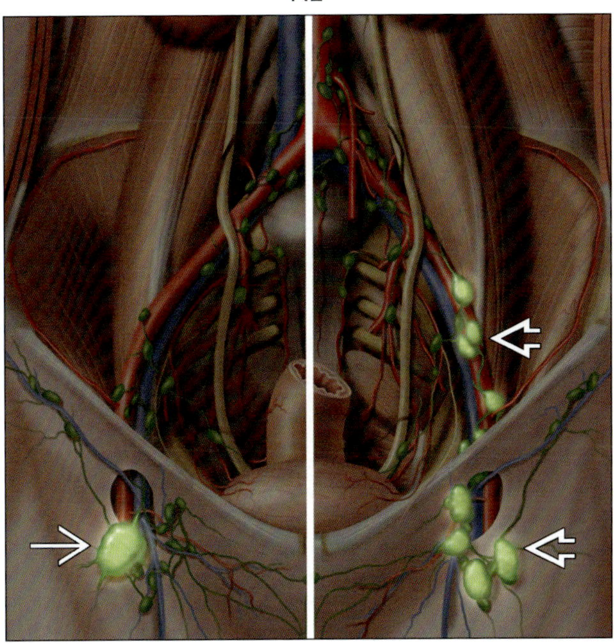

On the left, a single enlarged superficial inguinal node ➡ measures more than 2 cm. On the right, multiple nodes and multiple nodal stations are involved ➡. These are both examples of N2 disease. The presence of N2 disease upgrades disease severity to stage IV.

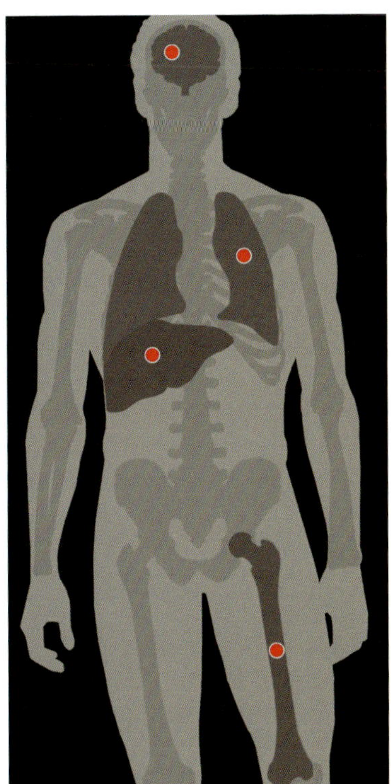

METASTASES, ORGAN FREQUENCY

Liver

Lung

Bone

Brain

Urethral carcinoma is so uncommon that the frequency distribution of metastases is unknown. Most metastatic disease is to local lymph nodes.

URETHRAL CARCINOMA

OVERVIEW

Classification
- Women: Location is **anterior** or **entire**
  - Anterior tumors exclusively in distal 1/3 of urethra
    - 46% of urethral tumors
    - Squamous cell carcinoma most common
  - Entire urethral tumors usually high grade and locally advanced
- Men: Location is **posterior** or **anterior**
  - Posterior: Prostatic urethra (10%)
  - Posterior: Bulbomembranous urethra (60%)
  - Anterior: Penile urethra (30%)

PATHOLOGY

Routes of Spread
- Local spread
  - In women: Local extension
    - Bladder neck, vagina, vulva
  - In men: Infiltrate via vascular spaces of corpus spongiosum and periurethral tissues
    - Anterior tumors may infiltrate to skin surface
    - Posterior/bulbomembranous tumors spread locally to perineum
- Lymphatic metastases to regional nodes
  - Anterior urethral cancer nodal distribution
    - Superficial and deep inguinal nodes
    - Occasionally external iliac nodes
  - Posterior urethral cancer nodal distribution
    - Pelvic nodes
  - Palpable inguinal nodes occur in 20%
    - Usually indicative of metastatic disease
  - Female cancer often spreads systemically without regional nodal disease
- Hematogenous spread uncommon except in
  - Primary transitional cell carcinoma (TCC) of prostatic urethra
  - Advanced local disease

General Features
- Comments
  - Prognosis depends on anatomic location and depth of invasion
    - Histology less important predictor
  - Superficial tumors may be resectable
- Etiology
  - Urethral stricture
    - Present in 1/2 of patients with primary urethral carcinoma
      - Insidious onset of disease
      - Requires high index of clinical suspicion
  - History of sexually transmitted diseases
    - ~ 1/4 of patients with primary urethral carcinoma
  - Chronic urinary tract infections
  - Age > 60 years
  - History of bladder cancer
    - If cystectomy done for bladder carcinoma → 10% will develop urethral cancer
    - Present in 30% of cystoprostatectomy specimens for bladder TCC
- Epidemiology & cancer incidence
  - Uncommon, < 1% of all urothelial malignancies
    - Associated with poor outcomes
  - M:F = 1:4
    - Only urologic malignancy more common in women
  - Usually occurs after 50 years of age

Gross Pathology & Surgical Features
- Anterior urethral lesions more amenable to surgical resection
- Localized, early stage tumor may present as papillary mass expanding urethra
- Large lesions may ulcerate

Microscopic Pathology
- H&E
  - Most common histologic subtypes are transitional cell carcinoma (TCC), squamous cell carcinoma (SCCa), and adenocarcinoma (AdenoCa)
    - In males
      - TCC most common in prostatic urethra
      - SCCa more common in bulbomembranous and penile urethra
      - Undifferentiated subtype associated with bulbomembranous urethra
      - AdenoCa from glands of Littré or Cowper
    - In females
      - SCCa > TCC > AdenoCa
      - Clear cell AdenoCa most common subtype in urethral diverticulum
      - Uncommon tumors include undifferentiated, sarcoma, melanoma, and metastases

IMAGING FINDINGS

Detection
- **Primary evaluation: Examination under anesthesia**
  - Cystoscopy
  - Bimanual examination
    - External genitalia, urethra, rectum, perineum
    - Flexible sigmoidoscopy if rectal involvement suspected
  - Transurethral or needle biopsy
- **Retrograde cystourethrography**
  - Standard imaging technique for morphologic and functional urethral evaluation
  - Tumor may be incidental finding during evaluation of stricture disease
    - Infiltrating lesions associated with tight stenoses
    - Often difficult or impossible to opacify urethral lumen above lesion
- **Voiding cystourethrogram**
  - Urethral strictures or filling defects
- **MR**
  - Best for depicting local extent of disease due to superior soft tissue resolution
- **Ultrasound**
  - Transperineal, transvaginal, or transrectal
    - Endourethral US with catheter-based transducer
  - Hypo- to isoechoic
  - Irregularly marginated urethral mass

Staging
- CECT
  - Limited utility for local disease

- Difficult to differentiate urethra from vagina/bladder base
- May appear as homogeneously or heterogeneously enhancing mass
  - ○ Local soft tissue extension
  - ○ Pelvic lymph node involvement
  - ○ Extension into adjacent bony structures
- **MR**
  - ○ T1WI
    - Low signal intensity mass, difficult to differentiate from urethra
  - ○ T2WI
    - Urethral wall: Signal intensity similar to muscle
    - Urethral cancer
      - Relatively high signal intensity mass disrupting female urethral "target-like" zonal anatomy
      - High signal intensity mass invading corpora cavernosa
  - ○ T1WI C+
    - Variable enhancement
    - Best for urethra and periurethral tissue evaluation

CLINICAL ISSUES

Presentation
- Urethral bleeding, serosanguineous discharge
- Palpable urethral mass
- Obstructive voiding symptoms
- Urethral fistula, periurethral abscess
- Perineal pain

Cancer Natural History & Prognosis
- Female: Anterior urethral cancer
  - ○ Much better prognosis, even with local nodal mets
- Female: Entire urethral cancer
  - ○ Commonly locally invasive with pelvic nodal mets
  - ○ Prospects for cure low unless lesions small
    - If < 2 cm, 5-year survival (60%)
    - If > 4 cm, 5-year survival (13%)
- Male: Anterior urethral cancer
  - ○ Potential for cure high with superficial disease
- Male: Posterior urethral cancer
  - ○ Prospects for cure low, high local recurrence rates
  - ○ 5-year survival from 15-20%

Treatment Options
- Major treatment alternatives
  - ○ Surgical treatment
    - Options depend on location and extent of disease
    - In men, no demonstrated benefit from prophylactic inguinal lymph node dissection
  - ○ Adjunctive or neoadjuvant radiation therapy
  - ○ Chemotherapy: In clinical trials for metastatic urethral cancer
    - Urethral TCC may respond to same chemotherapy regimens as advanced bladder TCC
- Treatment options by stage
  - ○ Female: Anterior urethral cancer
    - Stage 0/Tis, Ta: Open excision **or** electroresection and fulguration **or** laser vaporization-coagulation
    - Stage T1 and T2: External beam radiation therapy **or** interstitial radiation **or** combination **or** surgical resection of distal 1/3 of urethra

- T3/recurrent lesions: Anterior exenteration and urinary diversion ± preoperative radiation and urinary diversion
    - Palpable inguinal nodes: Frozen section tumor confirmation **then** ipsilateral node dissection
  - ○ Female: Entire urethral cancer
    - Preoperative radiation, anterior exenteration and urinary diversion with bilateral pelvic node dissection ± inguinal node dissection
    - If < 2 cm in greatest dimension, radiation alone **or** nonextensive surgery alone **or** the combination may be sufficient
  - ○ Male: Anterior urethral cancer
    - Stage 0/Tis, Ta: Open excision **or** electroresection and fulguration **or** laser vaporization-coagulation
    - T1, T2, T3: Partial penectomy, negative margins to 2 cm proximal to tumor
    - T1, T2, T3 (penectomy refused): Radiation
    - Palpable inguinal nodes: Frozen section tumor confirmation **then** ipsilateral node dissection
  - ○ Male: Posterior urethral cancer
    - Preoperative radiation, cystoprostatectomy, urinary diversion, and penectomy with bilateral pelvic node dissection ± inguinal node dissection
  - ○ Female/male: Recurrent urethral cancer
    - Local recurrence after radiation: Surgical excision
    - Local recurrence after surgery alone: Combination radiation and wider surgical resection

REPORTING CHECKLIST

T Staging
- Female
  - ○ Assess for tumor beyond periurethral muscle
  - ○ Assess for tumor in relation to bladder base
- Male
  - ○ Assess tumor extension beyond corpus spongiosum
  - ○ Determine relation of tumor to prostatic urethra
    - Tumor in prostatic urethra more likely prostate than urethral cancer

N Staging
- Size and number of nodes most significant

M Staging
- Lung, liver, bone, brain

SELECTED REFERENCES

1. American Joint Committee on Cancer: AJCC Cancer Staging Manual. 7th ed. New York: Springer, 2010
2. Gillitzer R et al: Single-institution experience with primary tumours of the male urethra. BJU Int. 101(8):964-8, 2008
3. Liedberg F et al: Prospective study of transitional cell carcinoma in the prostatic urethra and prostate in the cystoprostatectomy specimen. Incidence, characteristics and preoperative detection. Scand J Urol Nephrol. 41(4):290-6, 2007
4. Swartz MA et al: Incidence of primary urethral carcinoma in the United States. Urology. 68(6):1164-8, 2006
5. Kawashima A et al: Imaging of urethral disease: a pictorial review. Radiographics. 24 Suppl 1:S195-216, 2004

URETHRAL CARCINOMA

Stage I (T1 N0 M0)

Stage I (T1 N0 M0)

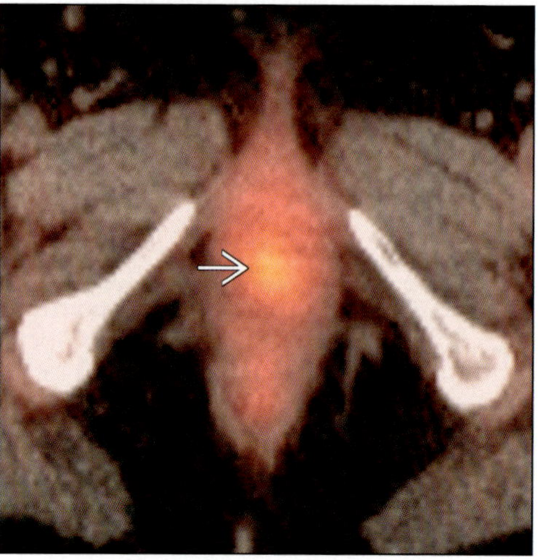

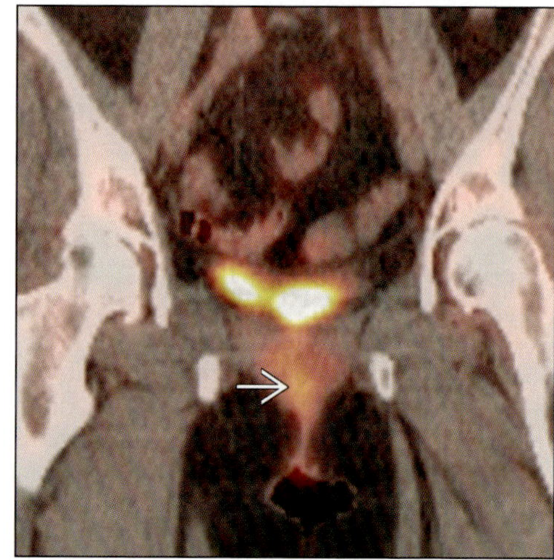

(Left) Axial PET/CT demonstrates minimal increased activity in the urethra ➡. Although this finding can be seen in normal mucosa, this patient had a < 1 cm anterior urethral mass, which was easily removed by local excision. *(Right)* Coronal PET/CT demonstrates minimally increased activity in the urethra ➡, corresponding to known site of disease. No discrete lesion was identified on imaging, nor were additional sites of disease identified.

Stage I (T1 N0 M0)

Stage II (T2 N0 M0)

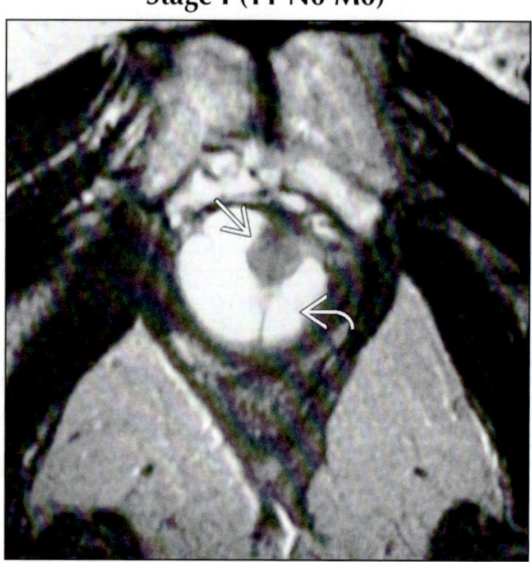

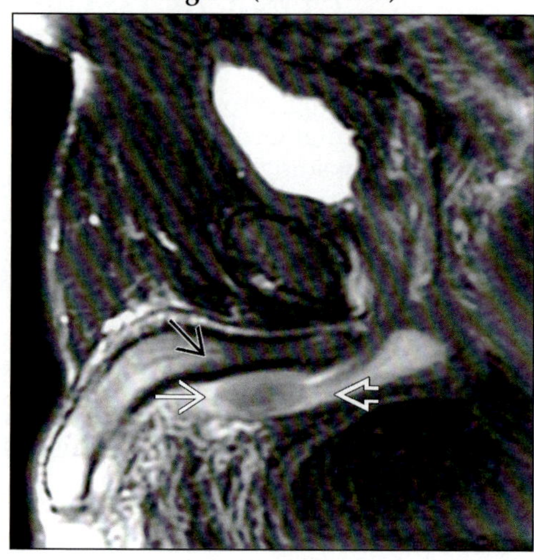

(Left) Axial T2WI MR demonstrates a soft tissue nodule ➡ within a urethral diverticulum ➡. The depth of invasion is difficult to assess. On resection the lesion depth was limited to the subepithelial connective tissue layer. *(Right)* Sagittal T2WI FS MR in a male patient demonstrates a low T2 SI expansile ureteral mass ➡ in the bulbous portion of the urethra. It involves the corpus spongiosum ➡, but the corpus cavernosum ➡ is spared. (Courtesy M. Lockhart, MD, MPH.)

Stage II (T2 N0 M0)

Stage II (T2 N0 M0)

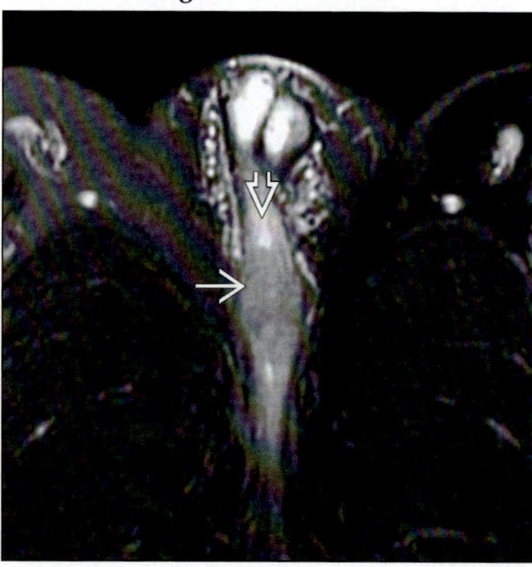

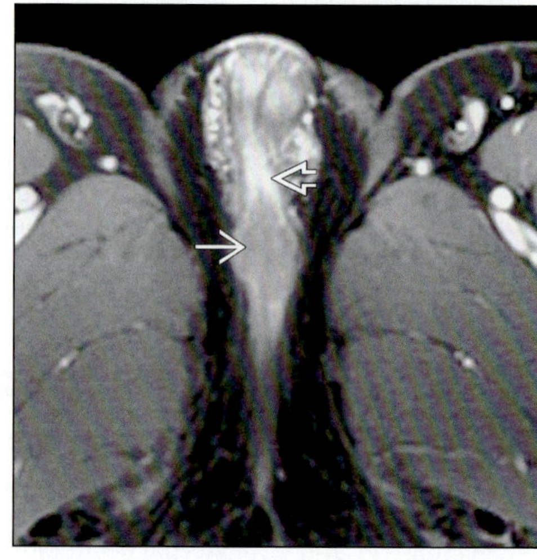

(Left) Axial T2WI FS MR in the same patient demonstrates a hypointense mass ➡ centered in the bulbous urethra with expansion into the surrounding corpus spongiosum ➡. (Courtesy M. Lockhart, MD, MPH.) *(Right)* Axial T1WI C+ FS MR demonstrates relatively poor enhancement of the tumor ➡ compared to the adjacent highly vascularized corpus spongiosum ➡. (Courtesy M. Lockhart, MD, MPH.)

Stage II (T2 N0 M0)

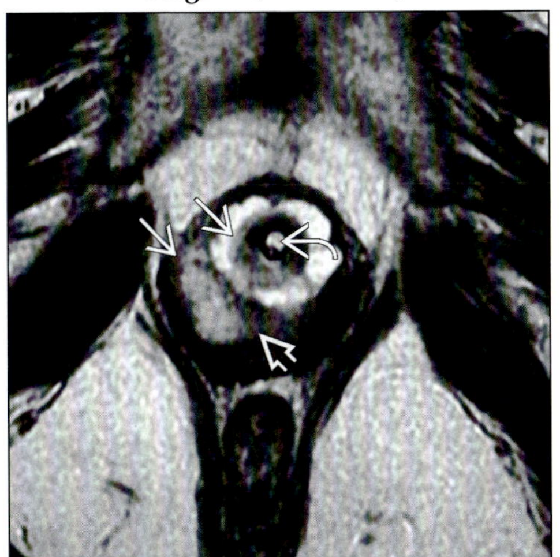

Stage II (T2 N0 M0)

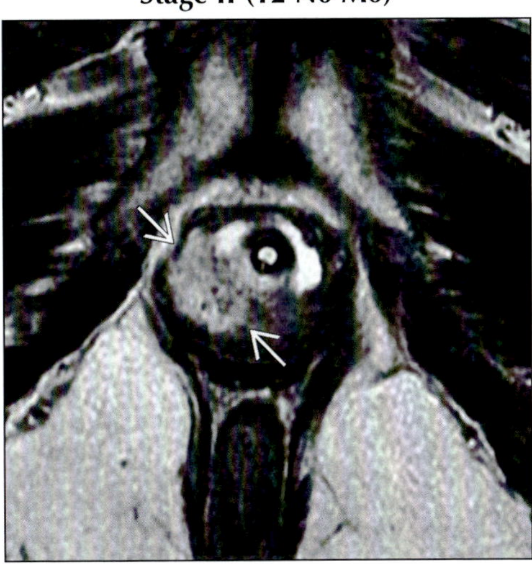

(Left) Axial T2WI MR demonstrates a relatively low T2 SI mass ➡ arising in a female urethral diverticulum, extending from the urethra into the periurethral tissues ➡. A Foley catheter is in place ➡. (Right) More caudal image in the same patient better demonstrates the extent of the relatively low T2 SI mass ➡ in the diverticulum.

Stage II (T2 N0 M0)

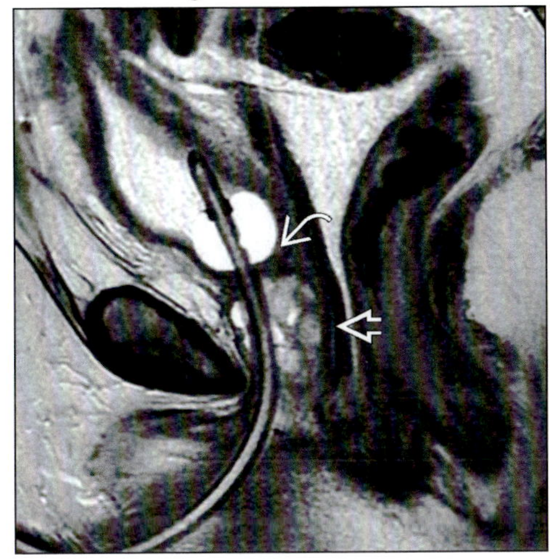

Stage II (T2 N0 M0)

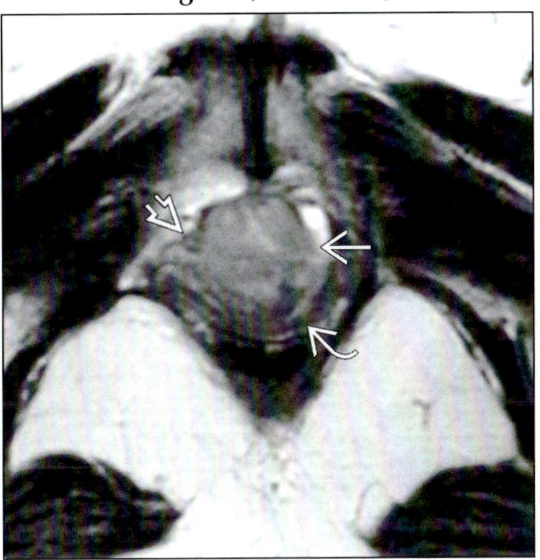

(Left) Sagittal image in the same patient demonstrates the mass's confinement to the urethral tissues with sparing of the bladder base ➡ and anterior vagina ➡. (Right) Axial T2WI MR in a different woman with urethral carcinoma shows a heterogeneously hypointense urethral mass ➡ with periurethral extension on the right ➡. The normally low T2 SI urethral wall ➡ appears to be intact adjacent to the vagina.

Stage III (T3 N0 M0)

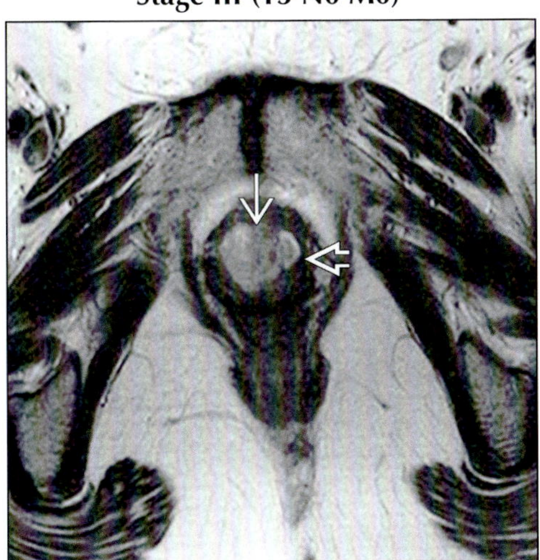

Stage III (T3 N0 M0)

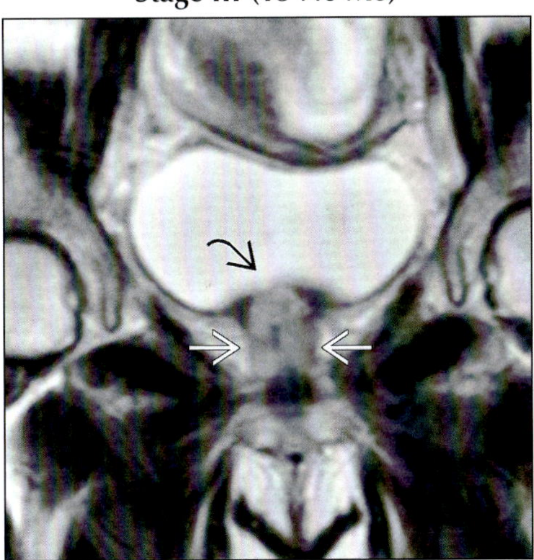

(Left) On axial T2WI MR an intermediate signal intensity urethral mass ➡ expands the urethra. The low T2 SI urethral muscular wall ➡ remains intact. (Right) Coronal image shows that the entire urethra is expanded by the mass ➡. Superior extension of the mass into the bladder neck ➡ upstages this to T3 disease.

URETHRAL CARCINOMA

Stage III (T3 N0 M0)

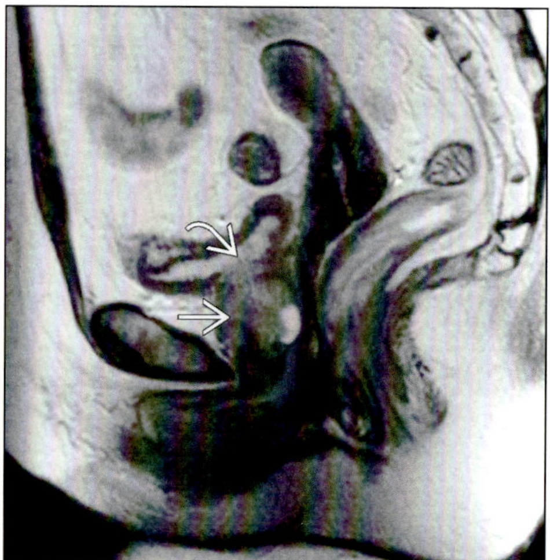

Stage III (T3 N0 M0)

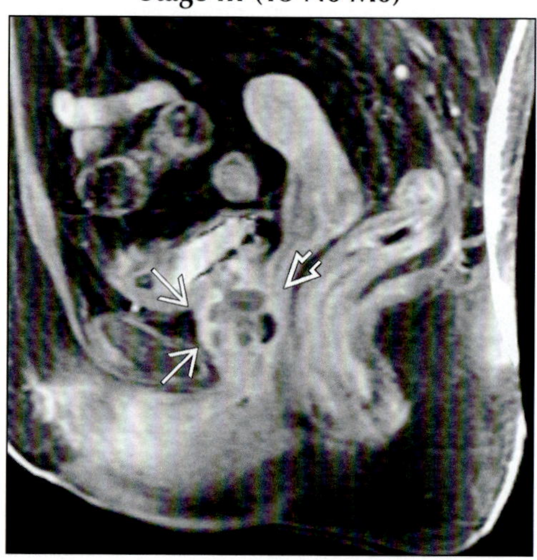

(Left) Sagittal T2WI MR in the same patient shows an intermediate signal intensity urethral mass ➡ that expands the urethra. The superior extension into the bladder neck is well depicted ➡. *(Right)* Post-contrast sagittal T1WI FS MR demonstrates a heterogeneously enhancing urethral mass ➡, with increased concern for involvement of the anterior vagina ➡.

Stage III (T2 N1 M0)

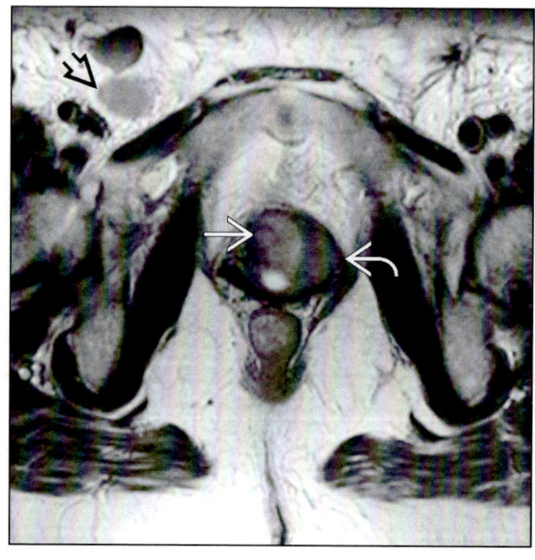

Stage III (T2 N1 M0)

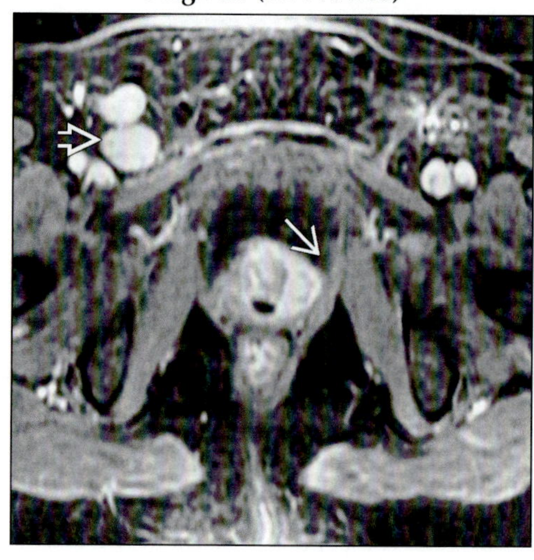

(Left) Axial T2WI MR demonstrates an intermediate signal intensity urethral mass ➡ expanding the female urethra. Periurethral muscle is thinned on left ➡. Deep periurethral muscle invasion is not seen. An enlarged right inguinal node is present ➡. *(Right)* Axial T1WI C+ FS MR shows the heterogeneously enhancing tumor contacting but not involving the left periurethral muscle ➡. Metastatic right inguinal adenopathy ➡ upstages the disease from stage II to stage III.

Stage IV (T2 N0 M1)

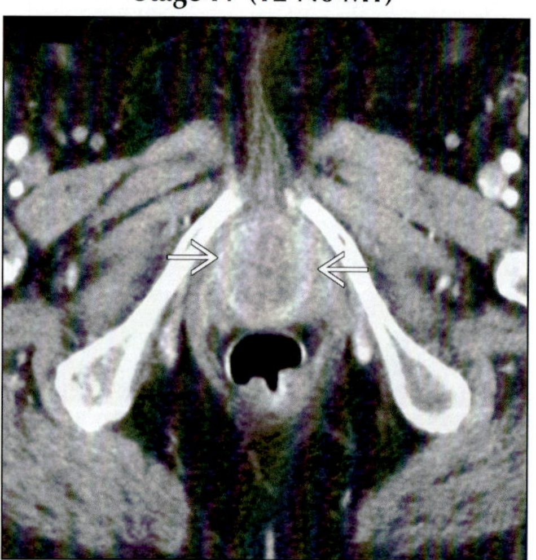

Stage IV (T2 N0 M1)

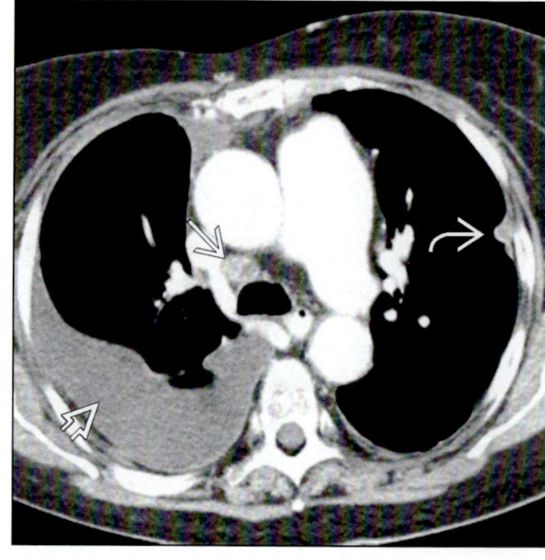

(Left) Axial CECT shows a heterogeneously enhancing urethral mass ➡; however, the integrity of periurethral tissue planes cannot be determined. Indeed, CT is of limited utility in assessing urethral T stage. *(Right)* Thoracic CECT in the same patient demonstrates an enlarged enhancing precarinal node ➡, a left pleural nodule ➡, and a right pleural effusion ➡. The extensive thoracic metastatic disease is best demonstrated on CT.

URETHRAL CARCINOMA

Stage IV (T4 N0 M0)

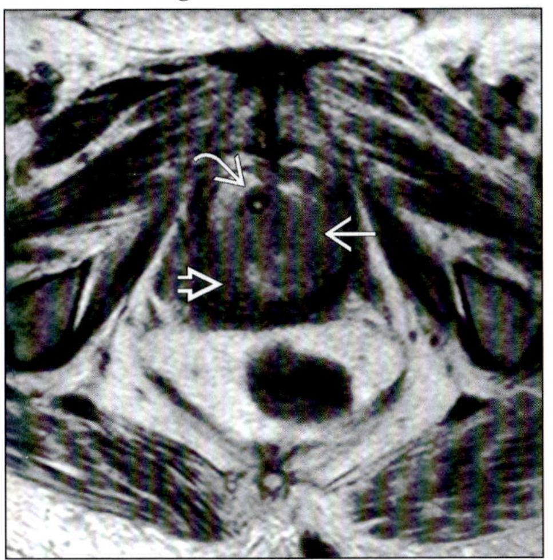

Stage IV (T4 N0 M0)

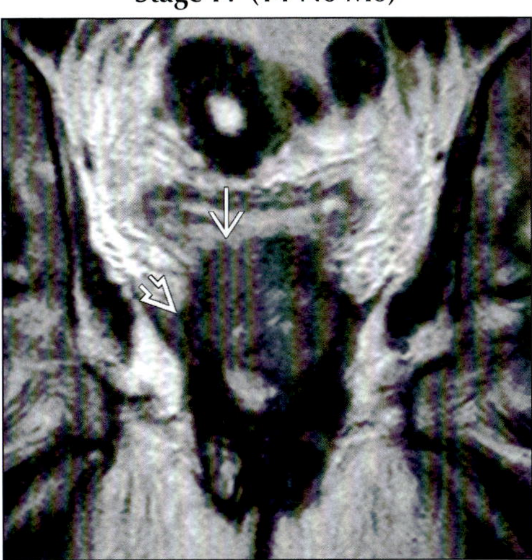

(Left) Axial T2WI MR demonstrates a heterogeneously hypointense mass ➡ expanding a female urethra with loss of a distinct high T2 SI plane in the vesicovaginal space ➡. A Foley catheter is in place ➡. (Right) Coronal T2WI MR in the same patient demonstrates infiltration beyond the periurethral tissue into the adjacent levator ani muscle complex on the right ➡. Additionally, the mass is seen invading the bladder base ➡.

Stage IV (T4 N0 M0)

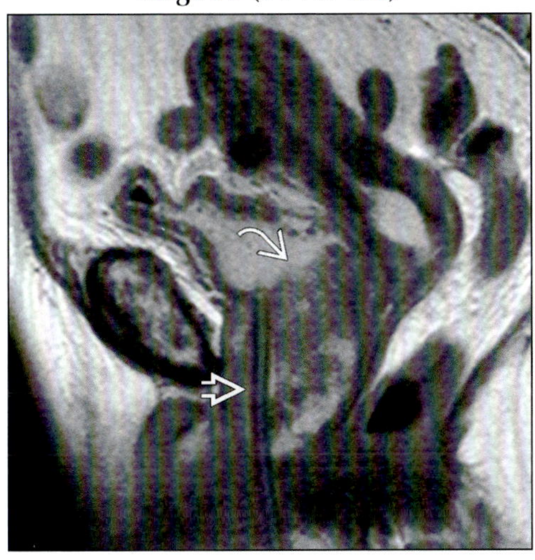

Stage IV (T4 N0 M0)

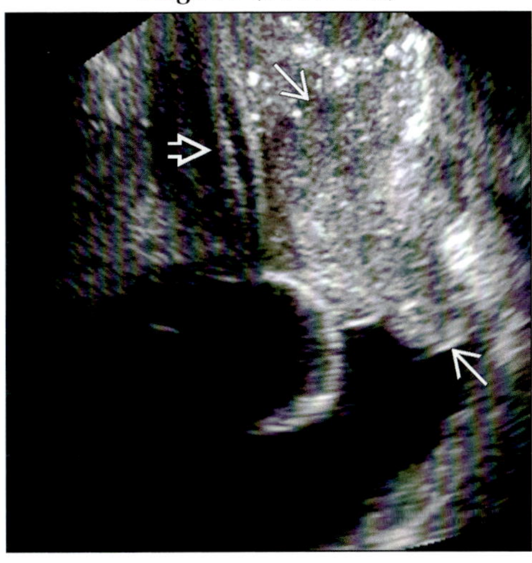

(Left) Sagittal T2WI MR in the same patient better demonstrates the heterogeneous low T2 SI mass involving the entire urethra and extending cranially to invade the bladder base ➡. A Foley catheter ➡ is present. (Right) Transperineal ultrasound in the same patient demonstrates the polypoid urethral mass ➡ extending into the bladder. A Foley catheter is well demonstrated within the urethra ➡ with the catheter balloon expanded in the bladder.

Postoperative Appearance

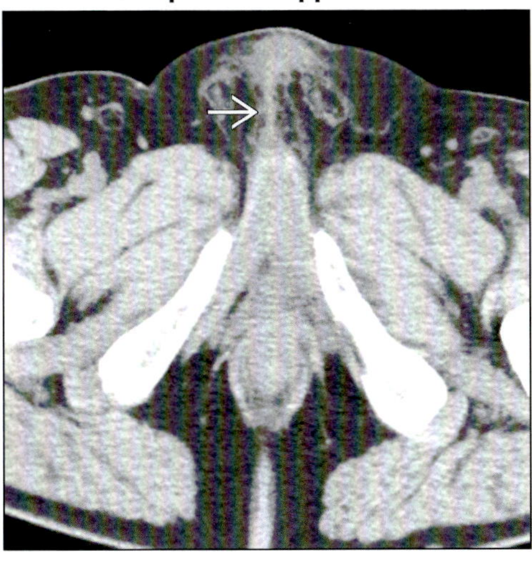

Postoperative Recurrence

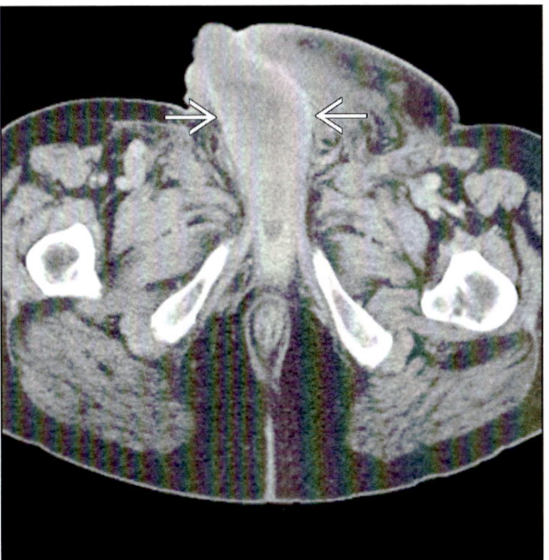

(Left) Axial CECT shows the postoperative appearance of a partial penectomy ➡ for anterior stage II disease. At this time, no local recurrence is present. Long-term survival has been reported in subjects who undergo this therapy. (Right) Axial NECT in a different patient demonstrates a local recurrence ➡ after partial penectomy. Recurrence developed along the bulbomembranous urethra.

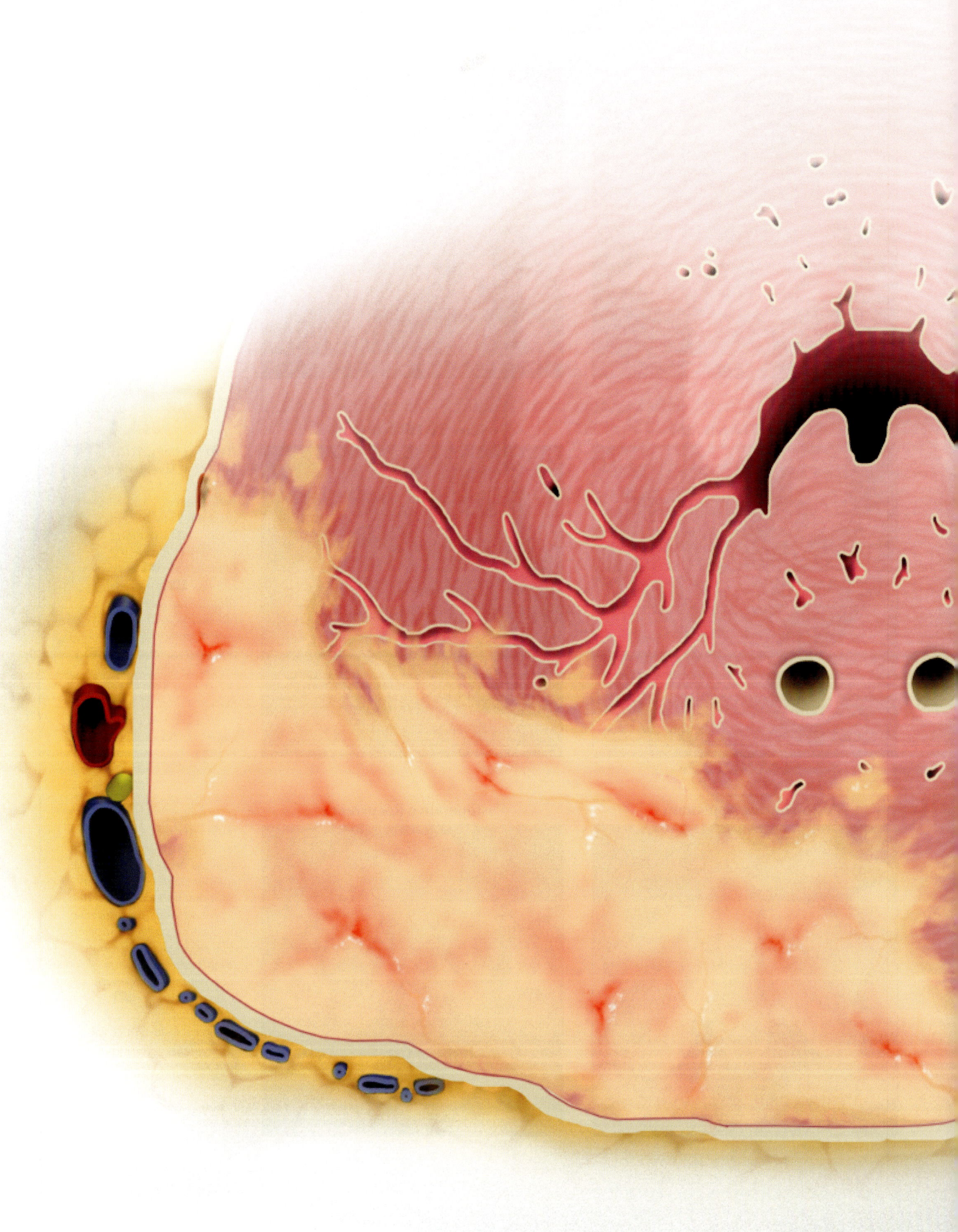

Prostate Carcinoma

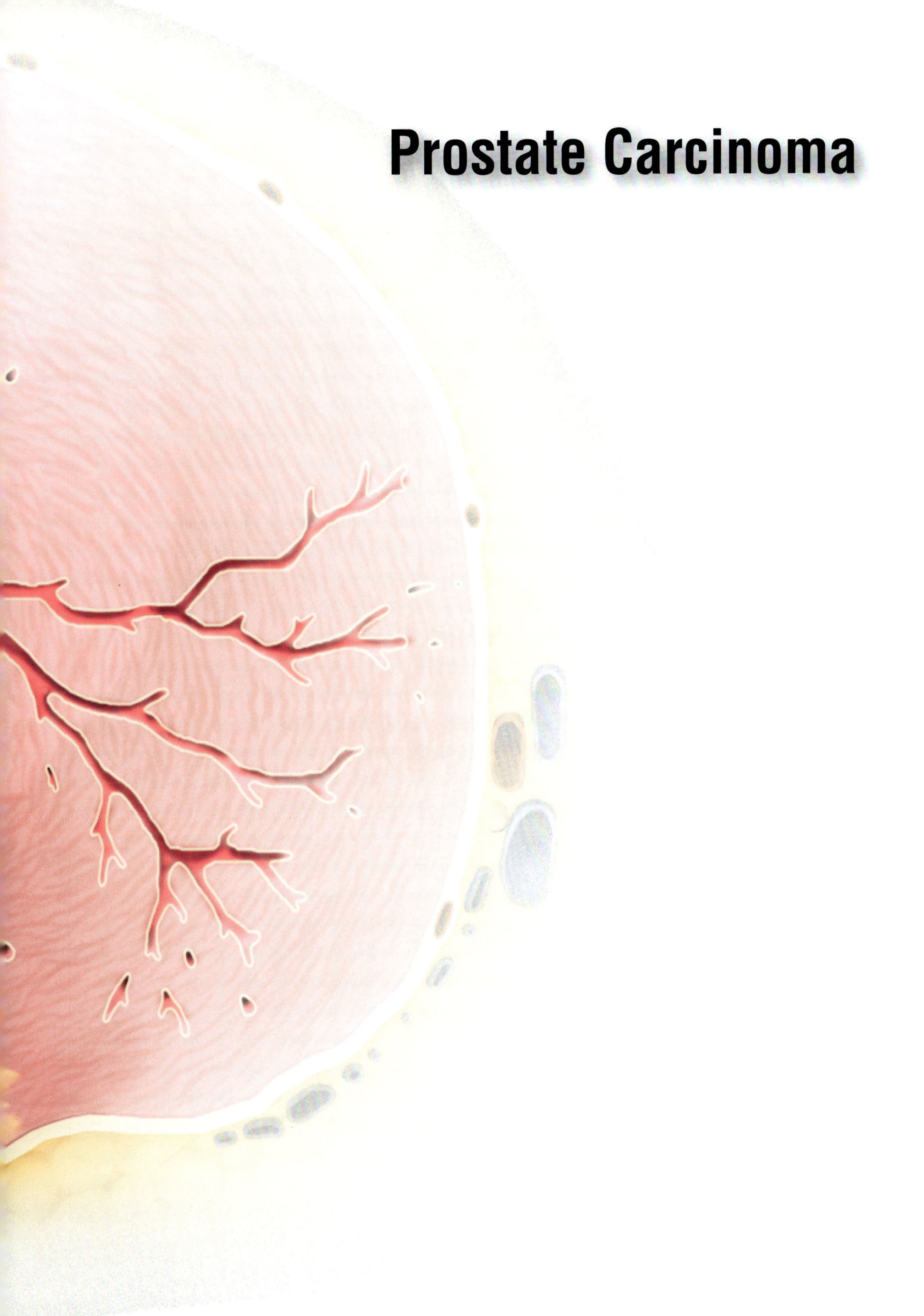

PROSTATE CARCINOMA

(T) Primary Tumor

Adapted from 7th edition AJCC Staging Forms.

TNM	Definitions
Clinical	
TX	Primary tumor cannot be assessed
T0	No evidence of primary tumor
T1	Clinically inapparent tumor neither palpable nor visible by imaging
T1a	Tumor incidental histologic finding in ≤ 5% of tissue resected
T1b	Tumor incidental histologic finding in > 5% of tissue resected
T1c	Tumor identified by needle biopsy (e.g., because of elevated PSA)
T2	Tumor confined within prostate[1]
T2a	Tumor involves ≤ 1/2 of 1 lobe
T2b	Tumor involves > 1/2 of 1 lobe but not both lobes
T2c	Tumor involves both lobes
T3	Tumor extends through the prostate capsule[2]
T3a	Extracapsular extension (unilateral or bilateral)
T3b	Tumor invades seminal vesicle(s)
T4	Tumor is fixed or invades adjacent structures other than seminal vesicles, such as external sphincter, rectum, bladder, levator muscles, &/or pelvic wall
Pathologic[3]	
pT2	Organ confined
pT2a	Unilateral, ≤ 1/2 of 1 side
pT2b	Unilateral, involving > 1/2 of 1 side but not both sides
pT2c	Bilateral disease
pT3	Extraprostatic extension
pT3a	Extraprostatic extension or microscopic invasion of bladder neck[4]
pT3b	Seminal vesicle invasion
pT4	Invasion of rectum, levator muscles, &/or pelvic wall

(N) Regional Lymph Nodes

Clinical	
NX	Regional lymph nodes were not assessed
N0	No regional lymph node metastasis
N1	Metastasis in regional lymph node(s)
Pathologic	
pNX	Regional nodes not sampled
pN0	No positive regional nodes
pN1	Metastases in regional node(s)

[1]*Tumor found in 1 or both lobes by needle biopsy, but not palpable or reliably visible by imaging, is classified as T1c.* [2]*Invasion into the prostatic apex or into (but not beyond) the prostatic capsule is classified not as T3 but as T2.* [3]*There is no pathologic T1 classification.* [4]*Positive surgical margin should be indicated by an R1 descriptor (residual microscopic disease).*

PROSTATE CARCINOMA

(M) Distant Metastasis

Adapted from 7th edition AJCC Staging Forms.

TNM	Definitions
M0	No distant metastasis
M1	Distant metastasis
M1a	Nonregional lymph node(s)
M1b	Bone(s)
M1c	Other site(s) with or without bone disease

When > 1 site of metastasis is present, the most advanced category is used (pM1c is most advanced).

(G) Histologic Grade

Adapted from 7th edition AJCC Staging Forms.

TNM	Definitions
GX	Gleason score cannot be processed
Gleason $\leq$ 6	Well differentiated (slight anaplasia)
Gleason 7	Moderately differentiated (moderate anaplasia)
Gleason 8-10	Poorly differentiated/undifferentiated (marked anaplasia)

AJCC Stages/Prognostic Groups

Adapted from 7th edition AJCC Staging Forms.

Stage	T	N	M	PSA	Gleason
I	T1a-c	N0	M0	PSA < 10	Gleason $\leq$ 6
	T2a	N0	M0	PSA < 10	Gleason $\leq$ 6
	T1-2a	N0	M0	PSA X	Gleason X
IIA	T1a-c	N0	M0	PSA < 20	Gleason 7
	T1a-c	N0	M0	10 $\leq$ PSA < 20	Gleason $\leq$ 6
	T2a	N0	M0	PSA < 20	Gleason $\leq$ 7
	T2b	N0	M0	PSA < 20	Gleason $\leq$ 7
	T2b	N0	M0	PSA X	Gleason X
IIB	T2c	N0	M0	Any PSA	Any Gleason
	T1-2	N0	M0	PSA $\geq$ 20	Any Gleason
	T1-2	N0	M0	Any PSA	Gleason $\geq$ 8
III	T3a-b	N0	M0	Any PSA	Any Gleason
IV	T4	N0	M0	Any PSA	Any Gleason
	Any T	N1	M0	Any PSA	Any Gleason
	Any T	Any N	M1	Any PSA	Any Gleason

When either PSA or Gleason is not available, grouping should be determined by T stage &/or either PSA or Gleason as available.

PROSTATE CARCINOMA

T1 (Gleason Score 3 + 3 = 6)

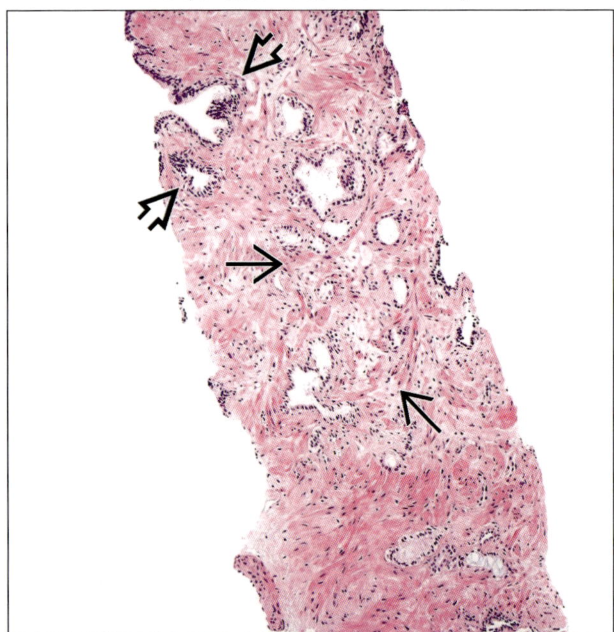

Low-power H&E stain from a core needle prostate biopsy sample shows a small focus of cancer ➡. Normal prostatic glands are also present ➡. The tumor represented < 5% of both the core biopsy and the final prostatectomy specimen. (Original magnification 100x.)

T1 (Gleason Score 3 + 3 = 6)

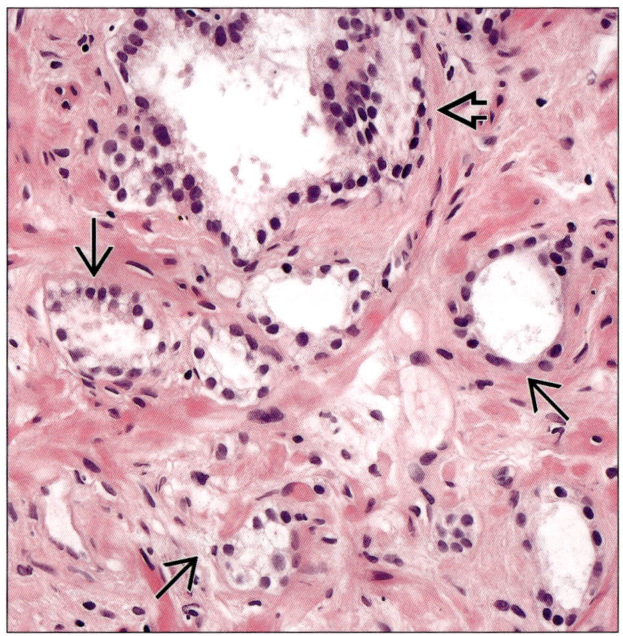

Higher magnification of the same sample shows the numerous invasive neoplastic glands ➡ lacking basal epithelial cells. Normal prostatic glandular tissue ➡ has normal benign luminal epithelial cells as well as basal epithelial layer. (Original magnification 400x.)

T1 (Gleason Score 3 + 3 = 6)

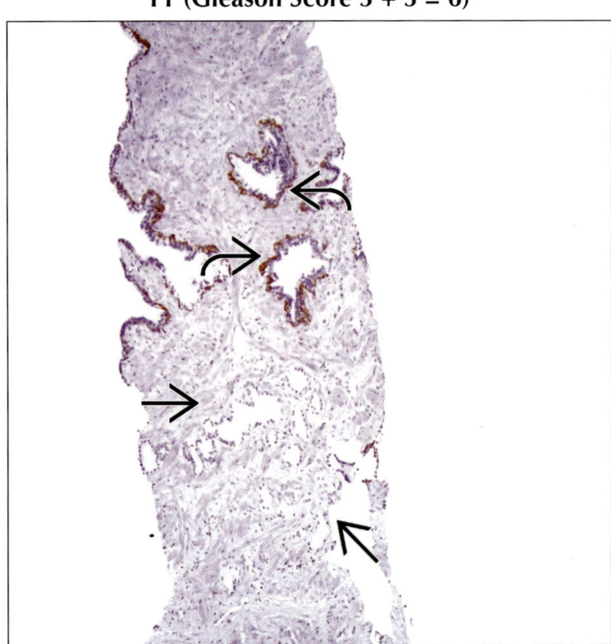

High molecular weight cytokeratin immunostain in the same case demonstrates absence of basal cell layer in the atypical glands ➡, supporting the diagnosis of adenocarcinoma. The benign glands ➡ show positive staining, which indicates intact basal cell layer. (Original magnification 100x.)

T1 (Gleason Score 3 + 3 = 6)

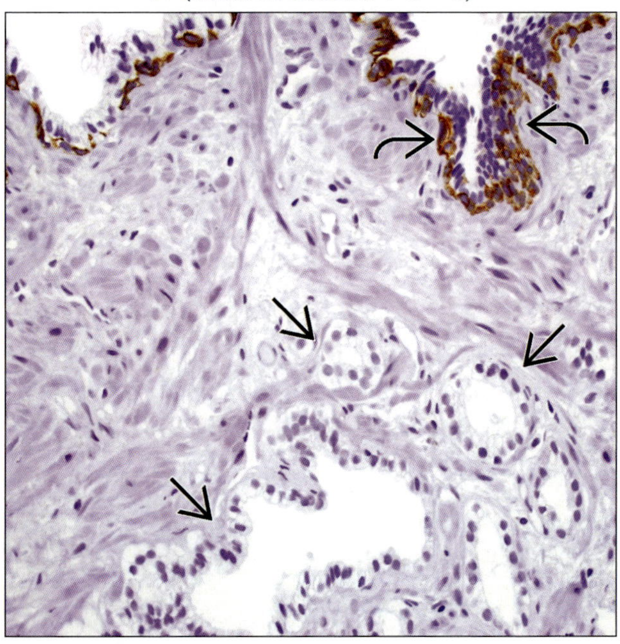

Higher magnification shows malignant glands ➡ and total absence of staining with keratin antibody. The basal cell layer is intact (brown staining) in benign glands ➡. (Original magnification 600x.)

T2b (Gleason Score 3 + 4 = 7)

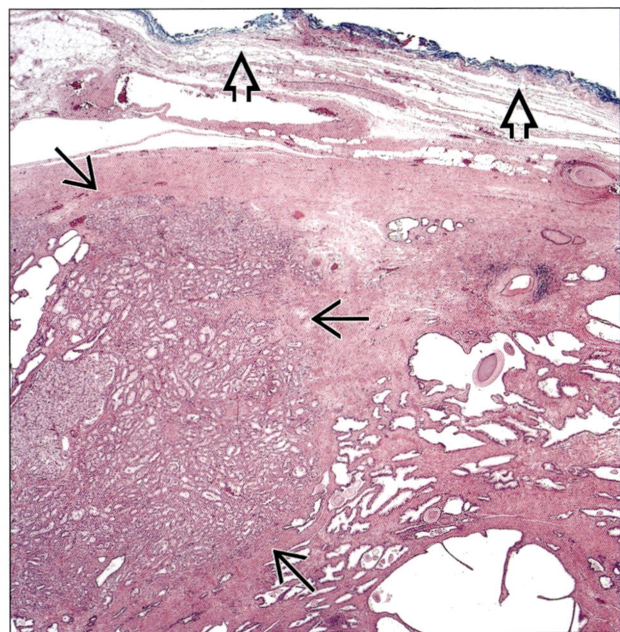

Low-power H&E stained section from a prostatectomy specimen shows sheets of invasive prostatic adenocarcinoma ➔ on the left. The adenocarcinoma is confined to the prostate tissue and is away from the prostatic capsule or the blue inked resection margin ▷. (Original magnification 40x.)

T2b (Gleason Score 3 + 4 = 7)

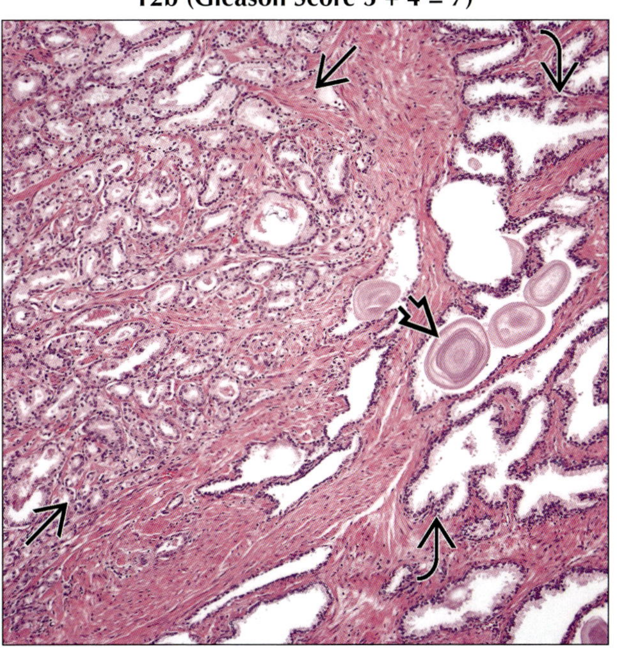

High-power view of the previous slide shows sheets of neoplastic glands in the left upper corner ➔ and benign prostatic glands ➔ with numerous pink round structures ▷, called corpora amylacea, representing laminated concretions of prostatic secretions within the glandular lumina. (Original magnification 400x.)

T3a (Gleason Score 4 + 3 = 7)

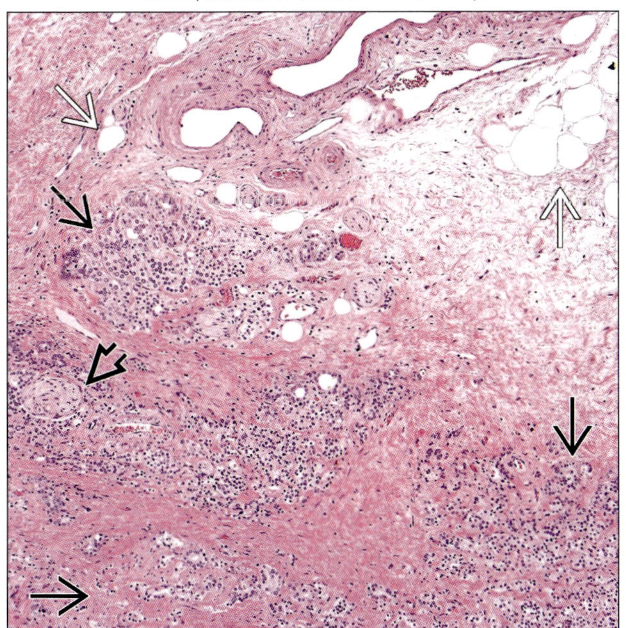

Low-power H&E stain from prostatectomy specimen shows the tumor ➔ extending into the periprostatic tissue in proximity to the periprostatic fat ➔. Note also the perineural invasion (tumor surrounding nerve tissue) ▷. (Original magnification 40x.)

T3b (Gleason Score 3 + 4 = 7)

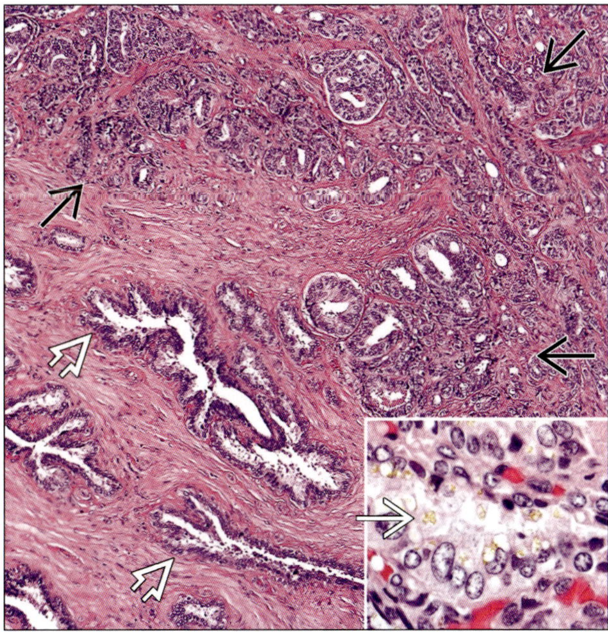

H&E stain of a tumor invading seminal vesicles shows the tumor ➔ and seminal vesicle tissue ▷. (Original magnification 400x.) The inset highlights the golden yellow pigment ➔ (lipofuscin) that is characteristically found abundantly in seminal vesicle tissue.

PROSTATE CARCINOMA

T2a

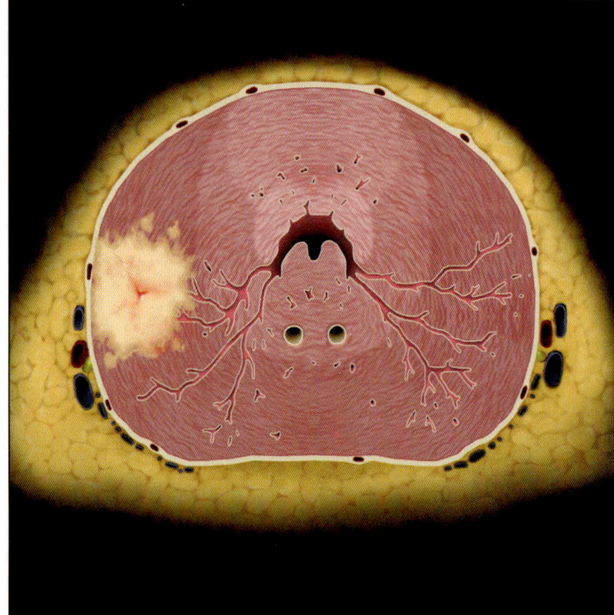

Axial graphic demonstrates a localized focus of peripheral zone tumor that involves less than 1/2 of 1 lobe of the prostate. This is consistent with T2a disease. T1 disease is neither clinically apparent nor visible on imaging.

T2b

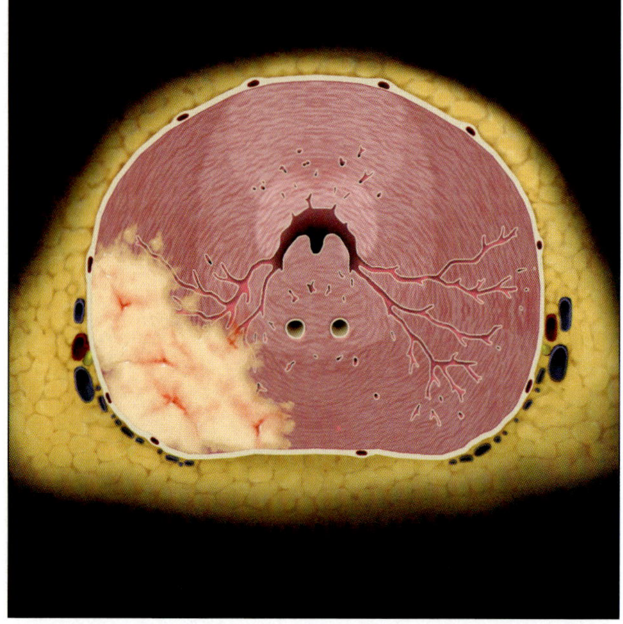

Axial graphic demonstrates a larger focus of peripheral zone tumor that involves more than 1/2 of 1 lobe of the prostate but does not cross the midline. The prostatic capsule is intact, and the neurovascular bundle is unaffected by tumor. This is consistent with T2b disease.

T2c

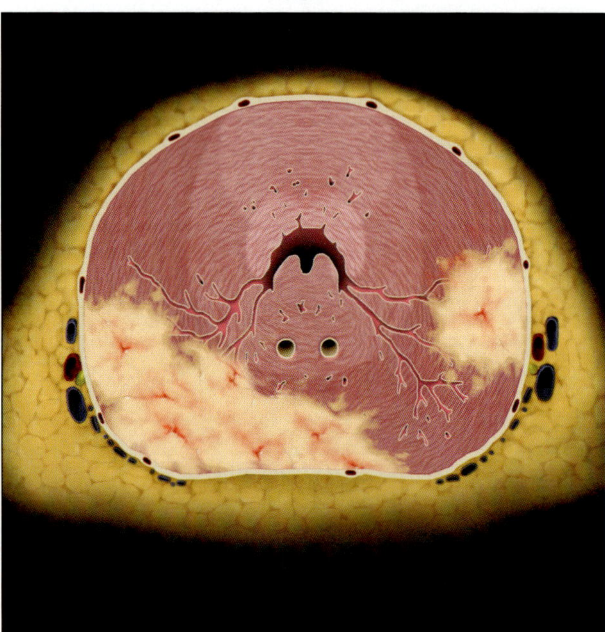

Axial graphic demonstrates a larger focus of peripheral zone tumor that involves more than 1/2 of 1 lobe of the prostate and crosses the midline. An additional focus of tumor is present on the contralateral side of the gland. Both of these findings fulfill the criteria for T2c disease.

T3a

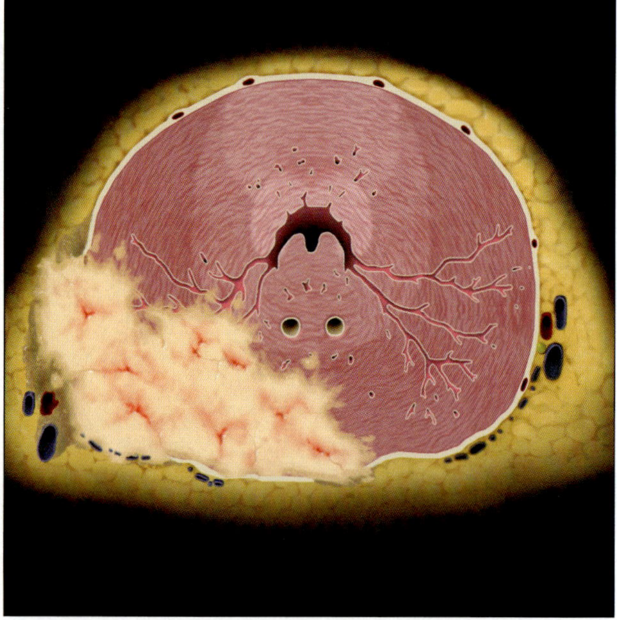

Axial graphic demonstrates a larger focus of peripheral zone tumor with focal bulging of the prostatic contour posteriorly. Additionally, in the posterolateral margin, the capsule is invaded and tumor spills into the surrounding periprostatic fat and surrounds the neurovascular bundle. This is consistent with T3a disease.

PROSTATE CARCINOMA

N1

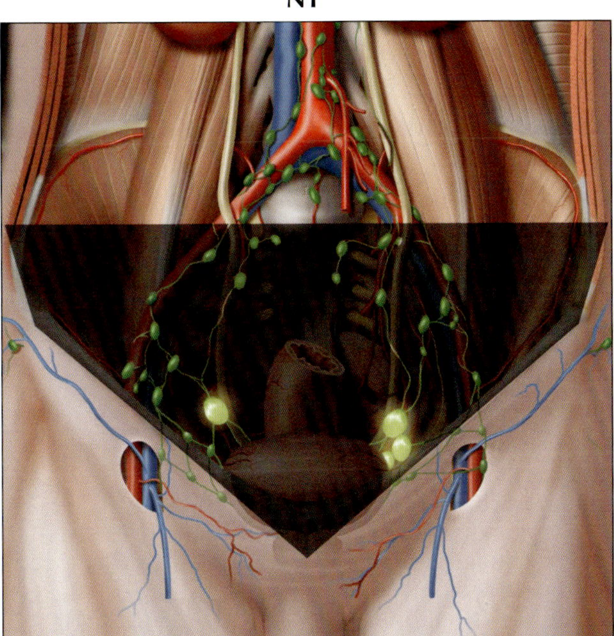

Coronal graphic shows regional lymph nodes shaded in black. Enlarged bilateral internal iliac nodes are present, indicating N1 disease. N1 disease is considered stage IV, regardless of the T stage.

M1a

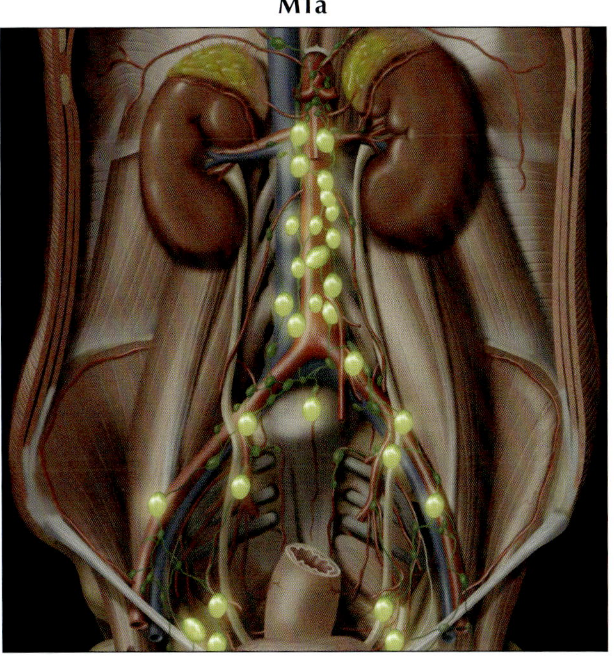

Coronal graphic shows enlarged regional lymph nodes in the pelvis and enlarged nonregional nodes in the common iliac and paraaortic lymph node stations. The presence of nonregional lymph node metastases upgrades disease to M1a.

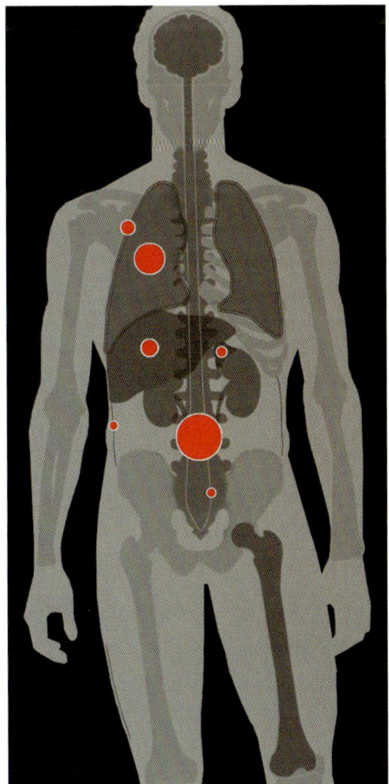

METASTASES, ORGAN FREQUENCY

Bone	90%
Lung	46%
Liver	25%
Pleura	21%
Adrenal gland	13%
Peritoneum	7%
Meninges	6%

Data from Bubendorf L et al: Metastatic patterns of prostate cancer: an autopsy study of 1,589 patients. Hum Pathol. 31(5):578-83, 2000.

PROSTATE CARCINOMA

OVERVIEW

General Comments
- Most common noncutaneous cancer in American men
- 1 in 6 men will develop prostate cancer in their lifetime
  - 80% of prostate cancer cases are detected while cancer is localized to prostate gland
  - Screening detects early stage disease well
    - Prostate-specific antigen (PSA) and digital rectal exam (DRE) common screening tests
    - Stage migration has occurred because of widespread PSA screening
      - Overall prevalence of patients with low-risk disease almost 2x greater now than in late 1980s
- Appropriate imaging utilization depends on clinical factors at presentation
  - PSA
  - Clinical stage based on DRE
  - Gleason score and disease volume on biopsy

Classification
- Adults: 95% of tumors are adenocarcinoma
- Children: Vast majority due to rhabdomyosarcoma

PATHOLOGY

Routes of Spread
- 2 different hematogenous routes of spread
  - Backwards venous spread most common source for osteoblastic metastases
    - Prostatic and vesicle venous plexus directly to vertebral (Batson) venous plexus
      - Lumbar spine mets 3x more common than cervical spine mets
      - This pathway may represent early pattern of hematogenous spread
  - Caval route may be later route of dissemination
    - Prostatic venous plexus to iliac veins
    - Inferior vena cava to lungs
    - Lung metastases followed by dissemination to pleura, liver, adrenal glands, etc.
      - Rarely hematogenous disease will bypass lungs
- Lymphatic route for nodal disease
  - Regional lymph nodes (N1 disease) include nodes of true pelvis; those nodes below bifurcation of common iliac arteries
    - Pelvic nodes NOS
      - 2nd most common site of nodal mets at autopsy
    - Iliac nodes (internal, external, or NOS)
    - Obturator nodes
    - Sacral nodes
    - Hypogastric nodes
  - Distant lymph nodes (M1a disease) are those outside true pelvis
    - Paraaortic nodal disease #1 most common site of nodal mets overall at autopsy
      - May result of direct nodal seeding from vertebral venous plexus in addition to lymphatic spread
      - Found more frequently when spinal mets are present than when spinal mets are absent
    - Common iliac nodes
    - Mediastinal
      - 3rd most common site of nodal mets
    - Inguinal, deep and superficial nodes
      - 4th most common site of nodal mets

General Features
- Comments
  - Optimal treatment decisions depend on risk assessment
    - Factors that have role in risk assessment include
      - How likely is cancer to be organ confined?
      - How likely is cancer to progress after treatment?
    - Prognosis can be estimated by incorporating clinical and laboratory factors
      - Clinical T stage based on DRE
      - Gleason score in biopsy specimen
      - Serum PSA
- Genetics
  - Hereditary prostate cancer accounts for approximately 10% of all prostate cancer cases
    - Unique genetics in early-onset disease (age < 55 years old)
      - Rare autosomal dominant prostate cancer susceptibility genes may account for almost 1/2 of early onset disease
    - Possible genetic hypotheses include X-linked or recessive inheritance
    - Hereditary prostate cancer 1 gene (*HPC1*) found on chromosome 1q23-25
  - Several candidate genes identified in pathway to development of prostate cancer
    - Occur in almost all aspects of cell regulation, including
      - Cell cycle control genes
      - Cell adhesion genes
      - Androgen receptor genes
      - Angiogenesis-related genes
      - Vitamin D pathway genes
- Etiology
  - Race
    - USA: African-American males have 60% higher incidence rate compared with white males
    - More common in Western world & rare in Asians (age-adjusted incidence rate 2-10/100,000 men)
    - Difficult to tease out specific risk related to race because of socioeconomic confounders
      - Access to health care
      - Income
      - Education
      - Insurance status
  - Family history
    - Relative risk (RR) if affected brothers = 3.4 (95% CI: 3.0-3.8)
    - RR if affected fathers = 2.2 (95% CI: 1.9-2.5)
    - Affected male with family history of prostate cancer may present at younger age (6-7 years) than male without such history
  - Age
    - Age < 44 years: Incidence approaches 0
    - Age 45-54 years: Incidence (8.6%)
    - Age 55-64 years: Incidence (28.0%)
    - Age 65-74 years: Incidence (36.1%)

PROSTATE CARCINOMA

- Age 75-84 years: Incidence (22.0%)
  - Diet
    - High-fat diet may increase risk
    - Soy-rich diet may be protective
  - Hormonal influence
    - Testosterone
    - 5-α-reductase
- Epidemiology & cancer incidence
  - Most common new cancer diagnosis in men in 2009
    - 25% of new cancer diagnoses in 2009
    - Estimated 192,280 new cases in 2009
    - Age-adjusted incidence rate: 159.3/100,000
    - Median age at diagnosis: 68 years
  - 2nd most common cause of death in men in 2009 (after lung cancer)
    - 9% of cancer deaths in 2009
    - Estimated 27,360 deaths in 2009
    - Age-adjusted death rate: 25.6/100,000
      - Rate has been declining annually since 1994
    - Median age at death: 80 years
  - Lifetime risk of developing prostate cancer approaches 16%

Gross Pathology & Surgical Features

- Usually more common in peripheral zone (PZ)
  - PZ accounts for ~ 80-85% of disease
    - More common in posterior portion of PZ
  - Transition zone (TZ) accounts for ~ 10-15% of disease
    - Site of origin of BPH
  - Central zone (CZ) accounts for ~ 5-10% of disease
    - CZ makes up most of base of prostate
- Localized, diffuse, or extracapsular extension (ECE)
  - Firm or "gritty" as result of fibrosis
- Extent of tumor contacting prostatic capsule
  - Stratifies surgical approaches between wide excision and attempted nerve-sparing procedures
  - Surgeon must balance oncologic control (disease free margins) and functional outcomes (incontinence & erectile dysfunction)

Microscopic Pathology

- H&E
  - Gleason score
    - Assignment of histologic grade to predominant (primary) and lesser (secondary) pattern of tumor
    - 2 Gleason grade numbers are summed for a Gleason score
  - Gleason score 1
    - Well-differentiated glandular pattern
    - Uniform epithelium, oval nuclei
    - Pale cytoplasm & rare mitotic figures
  - Gleason score 2
    - Well-differentiated glandular pattern
    - More intervening stroma between glands
  - Gleason score 3
    - Moderately differentiated glandular pattern
    - Distinctly infiltrative margins
  - Gleason score 4
    - Poorly differentiated glandular pattern
    - Irregular masses of neoplastic glands
  - Gleason score 5
    - Poorly differentiated/anaplastic glandular pattern
    - Only occasional gland formation
    - Sheets of tumor cells, mitoses, cellular atypia

- Histopathologic grading can be complex
  - Morphologic heterogeneity
  - Multifocality
- Special stains
  - Not required routinely
    - May be helpful in specific indications, including
      - Distinguishing prostate cancer from benign mimics and post-treatment changes
      - Distinguishing prostate cancer from nonprostatic malignancies that secondarily involve prostate
  - Broad categories of special stains include
    - Basal cell-associated markers
    - Prostate carcinoma-associated marker
    - Antibody stains
    - Epithelial lineage
    - Prostate lineage-specific markers

IMAGING FINDINGS

Detection

- **Transrectal ultrasound (TRUS) with biopsy** indicated after abnormal screening test (PSA or DRE)
  - Lesion may be identified in PZ, abutting adjacent normal tissue
    - Most commonly hypoechoic (60-70%)
    - Rarely hyperechoic (1-5%)
    - Isoechoic to normal PZ tissue is not uncommon (30-40%)
      - Most peripheral isoechoic lesions close to capsule
      - Look for asymmetrical contour + bulging along lateral aspect of prostate
    - Size of lesion important predictor for detection
      - < 5 mm tumor has 36% rate of detection
      - 16-20 mm tumor has 84% rate of detection
      - > 26 mm tumor has 92% rate of detection
    - May not be better than DRE for predicting extracapsular tumor extension or seminal vesicle involvement

Staging

- **Radionuclide bone scan** (Tc-99m whole body bone scan)
  - Most widely used for detecting bone metastases
  - Indication for use dependent on clinical scenario with specific calculated risk of metastatic disease
    - Highly indicated in intermediate- to high-risk patients (ACR appropriateness score = 9)
      - T1-2 & GS > 7 & PSA ≥ 20 or ≥ 50% positive core biopsy
      - Clinical T3, seminal vesicle, or bladder neck invasion
    - Indicated in intermediate-risk (ACR appropriateness score = 8)
      - T1-2 & GS ≤ 6 & PSA > 20 or ≥ 50% positive core biopsy
      - T1-2 & GS 8-10 & PSA < 20 and < 50% positive core biopsy
    - Consider for lower risk patients, including those with T1-2 & GS = 7 & PSA < 20 (ACR appropriateness score = 7)
      - If PSA in higher part of range or rapid rise in PSA

PROSTATE CARCINOMA

- If high-volume disease (≥ 50% positive core biopsy)
  - Consider for T1-2 and GS ≤ 6 and PSA 10-20 and ≥ 50% positive core biopsy (ACR appropriateness score = 6)
  - Consider for patients with symptomatic bone pain
  - Radiograph may be used to confirm abnormality seen on bone scan
- **CT**
  - Most indicated (ACR appropriateness score max = 7) in patients with high-range PSA or high-volume disease detected by biopsy
    - Very good for detecting pelvic and retroperitoneal disease in initial staging
      - Sensitivity (78%), specificity (97%)
  - Not accurate in detection of intraprostatic features
  - Some utility in detecting extracapsular extension
    - Obliteration of periprostatic fat plane
    - Abnormal enhancement of contiguous neurovascular bundle
    - Urinary bladder, rectal invasion
    - Distal lymphadenopathy
  - Of limited value for initial detection &/or local staging
    - Both false-positive and false-negative nodal diagnoses common
    - Poor sensitivity for detecting extracapsular extension (ECE) and seminal vesicles invasion (SVI)
- **MR**
  - Most indicated (ACR appropriateness score max = 7) for local staging and treatment planning in subjects who are intermediate to high risk for treatment failure
    - T1-2 & GS > 7 & PSA ≥ 20 or ≥ 50% positive core biopsy
    - Clinical T3
    - Helpful to surgeon for counseling patient regarding treatment choices and competing risks
  - Accuracy of MR in detection of ECE ranges between 60-90%
  - T2WI: Mainly used for local ECE and SVI
    - Best diagnostic clue: Nodular area of ↓ signal in normally high signal PZ
    - Signs of ECE
      - Obliteration of rectoprostatic angle
      - Encroachment of low signal area on neurovascular bundle (NVB)
      - Bulging prostatic outline
      - > 10 mm of low signal area contacting capsule margin suggests capsular invasion but may not be indicative of ECE
    - SVI: Low signal intensity extending into seminal vesicles
    - Urinary bladder or rectal invasion well depicted
  - Osteoblastic bone metastases
    - Low SI on both T1WI & T2WI
    - T1WI: Normal ↑ signal in fatty marrow is replaced by low-intermediate SI
  - Functional MR techniques
    - Diffusion-weighted imaging (DWI)

- Adjunct technique to T2WI with local prostate cancer appearing as areas of high signal on high-b-field DWI
- Corresponding apparent diffusion coefficient (ADC) is lower than normal tissue in areas of prostate cancer
- In small series, sensitivity and specificity between 57-93% and 57-100%, respectively
  - MR spectroscopy
    - Elevated choline peaks or elevated choline + creatine/citrate ratios are malignancy indicators
    - May have role in estimating grade of tumor
- **DRE**: Component of clinical staging
  - Cancer palpable on DRE, but organ confined classified as cT2
    - Tumor extending to adjacent structures is cT4
  - Cancer extending beyond capsule is cT3
    - Periprostatic NVB involvement
    - Seminal vesicle involvement
  - DRE alone is insufficient to determine stage because of low specificity for ECE
- **FDG PET/CT**
  - Little role in primary diagnosis or staging of prostate cancer
  - Difficult to differentiate prostate cancer from BPH and prostatitis
  - Major use is for detection and localization of distant mets in hormone-refractory prostate carcinoma
  - PPV of 98% for untreated visceral and nodal mets

Restaging

- Consider repeat imaging when PSA rises after therapy
  - Any detectable PSA level after radical prostatectomy is biochemical evidence of recurrence
    - However, survival is high even with biochemical recurrence
      - 10-year survival is 88% in subjects with rising PSA
      - 10-year survival is 93% in subjects with undetectable PSA
  - PSA kinetics (doubling time)
    - Long doubling time (> 6 months) suggests local recurrence
    - Rapid biochemical failure, high PSA velocity suggests distant metastases
- **TRUS and biopsy**
  - Hypoechoic lesion or fullness of vesico-urethral anastomosis suggests local recurrence
  - TRUS is unlikely to detect recurrence if PSA < 1 ng/ml
  - Limited utility since negative biopsy does not exclude metastatic &/or recurrent disease
- **CT**
  - Limited utility for assessment of local recurrence
    - Positivity rate < 15% in men with evidence of biochemical failure after prostatectomy
  - May have role in detecting extrapelvic nodal disease and bone mets
    - Extrapelvic nodal disease 2nd most common nonosseous metastases
    - Osteoblastic mets most common
- **MR**
  - Local recurrence may manifest as areas of enhancing soft tissue isointense to muscle on T1WI and hyperintense on T2WI

- ○ Some utility in detecting abnormal pelvic nodes in setting of rapidly rising PSA
- ○ Useful for detecting residual SVI
- ○ DCE-MR showing promise for detecting local recurrence in prostate bed
- ○ May also be useful for detecting bony mets when NM bone scan is equivocal
- **Radionuclide bone scan (Tc-99m whole body bone scan)**
  - ○ More likely to be positive if PSA doubling time is < 6 months
  - ○ Most likely to be helpful if symptomatic bone disease develops, very high baseline PSA (> 10 ng/mL) or high PSA velocity
- **FDG-PET**
  - ○ Interpretation of recurrence after radical prostatectomy or radiation therapy is difficult unless large mass lesions are present
- **In-111 capromab pendetide (ProstaScint)**
  - ○ Targets prostate-specific membrane antigen (PSMA) on prostate cancer cells
    - Look for nonphysiologic uptake of capromab, outside prostate bed
  - ○ Indication: Previous definitive treatment and rising PSA, but no obvious source of recurrence on CT &/or pelvic MR
  - ○ Limited utility because of sensitivity of 75% and specificity of 86%
    - Fusion with CT or MR may improve sensitivity

Screening

- American Cancer Society 2010 guidelines
  - ○ Prior to initiating prostate cancer screening, relative risks and benefits of screening and prostate cancer treatment should be discussed with patient
  - ○ For average-risk male with normal life expectancy (> 10-year overall survival) begin screening with PSA at age 50
  - ○ For high-risk male, begin screening with PSA at age 45
    - African-American males
    - Males with 1st-degree relative diagnosed with prostate cancer < age 65
  - ○ For even higher risk males, begin screening with PSA at age 40
    - Males with several 1st- and 2nd-degree relatives with prostate carcinoma
- DRE
  - ○ May be helpful for detection of abnormality
  - ○ Component of clinical staging/risk stratification
- PSA
  - ○ Challenges with false-negatives and false-positives
    - > 25% of biopsy-proven prostate carcinomas occur in patients with "normal" PSA
    - 70-80% of patients with "elevated" PSA do not have prostate carcinoma
      - May be elevated in BPH
  - ○ Upper limit of PSA levels at which to initiate more definitive testing for prostate cancer has not been established
- No imaging modality yet established as effective for screening

CLINICAL ISSUES

Presentation

- Most asymptomatic at presentation
- Usually detected by screening PSA &/or DRE
  - ○ Controversy exists in regard to benefit of disease detection compared to risk of treatment
- If other significant comorbidities, patient may succumb to death from competing diseases before metastatic prostate cancer
- Complicating feature of survival analysis after prostate cancer treatment is evidence of increasing diagnosis of nonlethal tumors
  - ○ PSA testing may detect disease 6-13 years before it would be clinically apparent

Cancer Natural History & Prognosis

- Early stage disease associated with excellent long-term survival
  - ○ 91% present in early stage with only regional nodal spread
    - 5-year survival approaches 100%
  - ○ 4% present with distant metastatic disease
    - 5-year survival reduced to 31.7%
  - ○ 5-year survival by race
    - White men (99.5%)
    - Black men (95.4%)
- Elderly patients, especially those with localized tumors, may die of other illnesses prior to suffering significant cancer-related disability
- Risk tables and nomograms may be helpful to predict individual patient risk of nodal disease &/or failure after therapy
  - ○ Example: Kattan nomogram
    - Predicts probability that patient will be progression-free after standard treatment
    - Predicts probability of 10-year survival after radical prostatectomy
    - Predicts likelihood of success for salvage radiation therapy if PSA rises after prostatectomy
    - Predicts 1- and 20-year survival after tumor becomes hormone refractory
- Mortality risk stratification
  - ○ Low risk ~ 80% 10-year PSA failure-free survival rate
    - 2002 AJCC clinical stage T1c or T2a; and
    - PSA ≤ 10 ng/mL; and
    - Gleason score ≤ 6
  - ○ Intermediate risk ~ 50% 10-year PSA failure-free survival rate
    - 2002 AJCC clinical stage T2b; or
    - PSA > 10 and ≤ 20 ng/mL; or
    - Gleason score = 7
  - ○ High risk ~ 33% 10-year PSA failure-free survival rate
    - 2002 AJCC stage T2c; or
    - PSA > 20 ng/mL; or
    - Gleason score ≥ 8

Treatment Options

- Major treatment alternatives
  - ○ Surgery
    - Radical prostatectomy for disease confined to prostate gland
    - Multiple approaches to surgery: Open, laparoscopic, robotic assisted

- Cryosurgery under clinical development
  - External beam radiation therapy (EBRT)
    - Confirmed pathological diagnosis of cancer, clinically confined to prostate &/or surrounding tissues
    - CT scan negative for metastases
    - Staging laparotomy and lymph node dissection not necessary
    - Good option for poor surgical candidates
  - Hormone therapy
  - Intersitial brachytherapy
    - Reserved for patients with favorable characteristics
      - Low Gleason score, low PSA, stage T1-T2
  - Careful observation without immediate treatment
- Major treatment roadblocks
  - Controversy over treatment for early stage disease
  - Serous side effects
    - Urinary incontinence
    - Sexual impotence
    - Urethral stricture
    - Fecal incontinence
  - Increasing perioperative morbidity and mortality with age
  - Radical prostatectomy may be difficult after transurethral resection of prostate (TURP)
- Treatment options by stage
  - **Stage I**
    - Careful observation without immediate treatment in selected patients
    - Radical prostatectomy and pelvic node dissection
      - If positive nodes on intraoperative frozen section, prostatectomy usually aborted
    - EBRT
    - Interstitial brachytherapy using imaging guidance for seed placement
  - **Stage II**
    - Radical prostatectomy and pelvic node dissection: If positive nodes on intraoperative frozen section, prostatectomy usually aborted
    - Careful observation without immediate treatment in selected patients
    - EBRT ± androgen-suppression therapy
    - Interstitial brachytherapy using imaging guidance for seed placement
    - Ultrasound-guided percutaneous cryosurgery under clinical evaluation
    - Neoadjuvant hormonal therapy followed by radical prostatectomy in clinical trials
  - **Stage III: Asymptomatic**
    - EBRT with hormonal therapy (LHRH agonist or orchiectomy)
    - Hormonal manipulations (orchiectomy or LHRH agonist)
    - Radical prostatectomy and pelvic node dissection with adjuvant radiation therapy
    - Careful observation without immediate treatment
  - **Stage III: Urinary symptoms**
    - EBRT
    - Hormonal manipulation
    - Palliative TURP
    - Trials of interstitial brachytherapy + EBRT
  - **Stage IV**
    - Hormonal manipulations as initial therapy

- EBRT ± hormonal manipulation
- Palliative radiation therapy for symptomatic bone metastases
- Palliative TURP
- Careful observation without immediate treatment

REPORTING CHECKLIST

T Staging

- Disease detectable by imaging is minimum T2
- Tumor contacting and invading prostatic capsule or prostatic apex (but not beyond) is T2 disease, not T3 disease
  - Capsular contact is different from extracapsular extension
- Most important factor affecting prognosis & choice of treatment is presence or absence of ECE & SVI (T3 disease)
  - Advanced imaging (MR) most sensitive imaging modality for detection of ECE

N Staging

- Metastases in regional nodes are N1 disease

M Staging

- Detection of nodal disease outside true pelvis is M1a
- Detection of osteoblastic lesions on plain radiograph in elderly male is prostate cancer until proven otherwise

SELECTED REFERENCES

1. American Joint Committee on Cancer: AJCC Cancer Staging Manual. 7th ed. New York: Springer, 2010
2. Beresford MJ et al: A systematic review of the role of imaging before salvage radiotherapy for post-prostatectomy biochemical recurrence. Clin Oncol (R Coll Radiol). 22(1):46-55, 2010
3. Albertsen PC: A challenge to contemporary management of prostate cancer. Nat Clin Pract Urol. 6(1):12-3, 2009
4. Dall'Era MA et al: Active surveillance for early-stage prostate cancer: review of the current literature. Cancer. 112(8):1650-9, 2008
5. Paner GP et al: Best practice in diagnostic immunohistochemistry: prostate carcinoma and its mimics in needle core biopsies. Arch Pathol Lab Med. 132(9):1388-96, 2008
6. Kundra V et al: Imaging in oncology from the University of Texas M. D. Anderson Cancer Center: diagnosis, staging, and surveillance of prostate cancer. AJR Am J Roentgenol. 189(4):830-44, 2007
7. Albertsen PC et al: 20-year outcomes following conservative management of clinically localized prostate cancer. JAMA. 293(17):2095-101, 2005
8. Albertsen PC et al: The positive yield of imaging studies in the evaluation of men with newly diagnosed prostate cancer: a population based analysis. J Urol. 163(4):1138-43, 2000
9. Bubendorf L et al: Metastatic patterns of prostate cancer: an autopsy study of 1,589 patients. Hum Pathol. 31(5):578-83, 2000

T2

T2

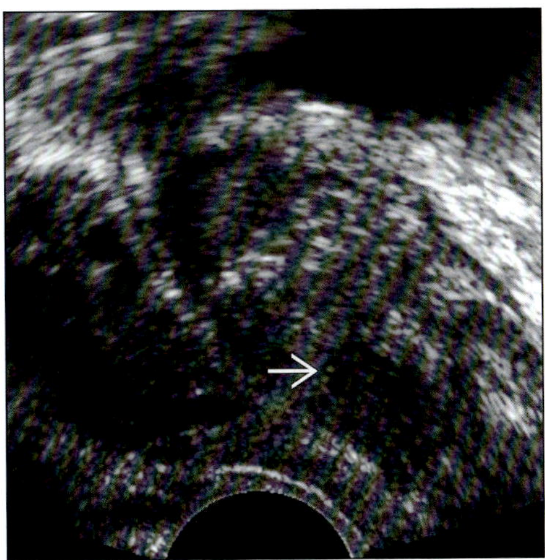

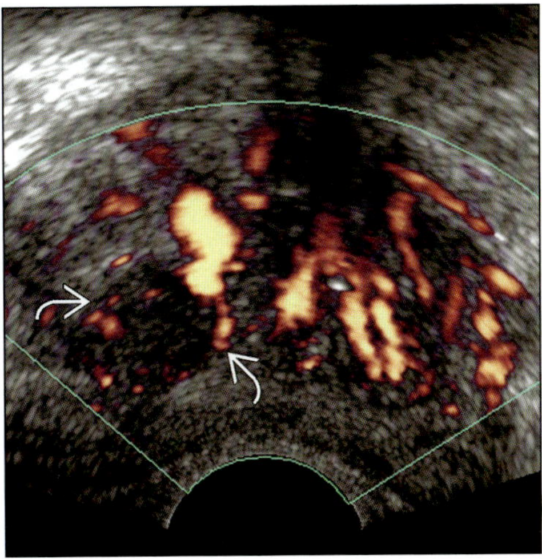

(Left) Grayscale transrectal ultrasound (TRUS) shows an ill-defined, hypoechoic, heterogeneous area ➡ in the right peripheral zone. The tumor appears confined to the limits of the prostatic capsule. However, TRUS is not sensitive enough to be used to exclude ECE or SVI. (Right) In the same patient the transducer is rotated to bring the nodule to the left side of the image. This power Doppler ultrasound shows neovascularization ➡ around the mass. A guided biopsy confirmed prostatic carcinoma.

Stage I (pT2a N0 M0, PSA 6, Gleason 6)

Stage I (pT2a N0 M0, PSA 6, Gleason 6)

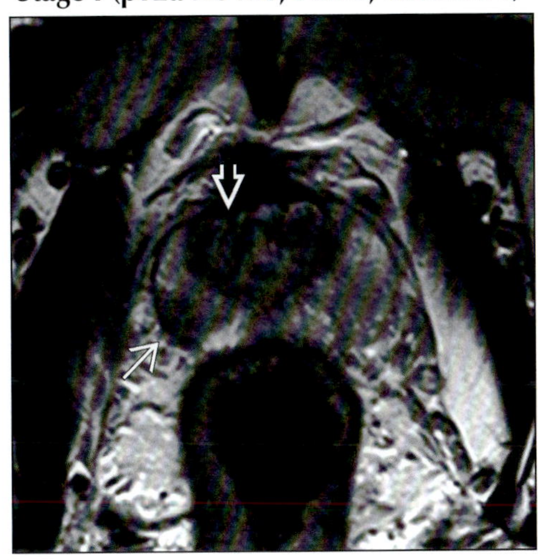

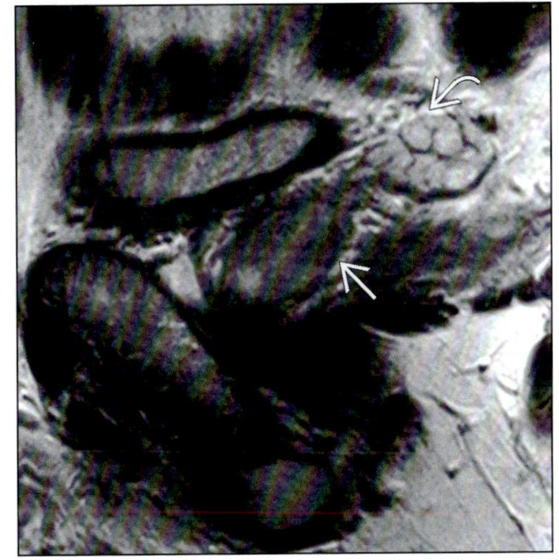

(Left) Axial T2WI MR without ER coil at 3.0T demonstrates a 9 mm focus of low T2 SI in the right peripheral zone ➡, with an intact sharply demarcated T2 dark fibrous band overlying the abnormal focus, suggesting an intact capsule. The normal heterogeneously low T2 SI of the central gland is well demonstrated ➡. (Right) Sagittal T2WI MR in the same patient shows the tumor focus ➡, although not as well. Normal high T2 SI is present in the right seminal vesicle ➡.

Stage IIA (T2b N0 M0)

Stage IIA (T2b N0 M0)

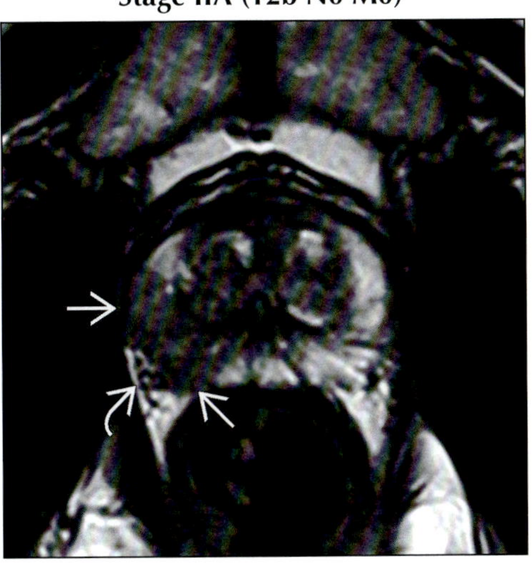

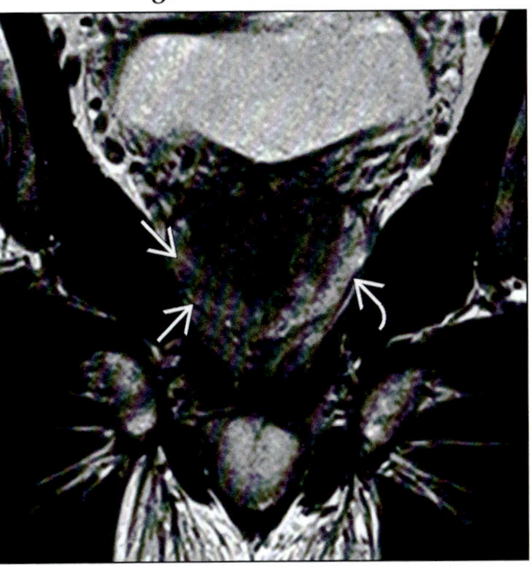

(Left) Axial T2WI MR without ER coil at 3.0T demonstrates low T2 SI in the right PZ mid gland spanning from 7 o'clock to 10:30 ➡. This area spans more than 1/2 of the left lobe, with normal heterogeneously high T2 SI in the right PZ. An intact neurovascular bundle ➡ is present. (Right) Coronal T2WI MR from the same patient demonstrates the PZ asymmetry, with abnormal low T2 SI in the right PZ ➡ and normal high T2 SI in the left PZ ➡.

PROSTATE CARCINOMA

Stage IIB (T2c N0 M0)

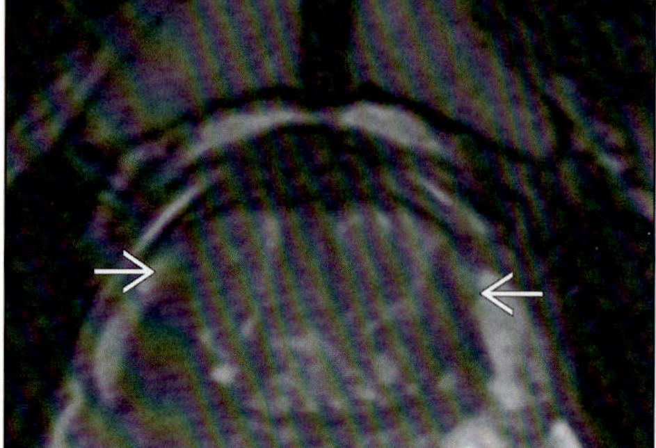

Stage IIB (T2c N0 M0)

(Left) Axial T2WI MR with ER coil at the prostate base shows a continuous band of low PZ T2 SI from 1 o'clock to 11 o'clock ➡. The band abuts both the prostate CZ and the T2 dark fibrous capsule ➡. The capsular margin appears intact. *(Right)* At the mid gland level in the same patient, a more focal nodule of disease is present on the left ➡ with a bulging rectoprostatic angle ➡. This is concerning for extracapsular extension. Right-sided low SI tumor is also seen at this level.

Stage III (pT3a N0 M0, PSA 6, Gleason 7)

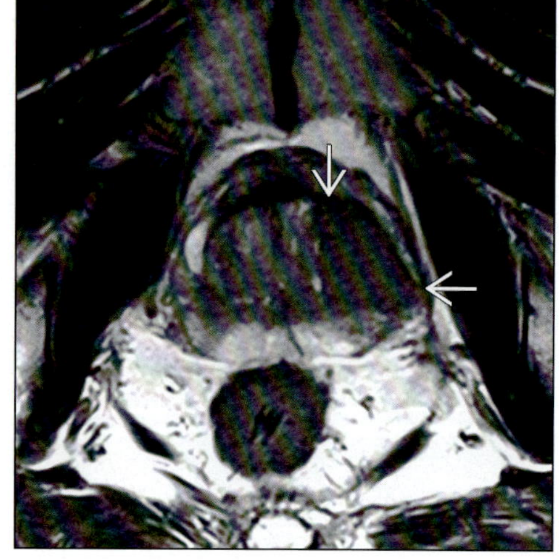
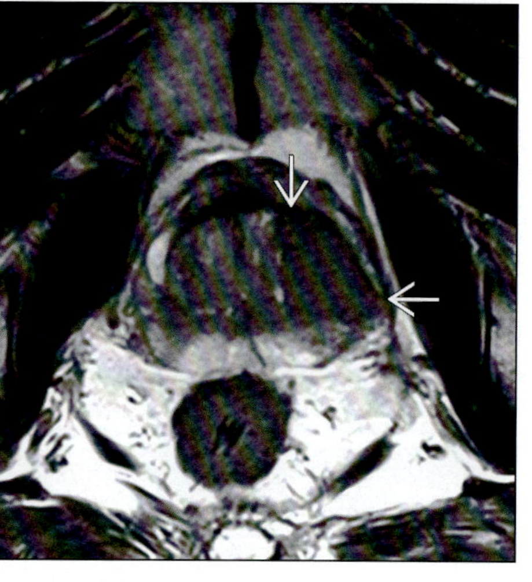

Stage III (pT3a N0 M0, PSA 6, Gleason 7)

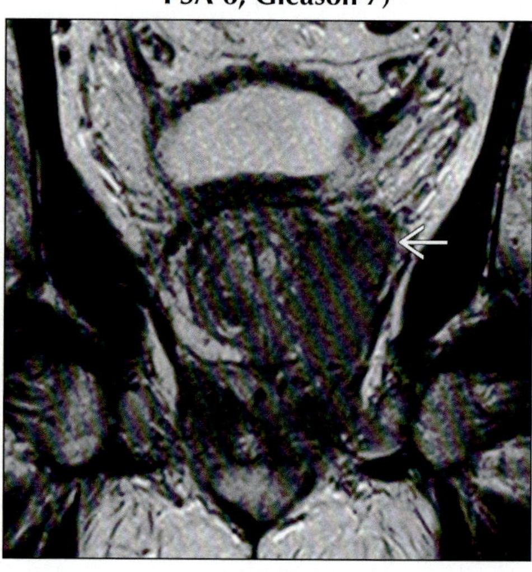

(Left) Axial T2WI MR without ER coil demonstrates large, homogeneously low T2 SI tumor in the left gland from 2 o'clock to 4 o'clock ➡. The mass involves the CZ and extends beyond the prostatic capsule. Because the bulk of the tumor is in the anterior portion of the gland, the neurovascular bundle may be spared. *(Right)* Coronal T2WI MR shows the focal bulge at the lateral base well ➡. This is consistent with extracapsular extension, which was confirmed at resection.

Stage III (pT3a N0 M0, PSA 6, Gleason 7)

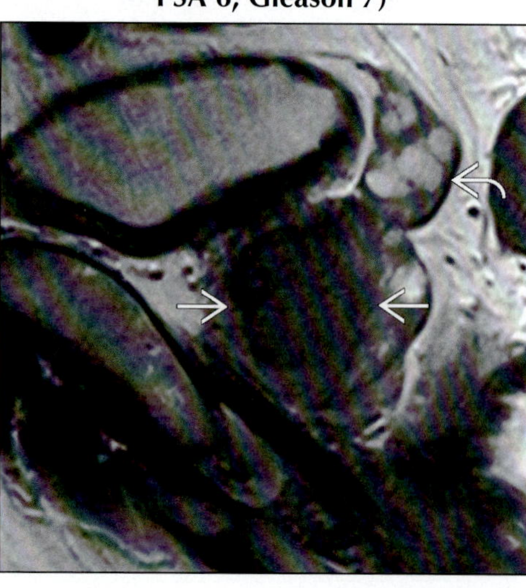

Stage III (pT3a N0 M0, PSA 6, Gleason 7)

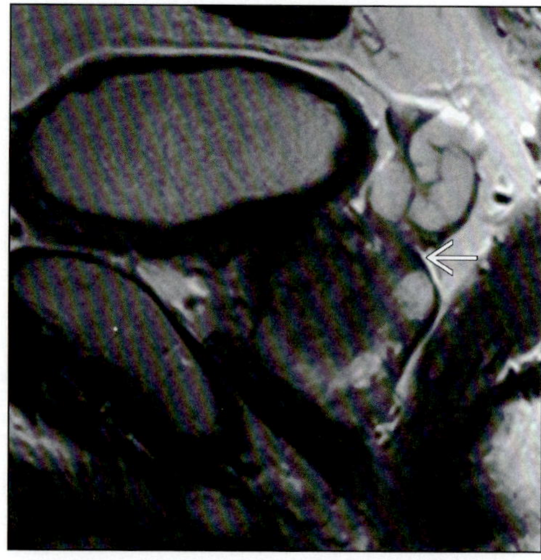

(Left) Sagittal T2WI MR in the same patient shows the focal low T2 SI area corresponding to tumor on the left ➡. No definite low SI is present in the seminal vesicle ➡. The bulk of the tumor is anterior in the prostate, decreasing the likelihood of direct seminal vesicles invasion. *(Right)* Sagittal T2WI MR on the right in the same patient shows the heterogeneously high PZ T2 SI. A focus of low T2 SI near the prostate base ➡ is concerning for an additional site of disease.

PROSTATE CARCINOMA

Stage III (T3a N0 M0)

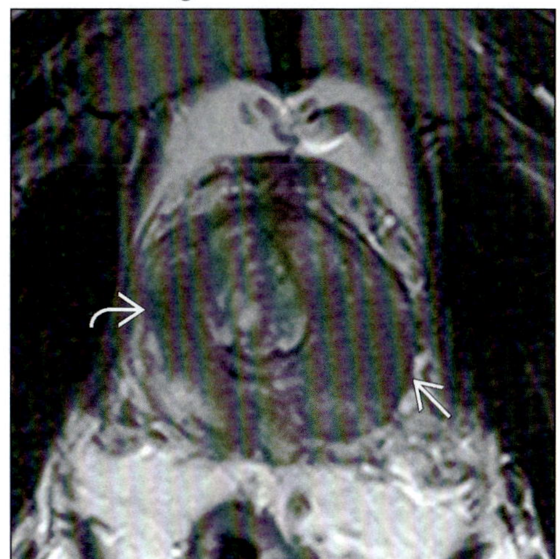

Stage III (T3a N0 M0)

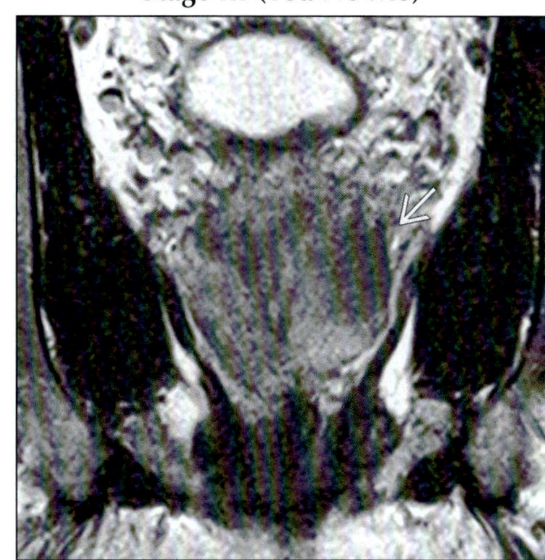

(Left) Axial T2WI MR shows diffuse low T2 SI throughout the PZ on the left ➡, with a rim of abnormal signal in the right TZ ➡. The capsule appears intact, but the low T2 SI area in the PZ contacts > 10 mm of the prostate margin. *(Right)* Coronal T2WI MR in the same patient shows the left-sided low T2 SI nodule with focal bulging and irregularity at the lateral base ➡. This is evidence of unilateral extracapsular extension. Seminal vesicles were uninvolved.

Stage III (T3b N0 M0)

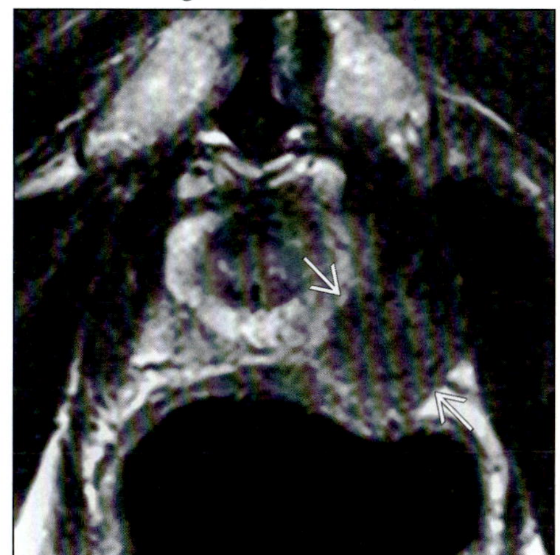

Stage III (T3b N0 M0)

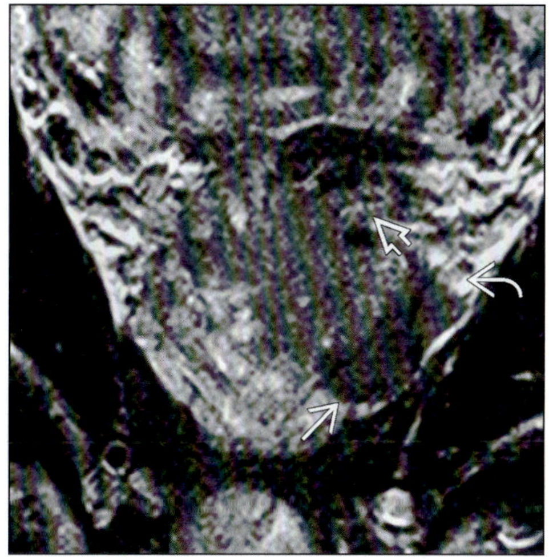

(Left) Axial T2WI MR shows a focal bulging low T2 SI mass ➡ in the left PZ. This is palpable on DRE as a firm nodule. *(Right)* Coronal T2WI MR in the same patient shows the focal area of very low T2 SI tumor ➡ extending from the left midgland to the left base. Extracapsular extension is seen at the base, where the tumor extends beyond the capsular margin ➡. Seminal vesicles invasion is present with heterogeneously low T2 SI extending into the SV ➡.

Stage III (T3b N0 M0)

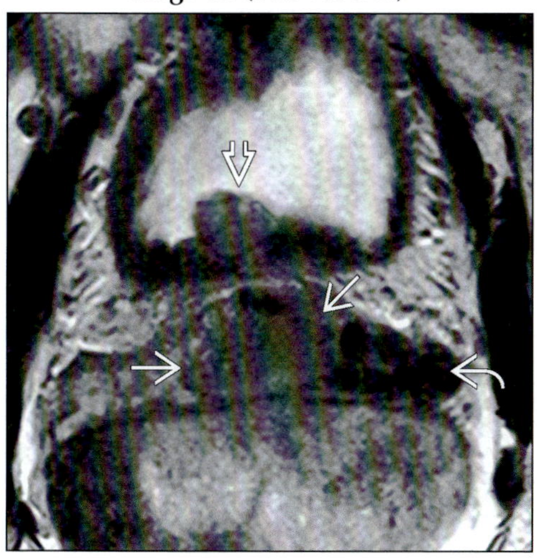

Stage III (T3b N0 M0)

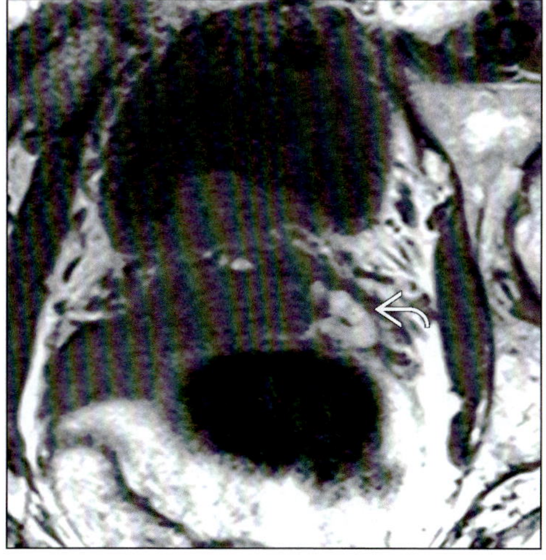

(Left) Axial T2WI more cranially at the level of the prostate base in the same patient shows the low T2 SI extending into the seminal vesicles ➡ related to patient's BPH. The tubules of the seminal vesicles on the left demonstrate very dark T2 SI ➡. A prostatic nodule from patient's BPH protrudes into the bladder base ➡. *(Right)* Axial T1WI MR at the same level confirms that the low T2 signal in the seminal vesicles on the left is due to hemorrhage, which is T1 bright ➡.

PROSTATE CARCINOMA

Stage IV (T3b N1 M0)

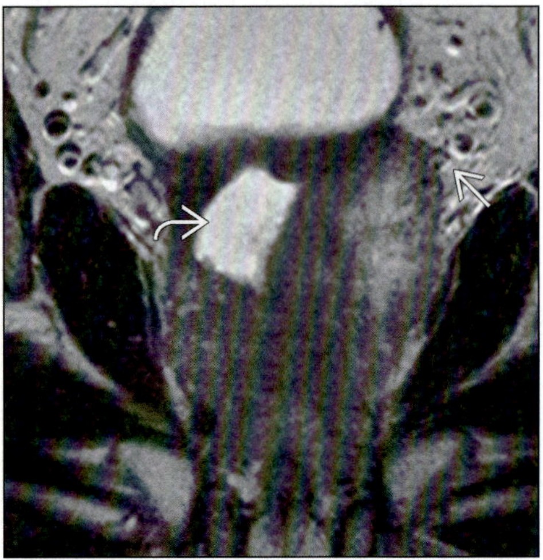

Stage IV (T3b N1 M0)

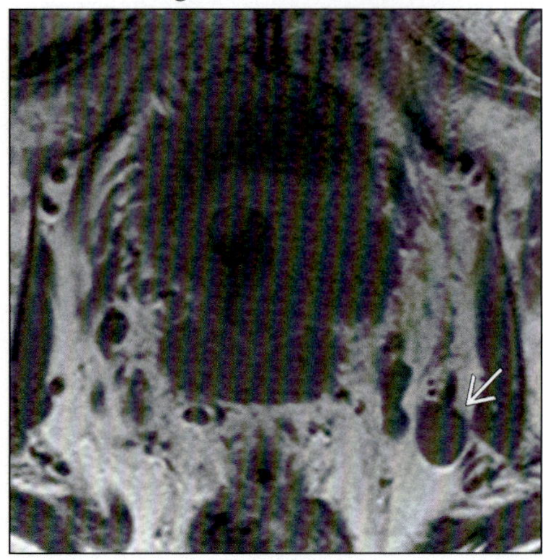

(Left) Coronal T2WI MR in a patient who had previously undergone a transurethral resection of the prostate (TURP) shows a large heterogeneous low T2 SI mass extending from the left side of the remaining prostate into the periprostatic fat, encasing vessels ➡. The surgical defect from the TURP is noted ➡. *(Right)* Axial T1WI MR in the same patient shows an enlarged left obturator node ➡, making this N1 disease.

Stage IV (T3b N1 M0, PSA 22, Gleason 9)

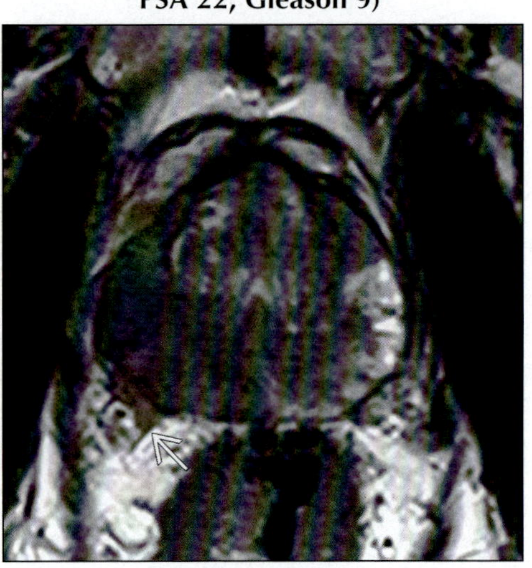

Stage IV (T3b N1 M0, PSA 22, Gleason 9)

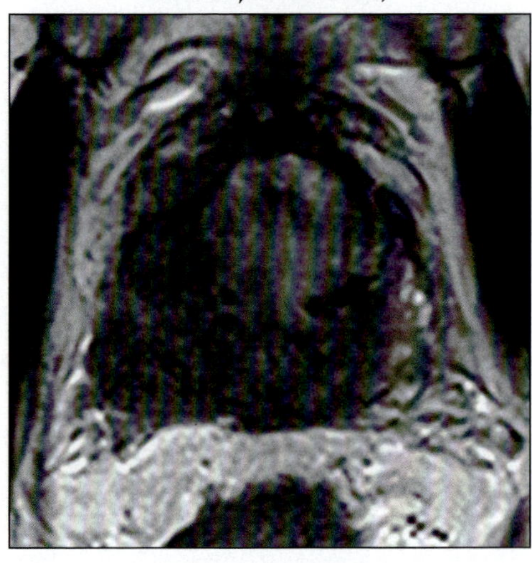

(Left) Axial T2WI MR at a mid gland level shows diffuse low T2 SI throughout the PZ. The margin between the PZ and CZ is obscured. The asymmetric bulge on the right, with low T2 SI infiltrating into the region of the neurovascular bundle ➡, is consistent with ECE and neurovascular bundle involvement. *(Right)* Axial T2WI MR shows mass-like confluent low T2 SI involving nearly the entire base of the prostate, with definite angularity at the right prostatic angle, evidence of ECE.

Stage IV (T3b N1 M0, PSA 22, Gleason 9)

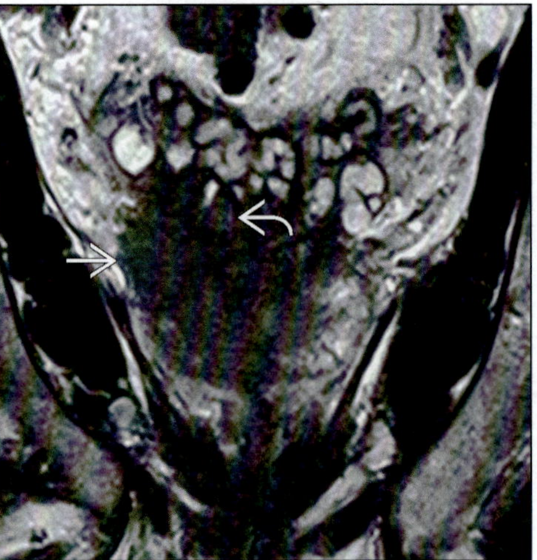

Stage IV (T3b N1 M0, PSA 22, Gleason 9)

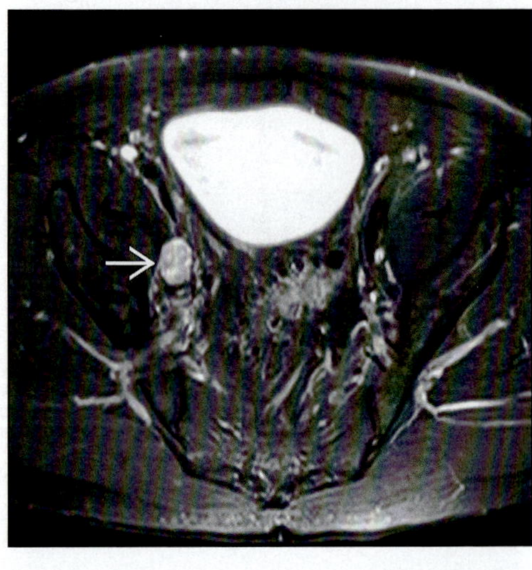

(Left) Coronal T2WI MR in the same patient shows the abnormal low T2 SI infiltrating from the left side of prostate ➡ into the left seminal vesicles, consistent with seminal vesicles invasion ➡. *(Right)* Axial T2WI FS MR in the same patient shows an abnormally enlarged right external iliac node ➡. The metastasis to a regional lymph node is N1 disease. Surgery is not indicated for this stage of disease.

PROSTATE CARCINOMA

Stage IV (T4 N0 M1b)

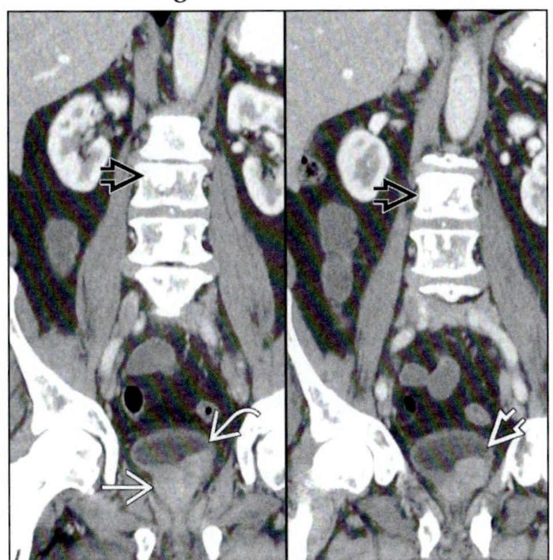

Stage IV (T4 N0 M1b)

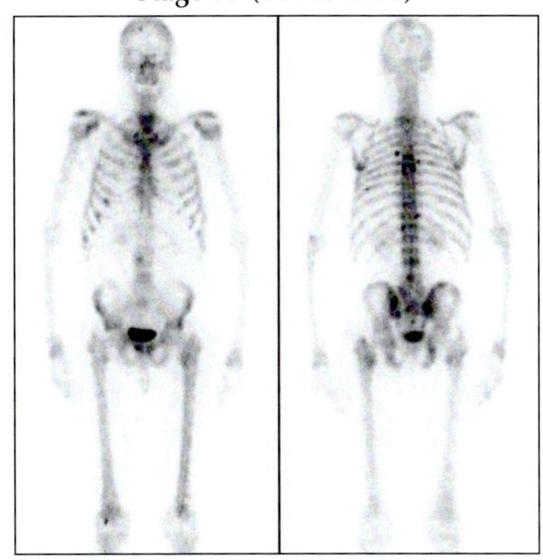

(Left) Coronal CECT images demonstrate a mass extending from the prostate ➡ into the bladder base ➡. The right image shows the intraluminal bladder component well ➡. Sclerotic lesions are seen in the lumbar spine ➡. *(Right)* Whole body bone scan in the same patient shows diffuse increased uptake in the spine and bony pelvis, as well as foci of increased uptake in many ribs. With little renal or soft tissue activity, this study approaches a "Superscan."

Stage IV (T2b N0 M1b, PSA 16.5, Gleason 7)

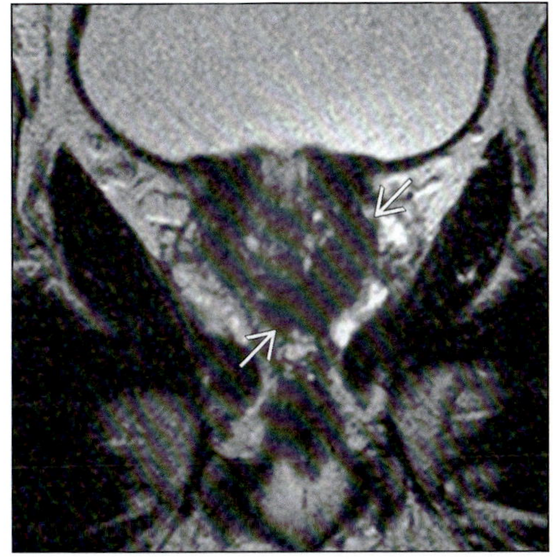

Stage IV (T2b N0 M1b, PSA 16.5, Gleason 7)

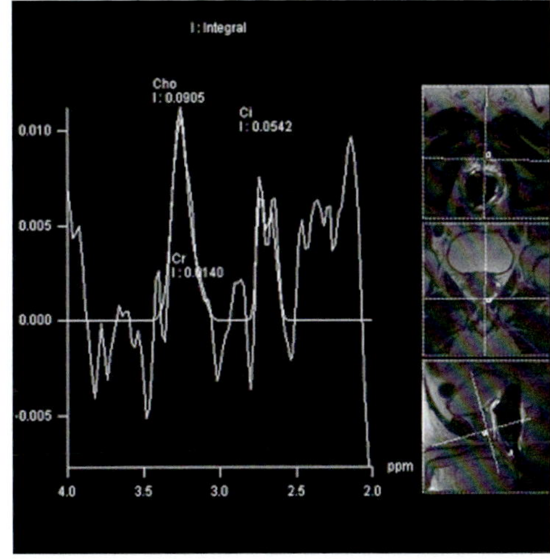

(Left) Coronal T2WI MR shows a band of low T2 SI extending from the apex to base on the left ➡. *(Courtesy S. Eberhardt, MD.)* *(Right)* Single voxel MR spectroscopy was performed in the same patient by placing a voxel over the area of tumor. This demonstrates a metabolic spectra of elevated choline + creatine/citrate. This spectra is consistent with malignancy. *(Courtesy S. Eberhardt, MD.)*

Stage IV (T2b N0 M1b, PSA 16.5, Gleason 7)

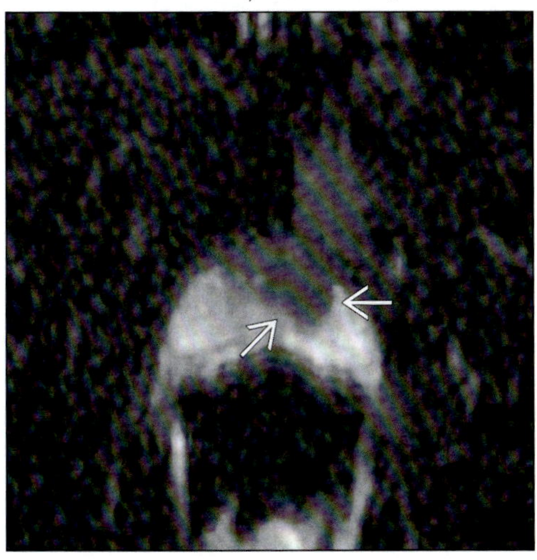

Stage IV (T2b N0 M1b, PSA 16.5, Gleason 7)

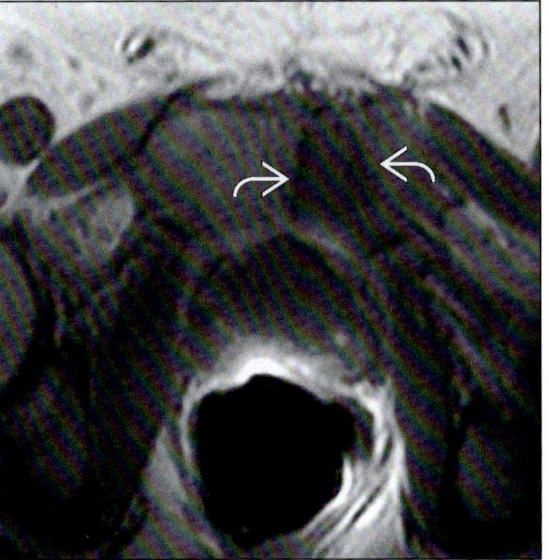

(Left) Axial ADC map from diffusion-weighted imaging in the same patient shows restricted diffusion corresponding to the area of decreased T2 SI ➡. *(Courtesy S. Eberhardt, MD.)* *(Right)* Coned down axial T1WI MR from the same patient demonstrates a focus of low T1 SI in the left pubis ➡. This is consistent with an osteoblastic bony metastasis. *(Courtesy S. Eberhardt, MD.)*

PROSTATE CARCINOMA

Stage IV (TX N1 M1a)

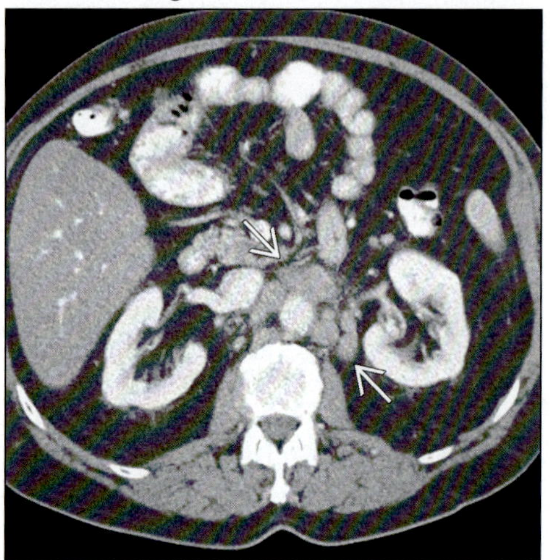

Stage IV (TX N1 M1a)

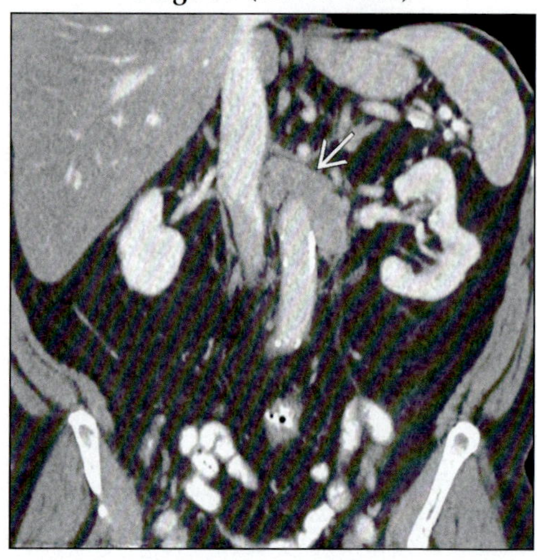

(Left) Axial CECT at the level of the right renal vein demonstrates significant periaortic lymphadenopathy ➡. *(Right)* Coronal CECT in the same patient demonstrates the confluent adenopathy ➡ crossing anterior to the aorta and between the aorta and IVC. Metastases to the paraaortic lymph nodes are the most common site of nonregional lymphatic spread of disease. These upstage the patient to M1a, while pelvic regional adenopathy is N1 disease.

Stage IV (TX N1 M1a)

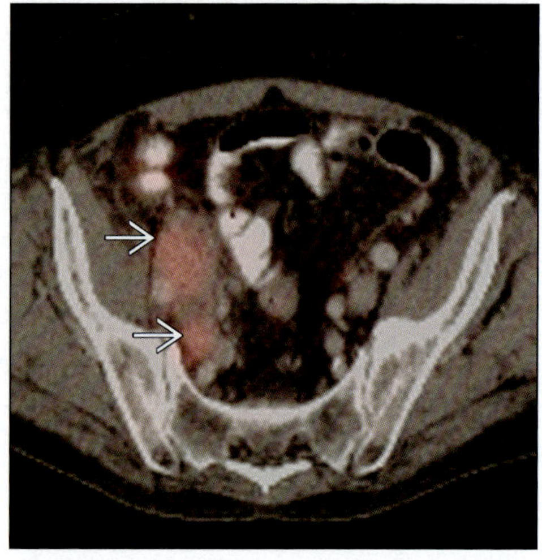

Stage IV (TX N1 M1a)

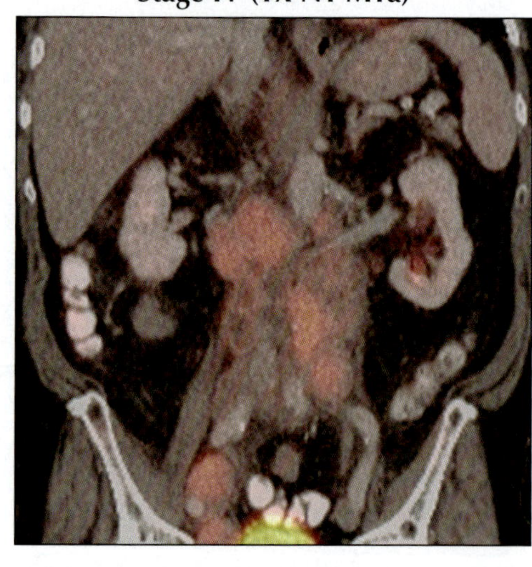

(Left) Axial fused PET/CT in the same patient shows the internal and external iliac adenopathy on the right ➡. This regional adenopathy is considered N1 disease. *(Right)* Coronal fused PET/CT in the same patient shows the extensive regional and distant lymphadenopathy. No bone lesions were identified on the PET.

Stage IV (TX NX M1c)

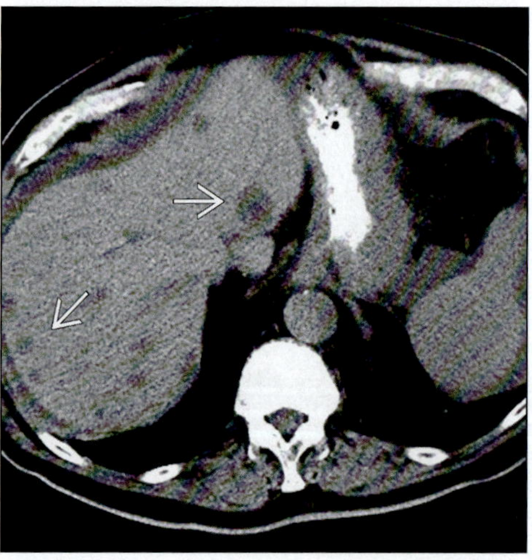

Stage IV (TX NX M1c)

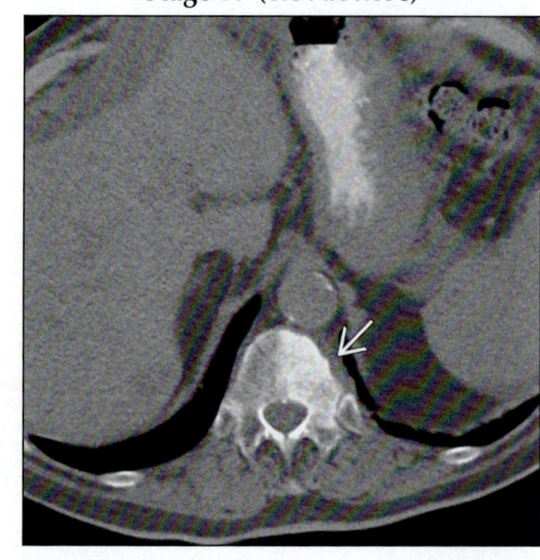

(Left) Axial NECT in a patient with a history of prostate cancer, treated more than 10 years prior who had a CT of his abdomen after abnormal liver function tests were found, shows multiple hypoattenuating hepatic lesions ➡. On percutaneous CT-guided biopsy, these were proven to be metastases from prostate cancer. *(Right)* Axial NECT shows that, in addition to the hepatic lesions, a sclerotic bone lesion in the T10 vertebral body ➡ is identified.

PROSTATE CARCINOMA

Stage IV (TX NX M1c)

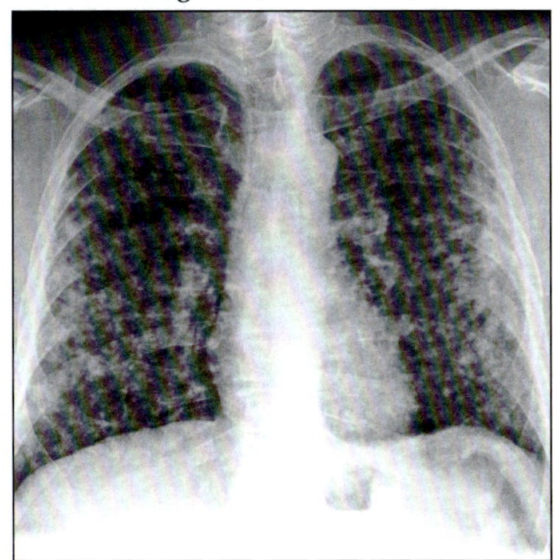

Stage IV (TX NX M1c)

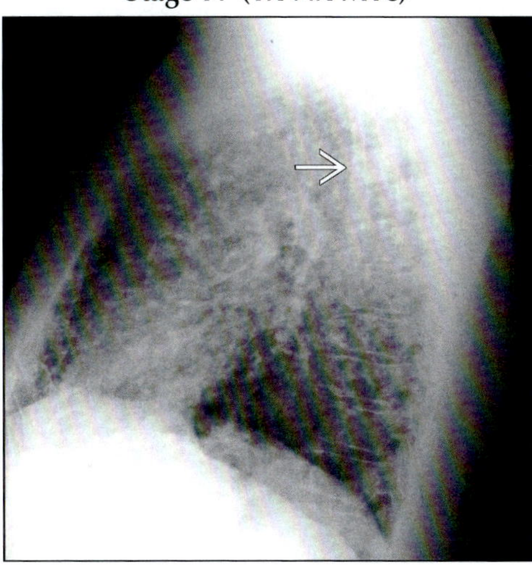

(Left) Frontal chest radiograph demonstrates diffuse pulmonary nodularity in an elderly man with known prostate cancer. *(Right)* Accompanying lateral radiograph demonstrates the innumerable pulmonary nodules. Additionally, there is the suggestion of sclerosis of the T4 vertebral body ➡. This appearance has been termed an "ivory vertebral body" and is due to near complete osteoblastic replacement of the vertebra.

Stage IV (TX NX M1c)

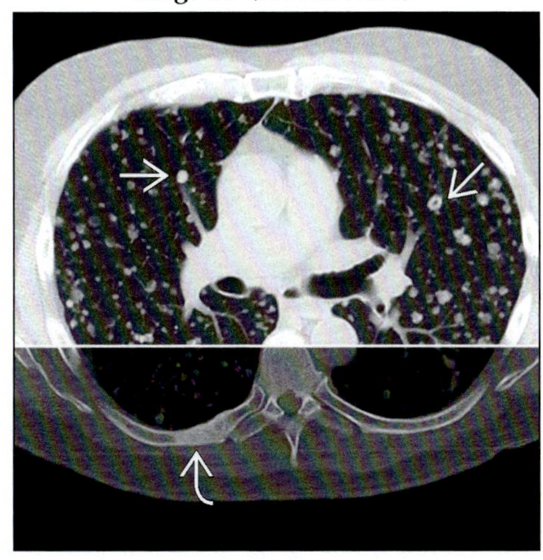

Stage IV (TX NX M1c)

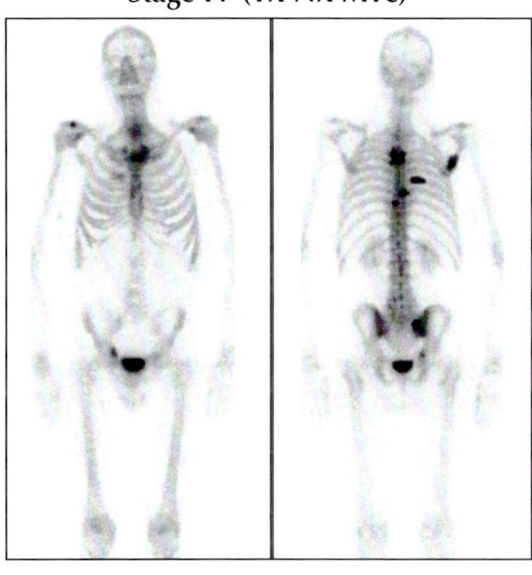

(Left) Axial NECT, lung window (top), in the same patient demonstrates the innumerable pulmonary nodules ➡. Bone window image (bottom) reveals a sclerotic lesion posteriorly in the right 6th rib ➡. *(Right)* Whole body bone scan in the same patient shows increased uptake in multiple vertebral bodies, including T4, as well as the right 6th rib, the right scapula, and the left pubis. These foci correspond to the sclerotic bone metastases seen on prior imaging.

Local Recurrence

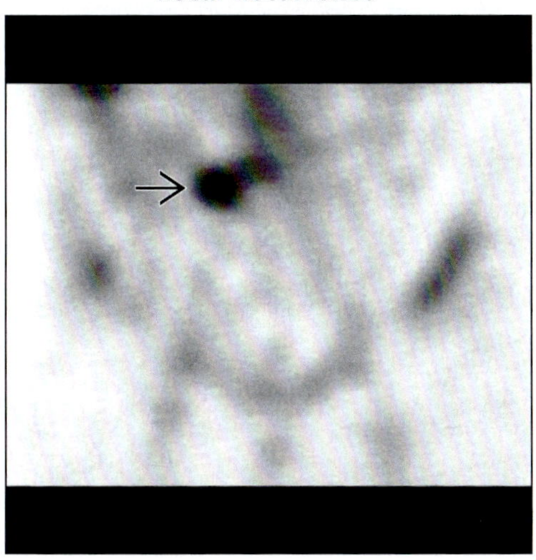

Local Recurrence

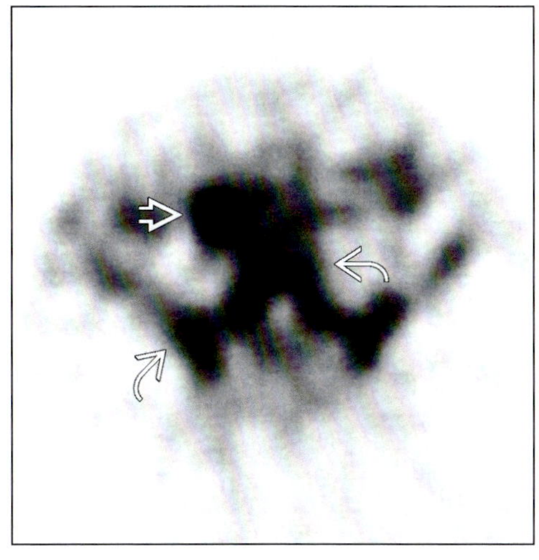

(Left) Coronal In-111 capromab (ProstaScint) SPECT image shows right proximal iliac focal uptake ➡ at the site of a 1.3 cm nodal metastasis. The patient had previously undergone a radical prostatectomy and had a rising PSA, with a PSA doubling time of approximately 6 months. *(Right)* Axial In-111 capromab (ProstaScint) image from the same patient again shows the node ➡. Normal marrow uptake ➡ is also noted in the iliac bones and vertebral bodies.

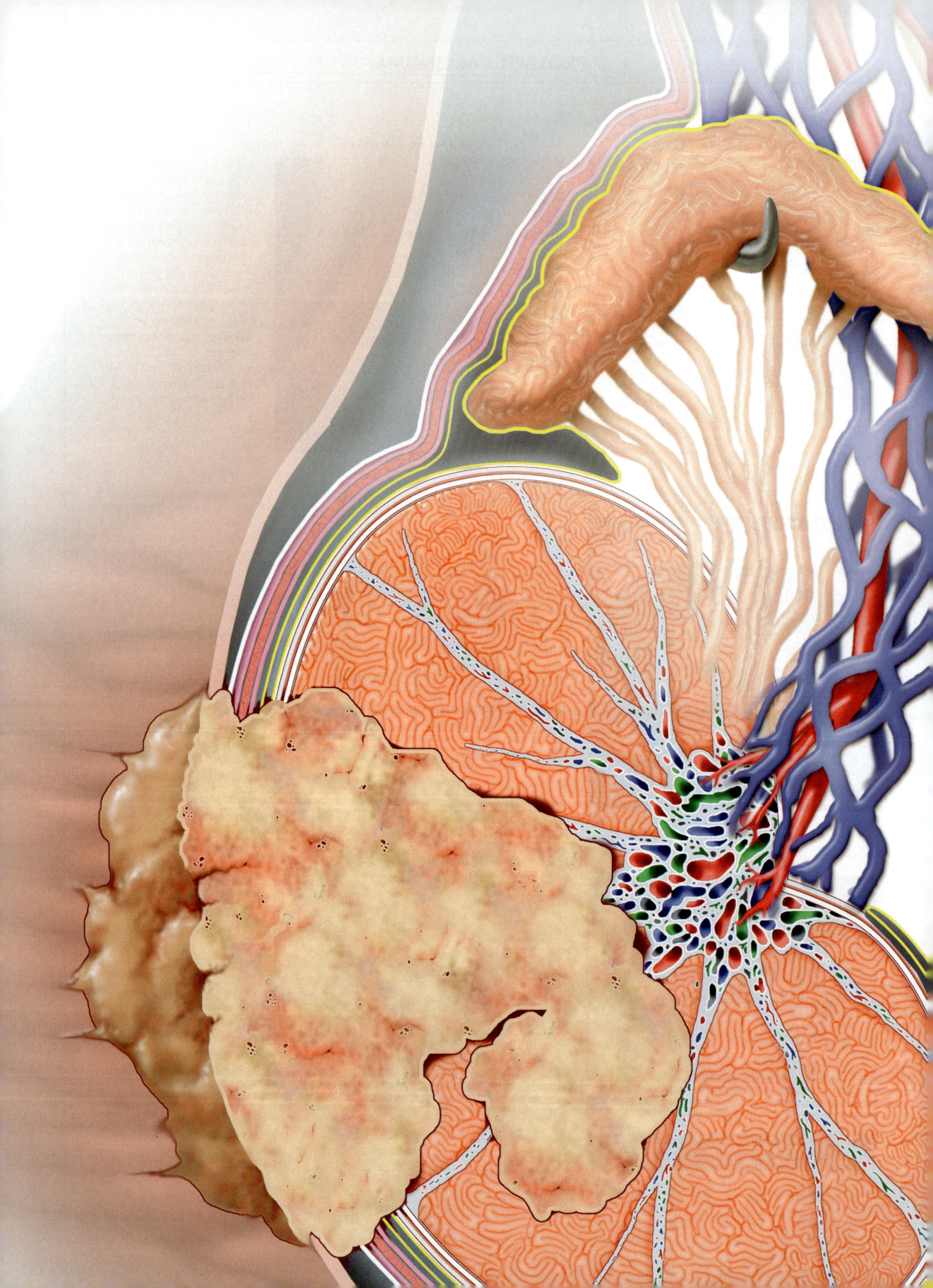

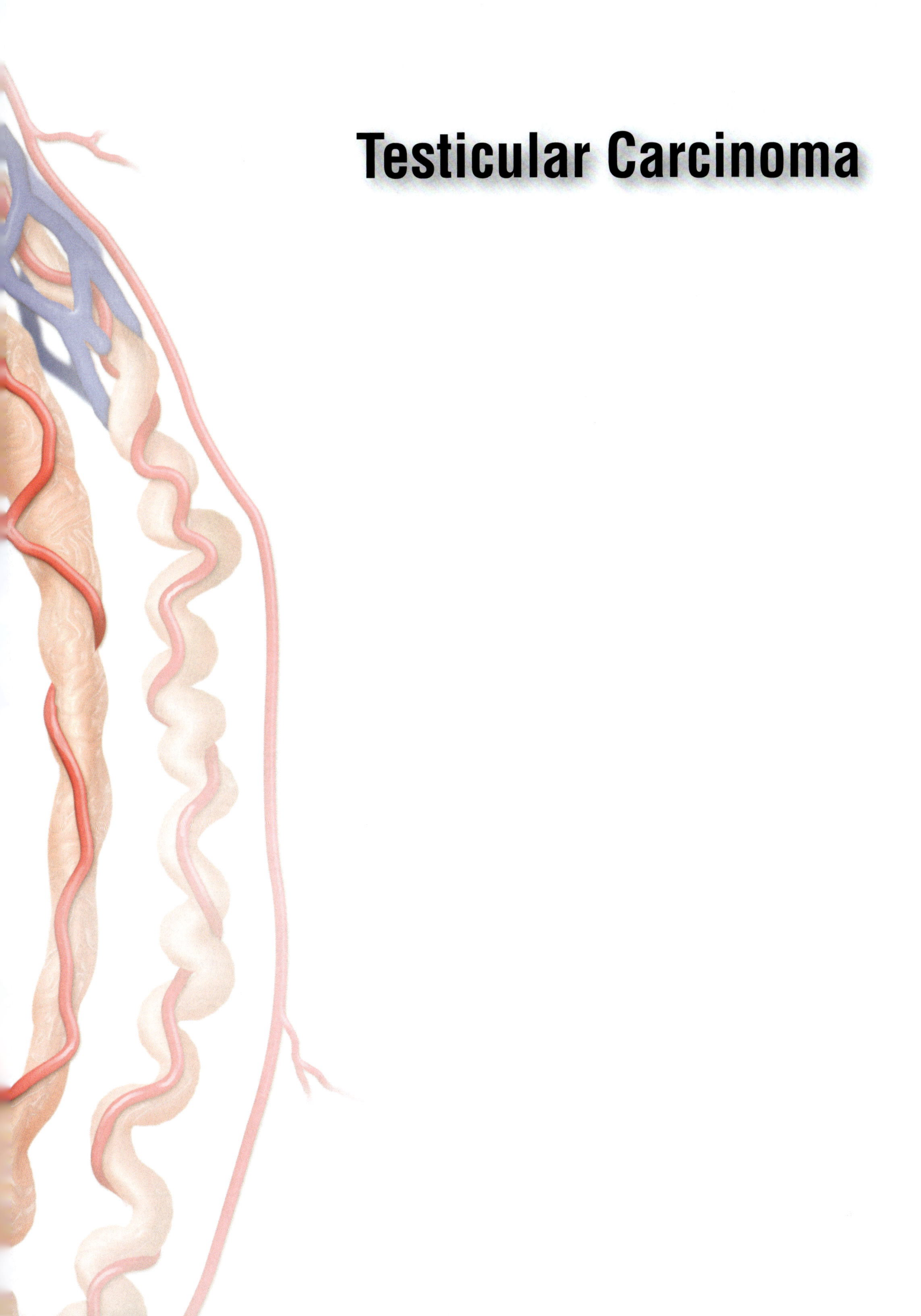

Testicular Carcinoma

TESTICULAR CARCINOMA

(T) Primary Tumor

Adapted from 7th edition AJCC Staging Forms.

TNM	Definitions
pTX	Primary tumor cannot be assessed (if no radical orchiectomy has been performed, TX is used)
pT0	No evidence of primary tumor (e.g., histologic scar in testis)
pTis	Intratubular germ cell neoplasia (carcinoma in situ)
pT1	Tumor limited to the testis and epididymis without vascular/lymphatic invasion; tumor may invade into the tunica albuginea but not the tunica vaginalis
pT2	Tumor limited to the testis and epididymis with vascular/lymphatic invasion, or tumor extending through the tunica albuginea with involvement of the tunica vaginalis
pT3	Tumor invades the spermatic cord with or without vascular/lymphatic invasion
pT4	Tumor invades scrotum with or without vascular/lymphatic invasion

(N) Regional Lymph Nodes

Clinical	
NX	Regional lymph nodes cannot be assessed
N0	No regional lymph node metastasis
N1	Metastasis with a lymph node mass $\leq$ 2 cm in greatest dimension; or multiple lymph nodes, none > 2 cm in greatest dimension
N2	Metastasis with a lymph node mass > 2 cm but $\leq$ 5 cm in greatest dimension; or multiple lymph nodes, any 1 mass > 2 cm but $\leq$ 5 cm in greatest dimension.
N3	Metastasis with a lymph node mass > 5 cm in greatest dimension
Pathological	
pNX	Regional lymph nodes cannot be assessed
pN0	No regional lymph node metastasis
pN1	Metastasis with a lymph node mass $\leq$ 2 cm in greatest dimension and $\leq$ 5 nodes positive, none > 2 cm in greatest dimension
pN2	Metastasis with a lymph node mass > 2 cm but $\leq$ 5 cm in greatest dimension; or > 5 nodes positive, none > 5 cm; or evidence of extranodal extension of tumor
pN3	Metastasis with a lymph node mass > 5 cm in greatest dimension

(M) Distant Metastasis

M0	No distant metastasis
M1	Distant metastasis
M1a	No regional nodal or pulmonary metastasis
M1b	Distant metastasis other than to nonregional lymph nodes and lungs

Except for pTis and pT4, extent of primary tumor is classified by radical orchiectomy. For this reason, a pathologic stage is usually assigned. TX may be used for other categories in the absence of radical orchiectomy.

Serum Tumor Markers (S)

TNM	Definitions
SX	Tumor marker studies not available or not performed
S0	Tumor marker study levels within normal limits
S1	LDH < 1.5x normal **and** β-hCG < 5,000 IU/L **and** AFP < 1,000 ng/mL
S2	LDH 1.5-10x normal **or** β-hCG 5,000-50,000 IU/L **or** AFP 1,000-10,000 ng/mL
S3	LDH >10x normal **or** β-hCG > 50,000 IU/L **or** AFP > 10,000 ng/mL

Serum tumor markers are used as part of tumor stage grouping in testicular cancer. LDH = lactate dehydrogenase, hCG = human chorionic gonadotropin, AFP = α-fetoprotein.

TESTICULAR CARCINOMA

AJCC Stages/Prognostic Groups

Adapted from 7th edition AJCC Staging Forms.

Stage	*T*	*N*	*M*	*S (Serum Tumor Markers)*
0	pTis	N0	M0	S0
I	pT1-4	N0	M0	SX
IA	pT1	N0	M0	S0
IB	pT2	N0	M0	S0
	pT3	N0	M0	S0
	pT4	N0	M0	S0
IS	Any pT/TX	N0	M0	S1-3 (measured post orchiectomy)
II	Any pT/TX	N1-3	M0	SX
IIA	Any pT/TX	N1	M0	S0
	Any pT/TX	N1	M0	S1
IIB	Any pT/TX	N2	M0	S0
	Any pT/TX	N2	M0	S1
IIC	Any pT/TX	N3	M0	S0
	Any pT/TX	N3	M0	S1
III	Any pT/TX	Any N	M1	SX
IIIA	Any pT/TX	Any N	M1a	S0
	Any pT/TX	Any N	M1a	S1
IIIB	Any pT/TX	N1-3	M0	S2
	Any pT/TX	Any N	M1a	S2
IIIC	Any pT/TX	N1-3	M0	S3
	Any pT/TX	Any N	M1a	S3
	Any pT/TX	Any N	M1b	Any S

TESTICULAR CARCINOMA

pTis (Intratubular Germ Cell Neoplasia)

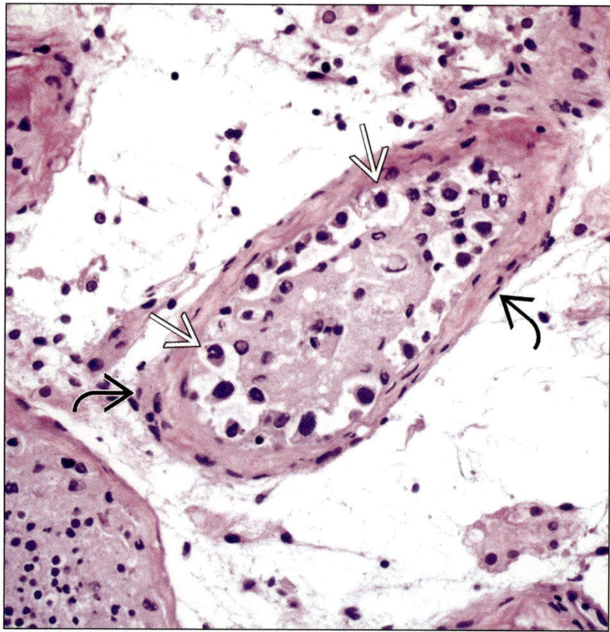

High-power magnification of an H&E stain shows a seminiferous tubule ➔ with neoplastic intratubular germ cells ➔. The neoplastic cells are large, pleomorphic with abundant vacuolated cytoplasm, and arranged in a single layer along the basement membrane. (Original magnification 400x.)

pT1

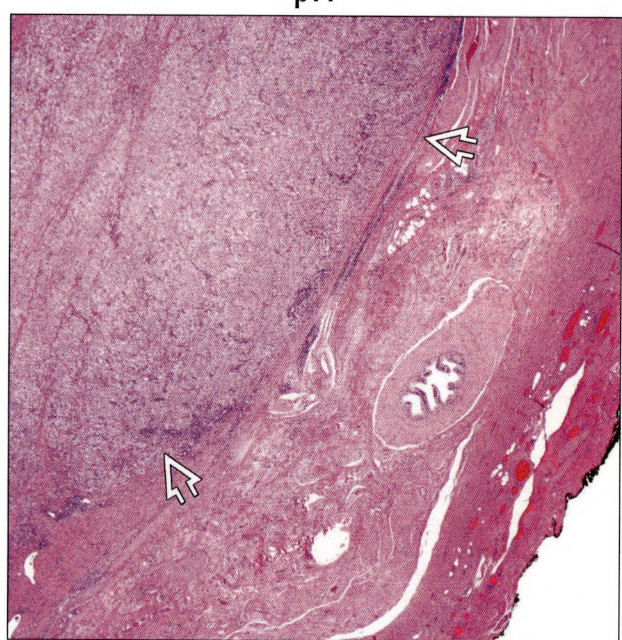

Low-power magnification of H&E stain shows sheets of seminoma ➔ that is replacing the testicular tissue but is limited to the testis without vascular or lymphatic invasion. (Original magnification 40x.)

pT1

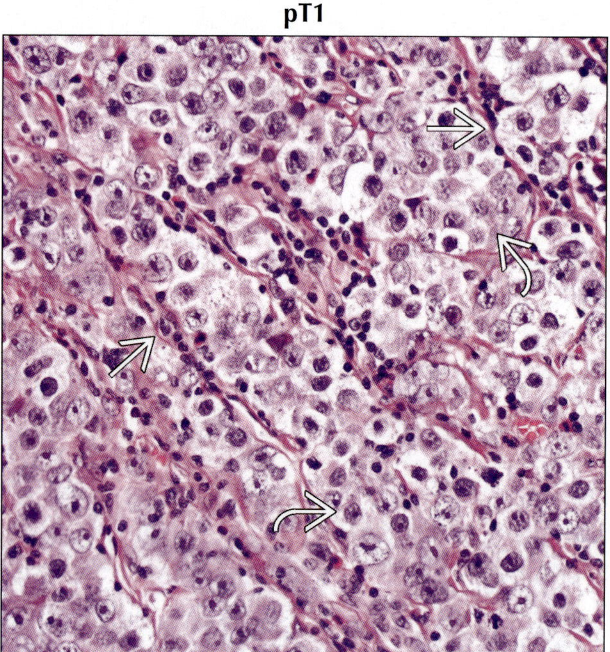

High-power magnification of an H&E stain of seminoma shows diffuse sheets of tumor cells ➔ with intervening branching fibrous septa ➔. The neoplastic cells are polyhedral and have pale to clear cytoplasm with round to oval nuclei and 1-2 prominent nuclei. (Original magnification 500x.)

pT1

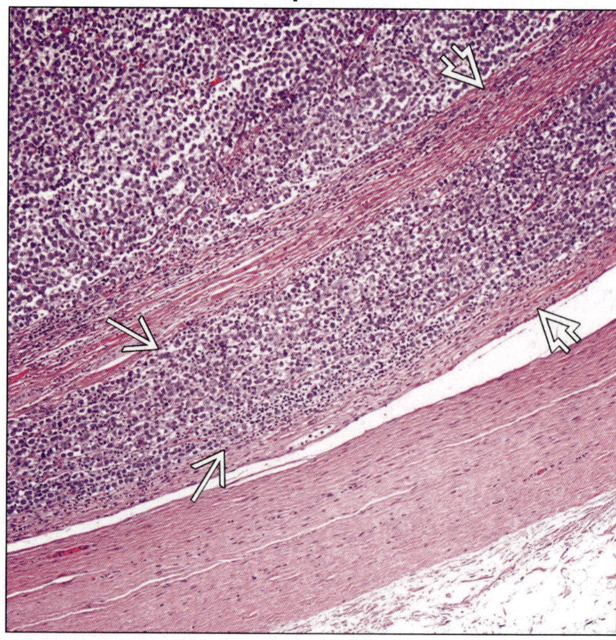

Intermediate-power magnification of H&E stain shows seminoma tumor cells ➔ that focally infiltrate into the tunica albuginea ➔ without involvement of the tunica vaginalis. (Original magnification 200x.)

TESTICULAR CARCINOMA

pT2

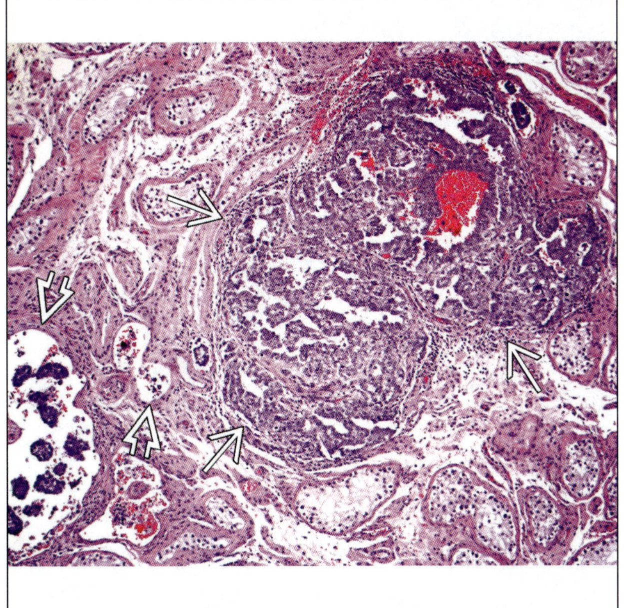

Intermediate-power magnification of H&E stain shows embryonal carcinoma component of germ cell tumor ➔ infiltrating the seminiferous tubules with intravascular invasion in lymphatic/blood vessel spaces ⮞. (Original magnification 200x.)

pT2

In an H&E-stained specimen from the same patient, other areas of the mixed germ cell tumor show yolk sac component. (Original magnification 400x.)

pT3

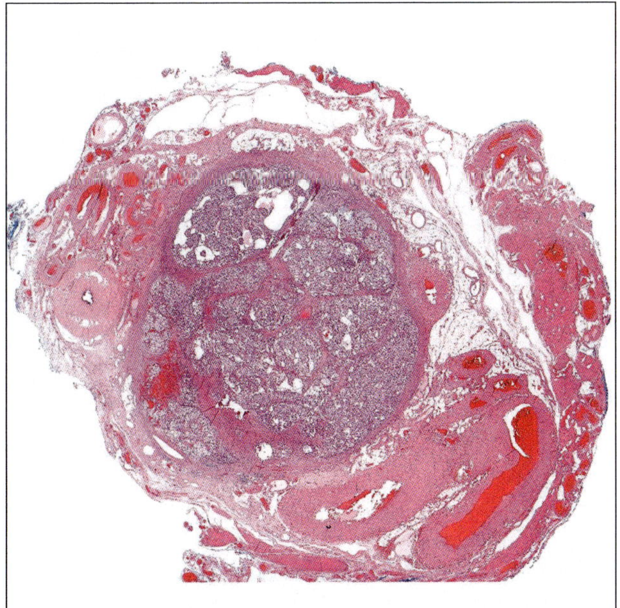

H&E stain of a cross section from a spermatic cord shows spermatic cord involvement by a testicular tumor. (Original magnification 20x.)

pT3

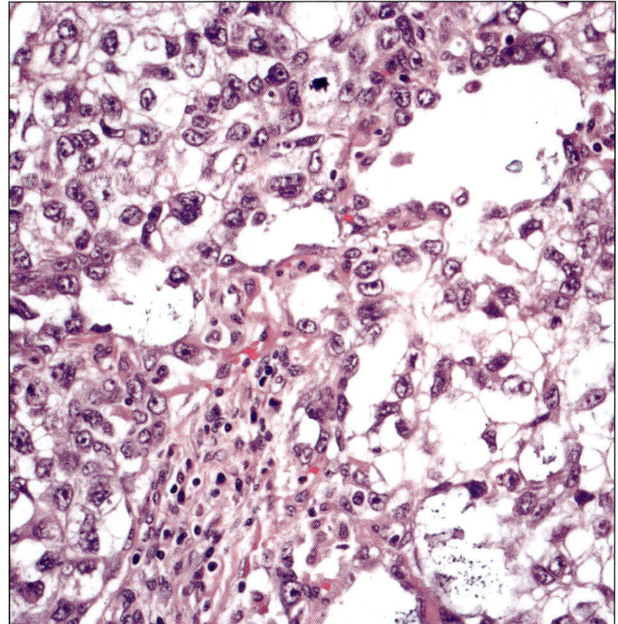

High-power magnification of the previous H&E stained section shows the yolk sac tumor, which expands the spermatic cord with a microcystic (most common) pattern giving a reticular or lace-like appearance. (Original magnification 400x.)

TESTICULAR CARCINOMA

T1

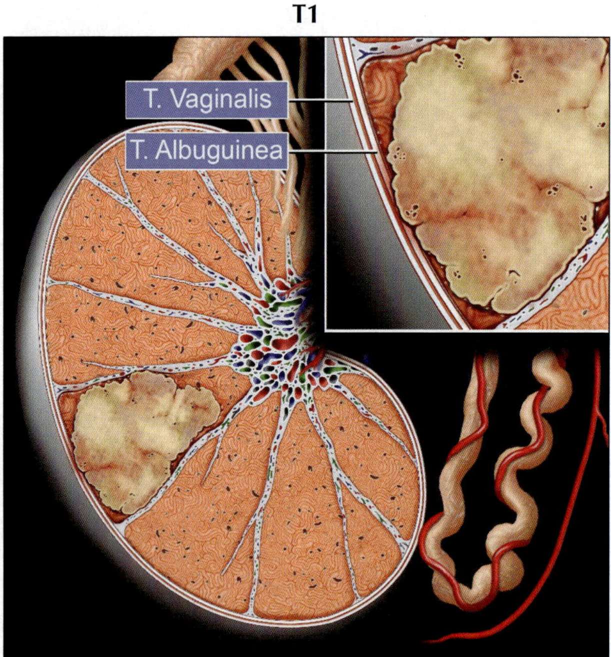

T2

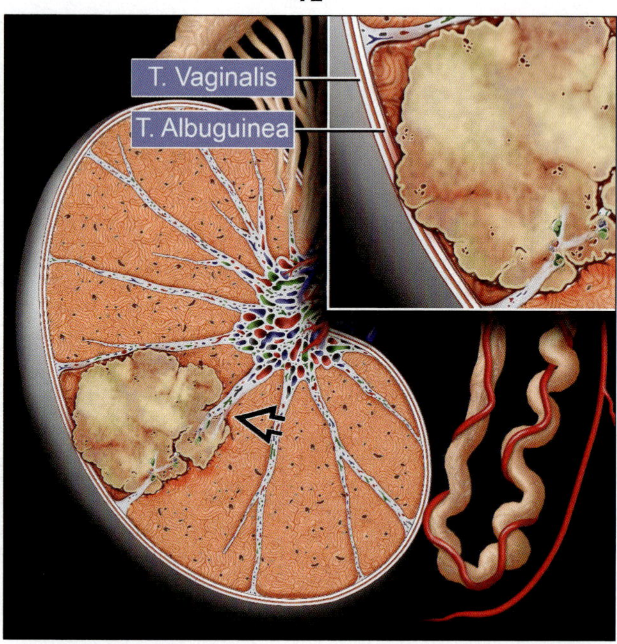

Graphic illustrates tumor limited to the testis and epididymis without vascular/lymphatic invasion. The tumor may invade into the tunical albuginea but not the tunica vaginalis (as seen in the inset). Both are classified as T1 disease.

Graphic illustrates tumor limited to the testis and epididymis with vascular/lymphatic invasion ➢. Tumor extending through tunica albuginea and involving tunica vaginalis (as seen in the inset) is also classified as T2 disease.

T3

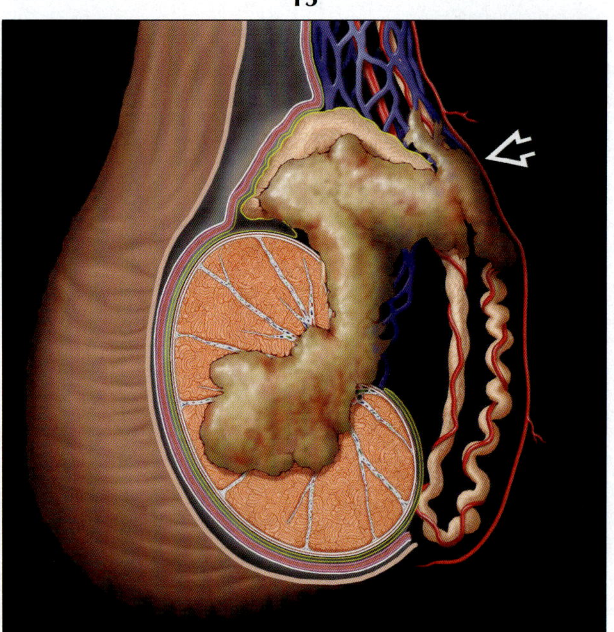

T4

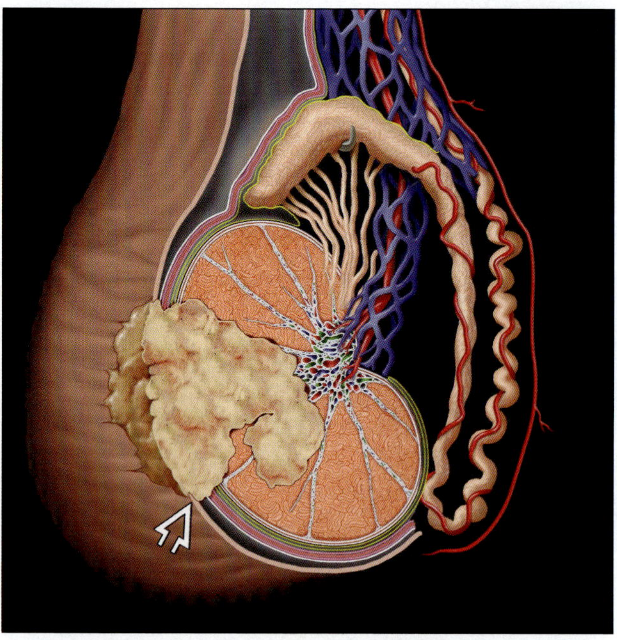

Graphic illustrates tumor invading the spermatic cord ➢ (with or without vascular/lymphatic invasion), compatible with T3 disease.

Graphic illustrates tumor invading the scrotum ➢ (with or without vascular/lymphatic invasion), which is considered T4 disease.

TESTICULAR CARCINOMA

- Seminoma stage IIB, IIC, and III status post chemotherapy
  - Chest, abdominal, and pelvic CT at least 4 weeks post treatment
    - If negative and tumor marker normal → surveillance
    - If residual mass and normal tumor markers → FDG PET
      - PET negative → surveillance
      - PET positive → surgery with biopsy, or biopsy and salvage therapy, or radiation therapy
      - If FDG PET not available, evaluate residual retroperitoneal mass on CT, if > 3 cm consider surgery or radiation therapy, if < 3 cm then surveillance
    - Progressive disease (growing mass or increasing tumor markers)
      - Salvage therapy (includes chemotherapy &/or radiation therapy)
    - Surveillance
      - Chest x-ray every 2 months for year 1, every 3 months for year 2, every 4 months for year 3, every 6 months for year 4, then annually
      - CT abdomen/pelvis at month 4 status post surgery or every 3 months until stable if no surgery option is used
      - FDG PET as indicated
- NSGCT stage IA and IB surveillance
  - Chest x-ray every 1-2 months in year 1, every 2 months in year 2, every 3 months in year 3, every 4 months in year 4, every 6 months in year 5, and then annually
  - Abdominal/pelvic CT every 2-3 months in year 1, every 3-4 months in year 2, every 4 months in year 3, every 6 months in year 4, then annually
- NSGCT any stage after complete response to chemotherapy &/or retroperitoneal lymph node dissection
  - Chest x-ray every 2-3 months in year 1, every 2-3 months in year 2, every 4 months in years 3 and 4, every 6 months in year 5, then annually
  - Abdominal/pelvic CT baseline postsurgical scan in setting of retroperitoneal lymph node dissection
  - Abdominal/pelvic CT status post chemotherapy every 6 months in year 1, every 6-12 months in year 2, every 12 months in years 3-5, every 12-24 months thereafter
- CECT
  - Restaging 4 weeks after chemotherapy treatment
    - Lesions > 3 cm have 30% chance of harboring residual tumor
- FDG PET/CT used for restaging and evaluation of response to therapy
  - Tumor marker elevation in absence of CT findings should prompt FDG PET evaluation for salvage surgery
  - FDG PET is best predictor of viable seminoma in residual masses after chemotherapy, may be useful in NSGCT
  - Masses with residual malignancy may remain negative on PET for up to 10-14 days after chemotherapy, "stunned" tumor
  - Difficult to differentiate mature teratoma vs. scar, as both have low FDG uptake
  - In multi-relapse seminoma patients, FDG PET has been shown to change treatment in 57% of cases

CLINICAL ISSUES

Presentation

- Majority of patients present with painless unilateral testicular mass
- Approximately 15% of patients have pain and a mass; can be mistaken for epididymoorchitis
- Diffuse testicular enlargement and evidence of metastatic disease can be seen in approximately 10% of patients
- 2-3% of testicular tumors are bilateral (synchronous or metachronous)

Cancer Natural History & Prognosis

- Testicular carcinoma is highly treatable, often curable cancer
- **NSGCT**
  - Good prognosis: All of following
    - AFP < 1,000 ng/mL and hCG < 5,000 IU/L (1,000 ng/mL) and LDH < 1.5x upper limit of normal (N)
    - Nonmediastinal primary
    - No nonpulmonary visceral metastases (NPVM)
    - 5-year progression-free survival (PFS) is 89%, 5-year survival is 92-94%
  - Intermediate prognosis: All of following
    - AFP 1,000–10,000 ng/mL, or hCG 5,000–50,000 IU/L, or LDH 1.5–10x N
    - Nonmediastinal primary site
    - No NPVM
    - 5-year PFS is 75%, 5-year survival is 80-83%
  - Poor prognosis: Any of following
    - AFP > 10,000 ng/mL or hCG > 50,000 IU/L or LDH > 10x N
    - Mediastinal primary site
    - NPVM
    - 5-year PFS is 41%, 5-year survival is 71%
- **Seminoma**
  - Good prognosis
    - Normal AFP, any hCG, any LDH
    - No NPVM
    - Any primary site
    - 5-year PFS is 82%, 5-year survival is 86%
  - Intermediate prognosis
    - NPVM present
    - 5-year PFS is 67%, 5-year survival is 72%
  - Poor prognosis: No seminomas are considered poor prognosis

Treatment Options

- Treatment options by stage
  - **Stage I seminoma**
    - Radical inguinal orchiectomy (RIO) with no retroperitoneal node radiation therapy, followed by frequent determination of serum markers, chest x-rays, and CT scans (surveillance)
    - RIO followed by single-dose carboplatin adjuvant therapy
    - RIO followed by radiation therapy
  - **Stage I nonseminoma**
    - RIO followed (in adults) by retroperitoneal lymph node dissection (RPLND)

- RIO with no RPLND followed by regular history (e.g., every 1–2 months), physical examination, determination of serum markers, and, during the 1st year, abdominal CT scan (surveillance)
  - **Stage II seminoma**
    - Nonbulky disease (retroperitoneal lymph nodes < 5 cm), RIO followed by radiation to retroperitoneal and ipsilateral pelvic lymph nodes
    - Bulky disease (retroperitoneal lymph nodes > 5 cm), RIO followed by combination chemotherapy (with cisplatin based regime) or radiation to retroperitoneal and pelvic lymph nodes
  - **Stage II nonseminoma**
    - RIO with RPLND followed by monthly physical exam, chest x-ray, and serum markers
    - RIO with RPLND followed by chemotherapy and monthly check-ups
    - RIO followed by chemotherapy and delayed surgery for removal of residual lymph node masses (if present) and monthly check-ups
  - **Stage III seminoma**
    - RIO with multidrug chemotherapy regime
      - Some advocate resection of residual masses > 3 cm or empiric radiation
      - Viable alternative is serial serum markers and CT exam
  - **Stage III nonseminoma**
    - RIO with multidrug chemotherapy regime

REPORTING CHECKLIST

T Staging

- Intratesticular mass vs. extratesticular mass
  - Ultrasound used to differentiate
- Invasion of tunica albuginea/vaginalis, spermatic cord, and scrotum
  - MR may be helpful
    - Little clinical relevance as appropriate management requires orchiectomy with detailed pathologic analysis

N Staging

- Particularly retroperitoneal nodes, including left paraaortic and right paracaval and aortocaval
- Inguinal adenopathy in setting of prior lymphatic disruption from scrotal or inguinal surgery
- Size of nodes is important in staging, number of nodes is not

M Staging

- Common sites include lung, liver, brain, bone, kidney, and adrenal glands
- Inguinal adenopathy without history of lymphatic disruption from scrotal or inguinal surgery or scrotal tumor invasion

SELECTED REFERENCES

1. American Joint Committee on Cancer: AJCC Cancer Staging Manual. 7th ed. New York: Springer, 2010
2. National Comprehensive Cancer Network (NCCN): Clinical Practice Guidelines in Oncology, Testicular Cancer. www.nccn.org, v.2, 2009
3. DeCastro BJ et al: A 5-year followup study of asymptomatic men with testicular microlithiasis. J Urol. 179(4):1420-3; discussion 1423, 2008
4. Hinz S et al: The role of positron emission tomography in the evaluation of residual masses after chemotherapy for advanced stage seminoma. J Urol. 179(3):936-40; discussion 940, 2008
5. Sohaib SA et al: The role of imaging in the diagnosis, staging, and management of testicular cancer. AJR Am J Roentgenol. 191(2):387-95, 2008
6. Huddart RA et al: 18fluorodeoxyglucose positron emission tomography in the prediction of relapse in patients with high-risk, clinical stage I nonseminomatous germ cell tumors: preliminary report of MRC Trial TE22--the NCRI Testis Tumour Clinical Study Group. J Clin Oncol. 25(21):3090-5, 2007
7. Kim W et al: US MR imaging correlation in pathologic conditions of the scrotum. Radiographics. 27(5):1239-53, 2007
8. Becherer A et al: FDG PET is superior to CT in the prediction of viable tumour in post-chemotherapy seminoma residuals. Eur J Radiol. 54(2):284-8, 2005
9. Kim B et al: Testicular microlithiasis: clinical significance and review of the literature. Eur Radiol. 13(12):2567-76, 2003
10. Woodward PJ et al: From the archives of the AFIP: tumors and tumorlike lesions of the testis: radiologic-pathologic correlation. Radiographics. 22(1):189-216, 2002
11. Walsh PC. Campbell's Urology. 7th ed. Philadelphia: Saunders. 3430, 1998
12. Horwich A. Testicular Cancer: Investigation and Management. 2nd ed. New York: Chapman and Hall Medical. 427, 1996
13. Brown LM et al: Testicular cancer in young men: the search for causes of the epidemic increase in the United States. J Epidemiol Community Health. 41(4):349-54, 1987
14. Bredael JJ et al: Autopsy findings in 154 patients with germ cell tumors of the testis. Cancer. 50(3):548-51, 1982
15. Beard CM et al: The incidence and outcome of mumps orchitis in Rochester, Minnesota, 1935 to 1974. Mayo Clin Proc. 52(1):3-7, 1977

TESTICULAR CARCINOMA

Stage I (T1 N0 M0)

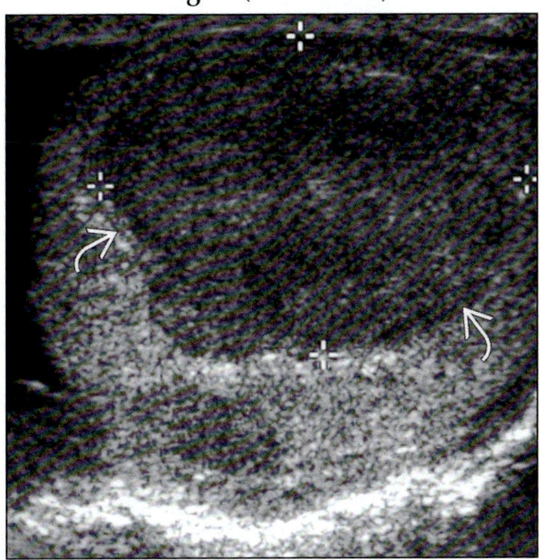

Stage I (T1 N0 M0)

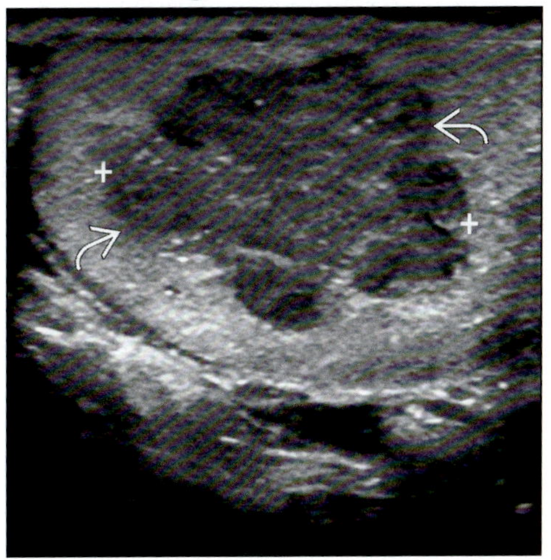

(Left) Longitudinal grayscale ultrasound shows circumscribed, homogeneously hypoechoic mass ⇗ found to be seminoma. This is a characteristic ultrasound appearance of seminoma. Ultrasound is not sensitive for evaluating tunica vaginalis, spermatic cord, or scrotal invasion. (Right) Longitudinal grayscale ultrasound shows lobulated, heterogeneous, predominately hypoechoic mass ⇗. The sonographic appearance is nonspecific and proved to be embryonal cell carcinoma.

Stage I (T1 N0 M0)

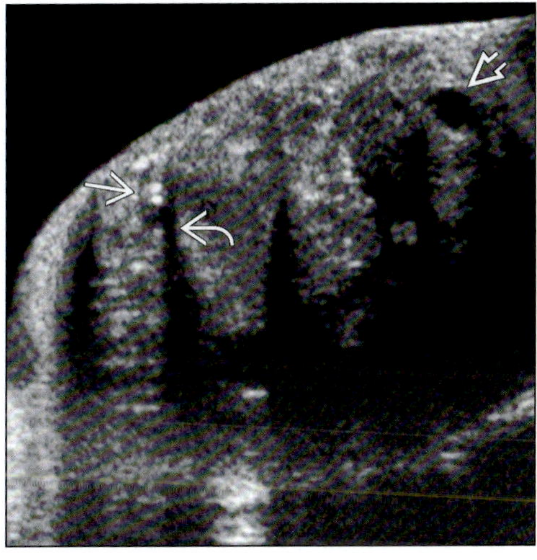

Stage I (T1 N0 M0)

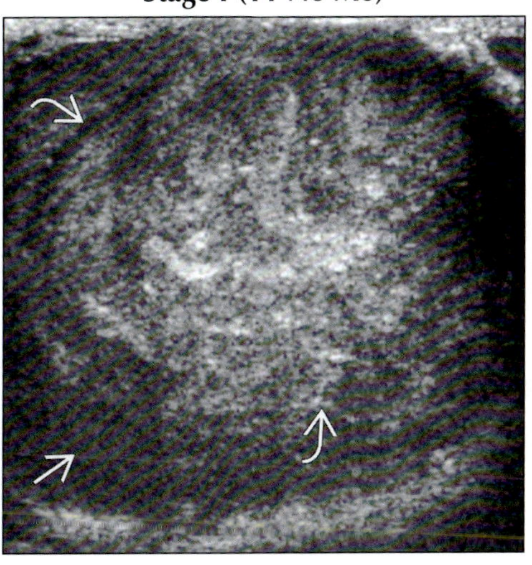

(Left) Longitudinal grayscale ultrasound demonstrates heterogeneous, poorly defined mass. Mass contains foci of calcification ➡ with shadowing ⇗ and cystic areas ⇗. Pathology revealed mature teratoma without invasion of the tunica or spermatic cord. (Right) Longitudinal grayscale ultrasound shows a poorly circumscribed heterogeneous testicular mass ⇗. Pathology revealed a yolk sac tumor. It can be difficult to differentiate tumor from normal testicle ➡.

Stage I (T1 N0 M0)

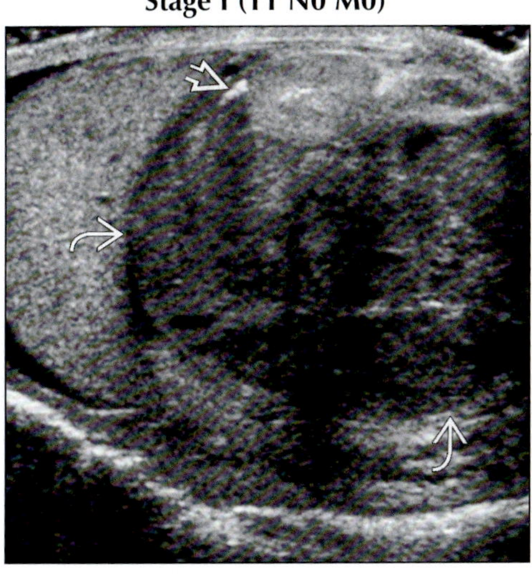

Stage I (T1 N0 M0)

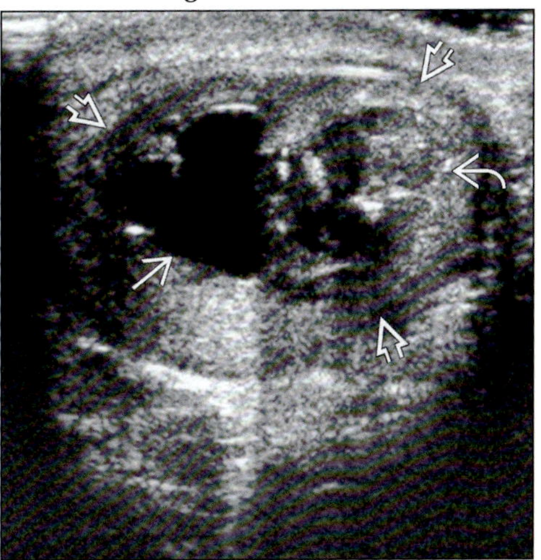

(Left) Longitudinal grayscale ultrasound shows circumscribed mass ⇗ with foci of calcification ⇗. This mass proved to be Sertoli cell tumor, although imaging findings are nonspecific. (Right) Longitudinal grayscale ultrasound demonstrates a heterogeneous mass ⇗ with solid ⇗ and cystic ➡ components. Pathology revealed mixed germ cell tumor with seminoma and embryonal cell components that developed in this patient with cryptorchidism.

TESTICULAR CARCINOMA

Stage I (T1 N0 M0)

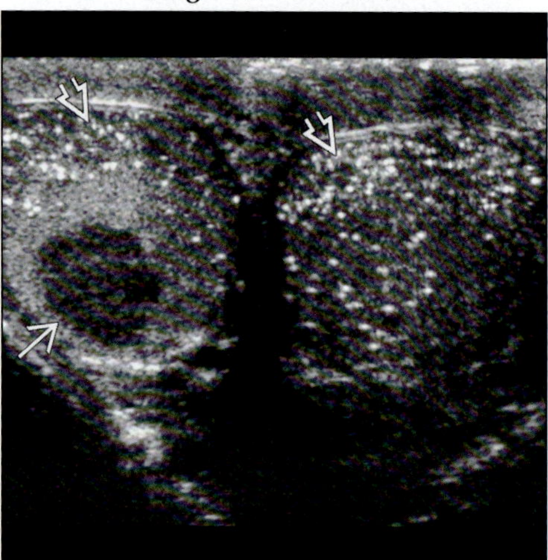

Stage I (T1 N0 M0)

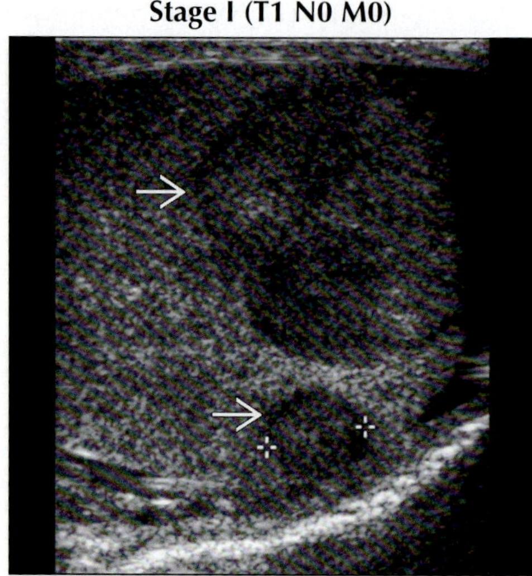

(Left) Longitudinal grayscale ultrasound shows a circumscribed, homogeneous, hypoechoic right testicular mass ➡ in a patient with bilateral testicular microlithiasis ⇨. Mass proved to be seminoma at orchiectomy. *(Right)* Longitudinal grayscale ultrasound shows 2 homogeneous, hypoechoic, circumscribed masses ➡ found to be multifocal seminoma.

Stage I (T1 N0 M0)

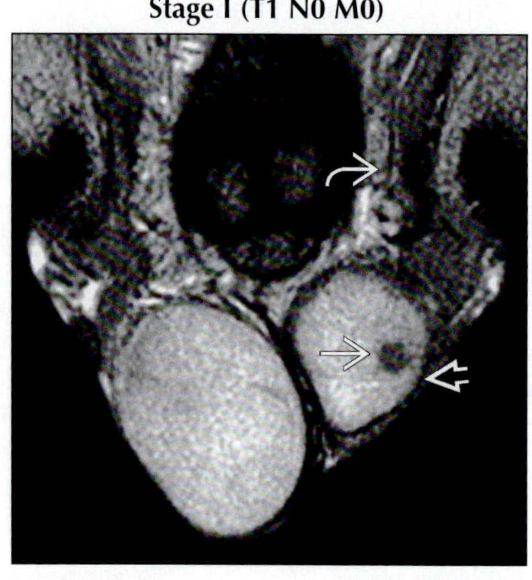

Stage I (T1 N0 M0)

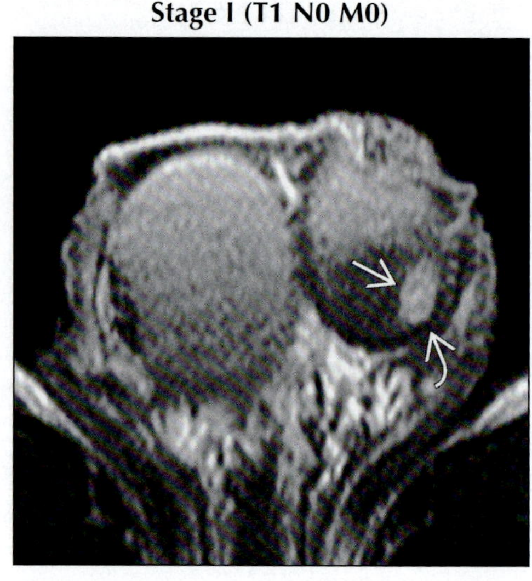

(Left) Coronal T2WI MR shows a circumscribed, T2 homogeneously hypointense mass in the left testicle ➡. MR is best imaging modality to evaluate for tunica ⇨ and spermatic cord ➡ involvement, neither of which were involved in this case. Pathology revealed seminoma. *(Right)* Axial T1WI C+ MR in the same patient shows homogeneous enhancement in left testicular mass ➡ with sparing of the low signal tunica ➡.

Stage I (T1 N0 M0)

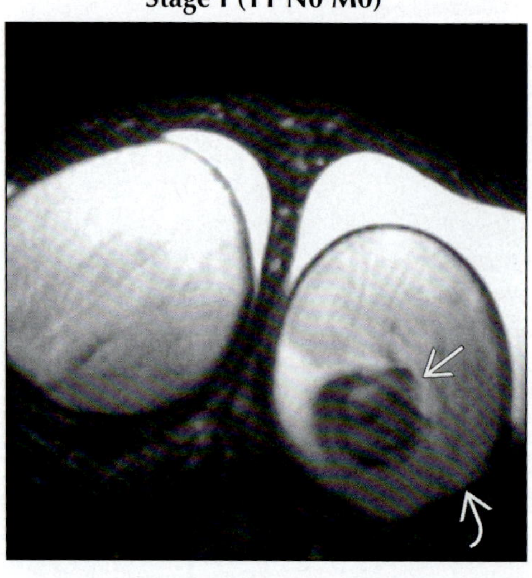

Stage I (T1 N0 M0)

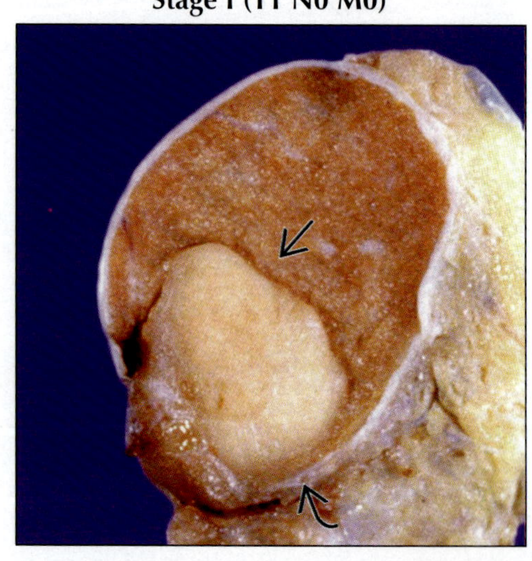

(Left) Axial T2WI MR shows a circumscribed, mildly heterogeneous, hypointense mass in left testicle ➡. Tunica vaginalis ➡ is not invaded. *(Right)* Gross pathology in sagittal plane from the same patient demonstrates testicular mass ➡, which was pure seminoma. Tunica vaginalis is intact ➡, corresponding to imaging findings.

TESTICULAR CARCINOMA

Stage IB (T2 N0 M0)

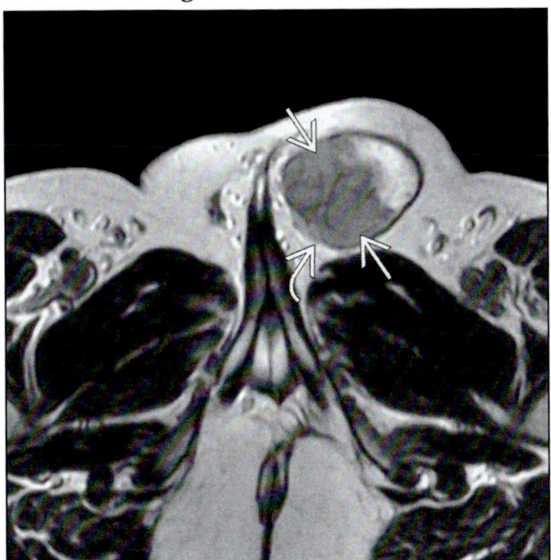

Stage IB (T2 N0 M0)

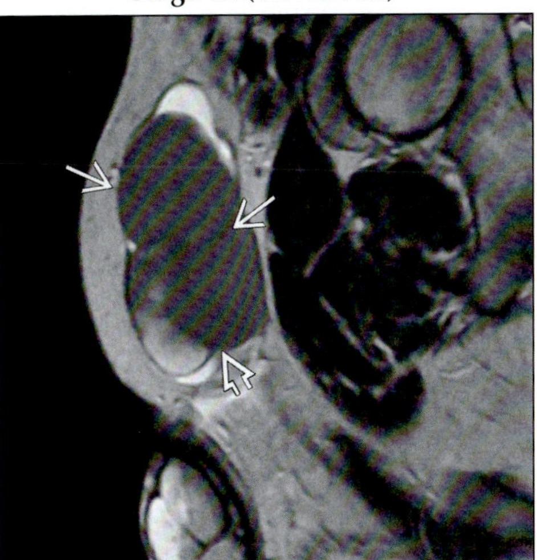

(Left) Axial T2WI MR shows a heterogeneous hypointense mass ➡ replacing the majority of normal testicular tissue of this left side undescended testicle. Tunica vaginalis has been invaded ➡. (Right) Sagittal T2WI MR in the same patient shows a large hypointense mass ➡ replacing the majority of normal testicular tissue in this undescended testicle. Disruption of tunica vaginalis is again demonstrated ➡.

Stage IB (T2 N0 M0)

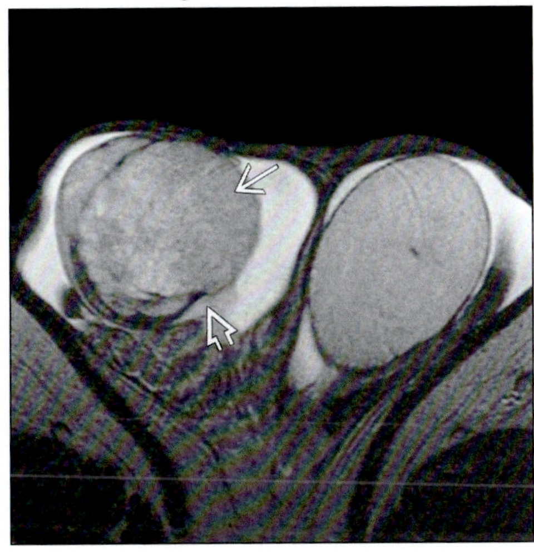

Stage IB (T2 N0 M0)

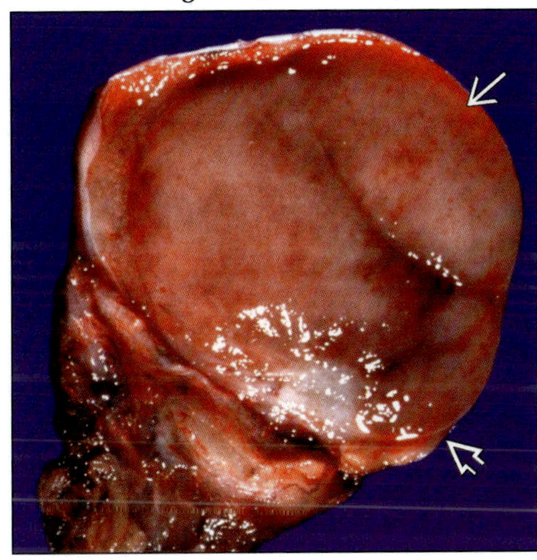

(Left) Axial T2WI MR shows a large, heterogeneous, predominately isointense mass ➡ replacing the majority of normal right testicle. Tunica vaginalis is invaded ➡. (Right) Gross pathology from the same patient correlates to imaging findings showing mass ➡ replacing the majority of testicular tissue, as well as invasion through tunica vaginalis ➡.

Stage IB (T3 N0 M0)

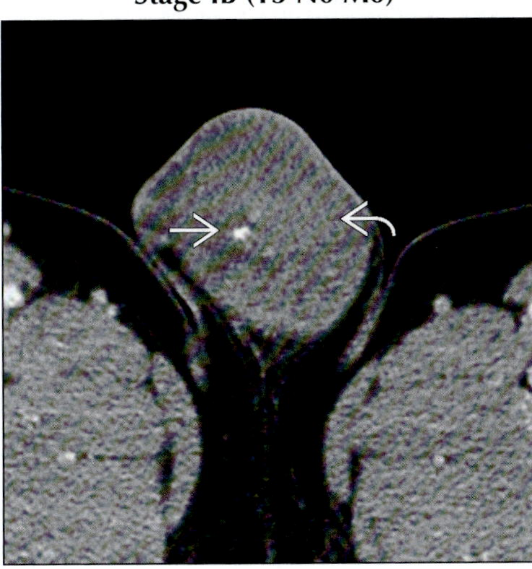

Stage IB (T3 N0 M0)

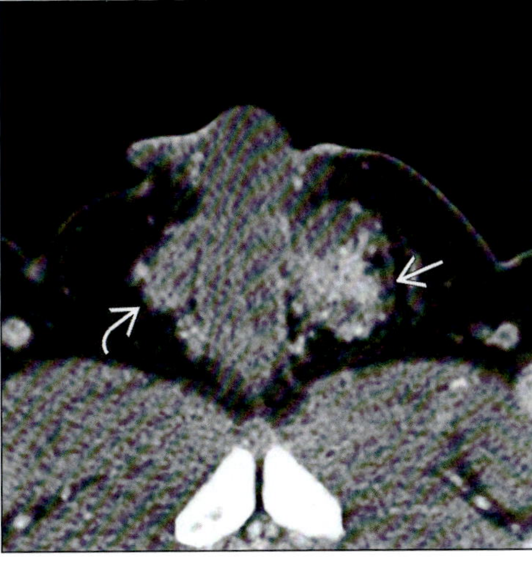

(Left) Axial CECT shows a heterogeneous left testicular mass ➡ with foci of calcification ➡. Pathology demonstrated invasion of tunica vaginalis. (Right) Axial CECT in the same patient shows tumor involvement in the left spermatic cord ➡. Compare the appearance to that of the normal right spermatic cord ➡.

TESTICULAR CARCINOMA

Stage IIA (T3 N1 M0)

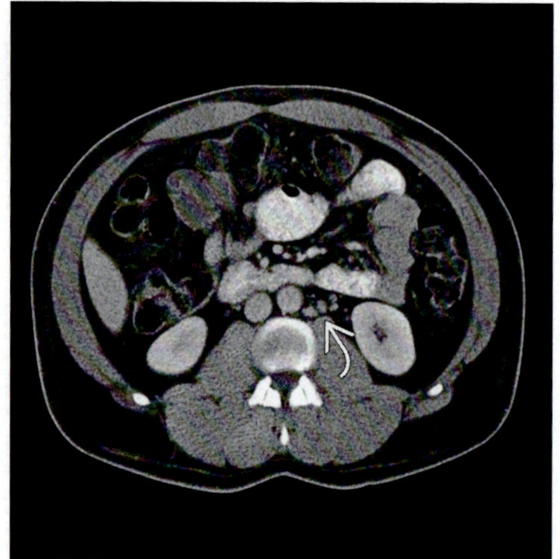

Stage IIA (T3 N1 M0)

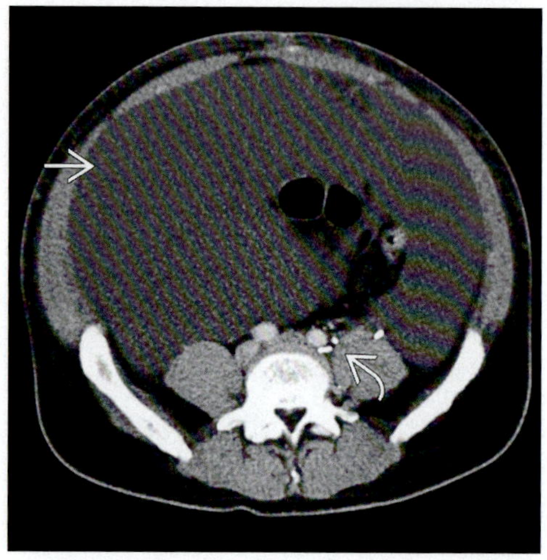

(Left) Axial CECT in a patient with a mixed germ cell tumor shows left-sided paraaortic adenopathy ➔. Nodes measure less than 2 cm in size. *(Right)* Axial CECT in the same patient status post orchiectomy and retroperitoneal lymph node resection ➔ reveals chylous ascites ➔, which developed post surgery.

Stage IIB (T2 N2 M0)

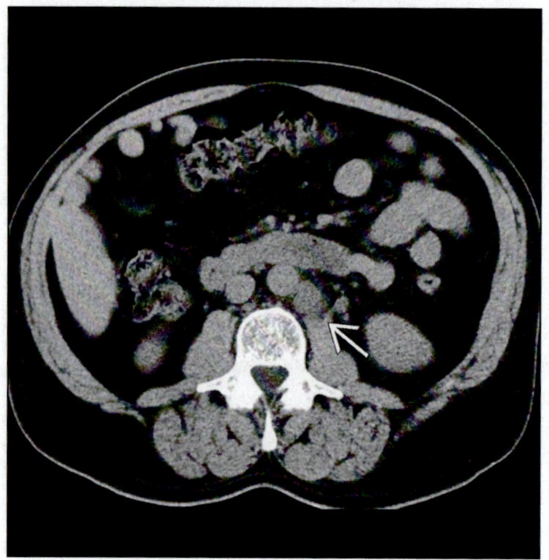

Stage IIB (T2 N2 M0)

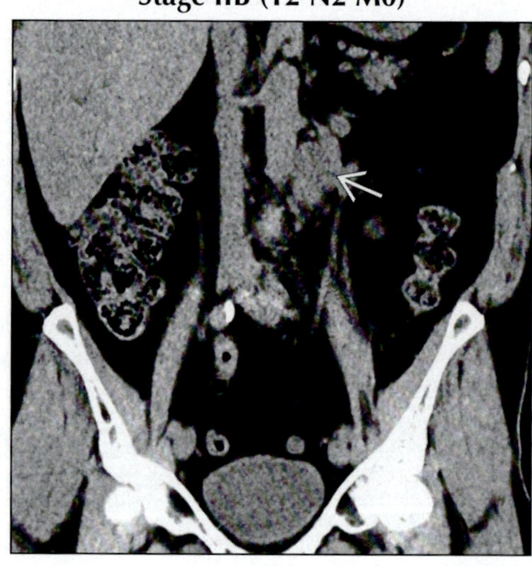

(Left) Axial NECT in a patient with left side seminoma shows left paraaortic lymph node with hazy border ➔, concerning for extranodal extension. Pathology post orchiectomy demonstrated vascular and lymphatic invasion, making this testicular mass T2 disease. *(Right)* Coronal NECT in the same patient demonstrates left paraaortic lymph node conglomeration measuring up to 4 cm ➔, making this N2 disease.

Stage IIC (T1 N3 M0)

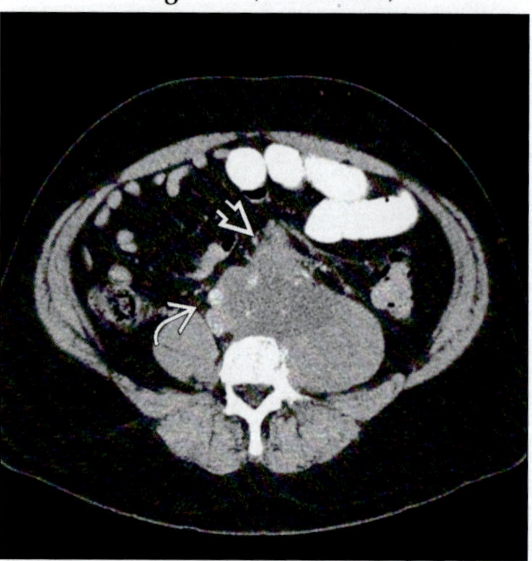

Stage IIC (T1 N3 M0)

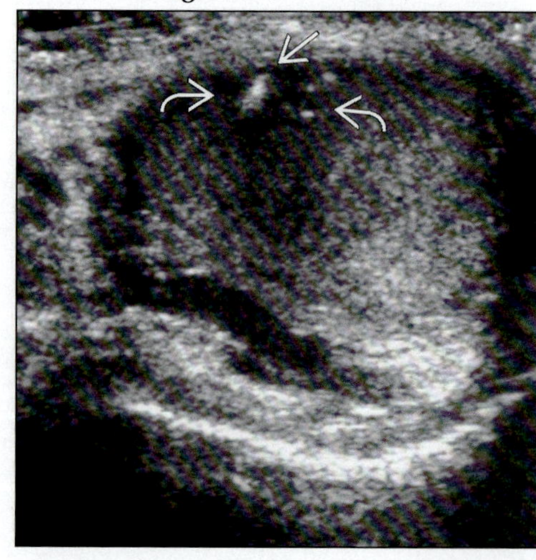

(Left) Axial CECT shows a retroperitoneal mass ➔ with displacement of infrarenal abdominal aorta ➔. Biopsy revealed poorly differentiated carcinoma. Tumor staining indicated positive germ cell markers. Retroperitoneal mass is greater than 5 cm, making this N3 stage. *(Right)* Subsequent ultrasound in the same patient shows foci of calcification ➔ within a small hypoechoic testicular mass ➔ due to a "burned-out" germ cell tumor.

TESTICULAR CARCINOMA

Stage IIIB (T2 N3 M1a)

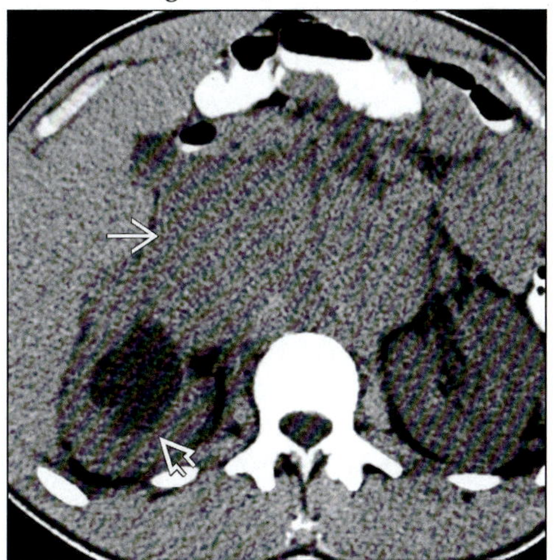

Stage IIIB (T2 N3 M1a)

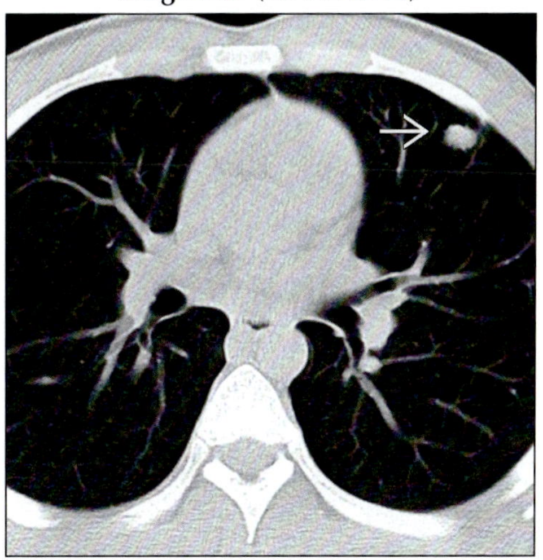

(Left) Axial NECT in a patient with testicular seminoma shows a large retroperitoneal mass →. Right hydronephrosis ⇒ is related to ureteric obstruction by the nodal mass. (Right) Axial NECT in the same patient shows pulmonary parenchymal metastatic lesion in the chest →, making this M1a stage.

Stage IIIC (T2 N3 M1b)

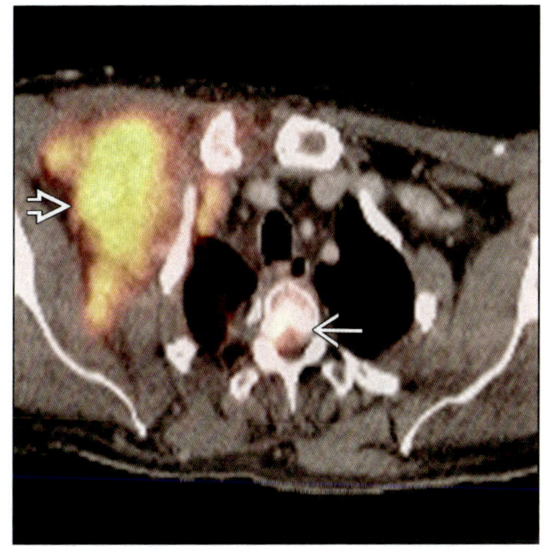

Stage IIIC (T2 N3 M1b)

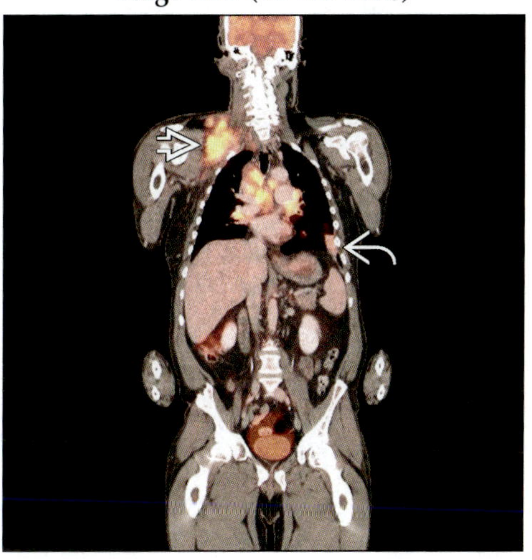

(Left) Axial fused PET/CT demonstrates FDG-avid supraclavicular adenopathy ⇒ and FDG-avid vertebral body lesion → in a patient with testicular seminoma. (Right) Coronal PET/CT in the same patient shows supraclavicular adenopathy ⇒ and left lower lobe lung lesion →.

Stage IIIC (T2 N3 M1b)

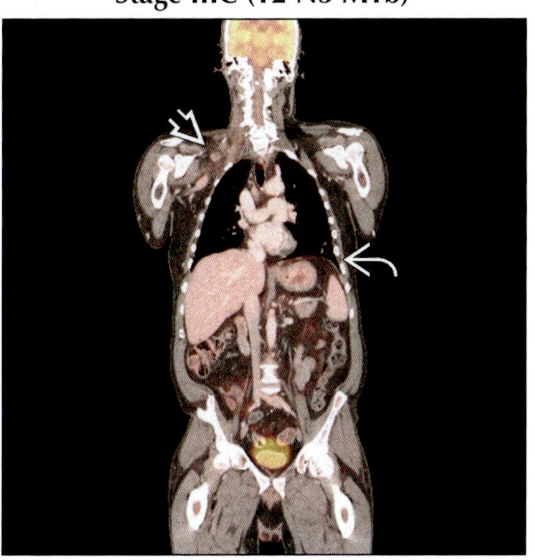

Stage IIC (T1 N3 M0)

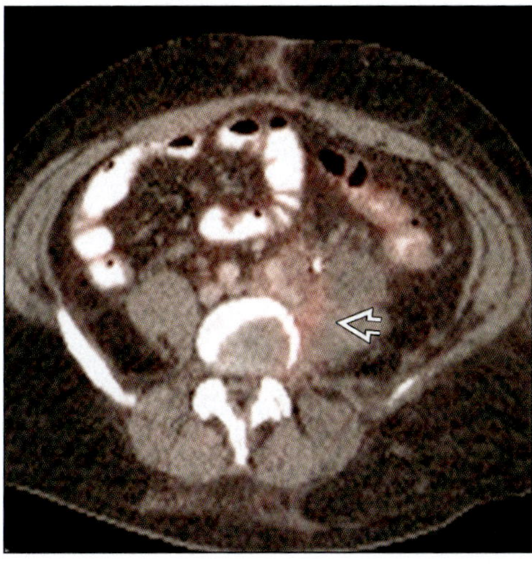

(Left) Coronal PET/CT for restaging in the same patient after treatment shows significant decrease in supraclavicular adenopathy ⇒ and resolution of lung nodule →. (Right) Axial fused PET/CT for restaging in a patient with "burned-out" germ cell tumor post tumor resection and chemotherapy demonstrates residual retroperitoneal mass with FDG uptake ⇒. This is consistent with residual viable tumor.

TESTICULAR CARCINOMA

Stage IIIC (T1 N3 M1b)

Stage IIIC (T1 N3 M1b)

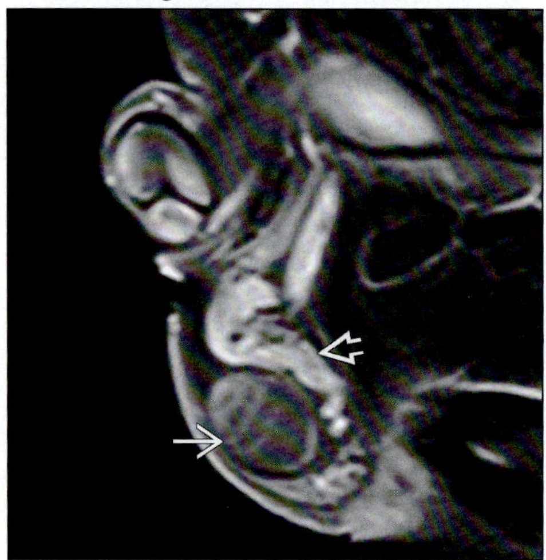

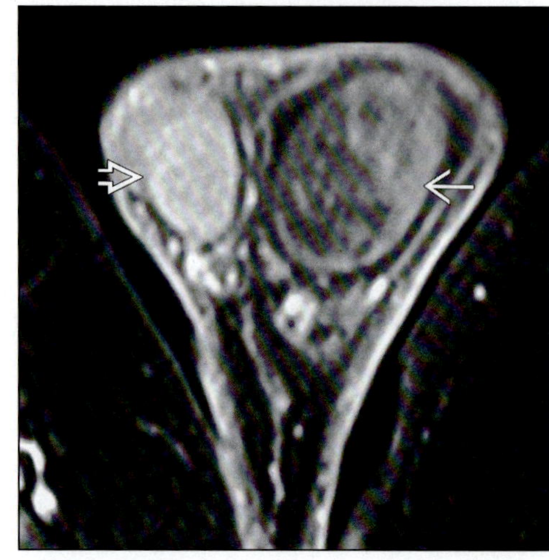

(Left) Sagittal T1WI C+ MR shows mild irregular heterogeneous enhancement ➡ throughout an enlarged left testicle. No focal mass lesion is identified. Left spermatic cord is spared ➡. (Right) Axial T1WI C+ MR in the same patient shows an enlarged, heterogeneous, enhancing left testicle ➡ compared to a normal right testicle ➡.

Stage IIIC (T1 N3 M1b)

Stage IIIC (T1 N3 M1b)

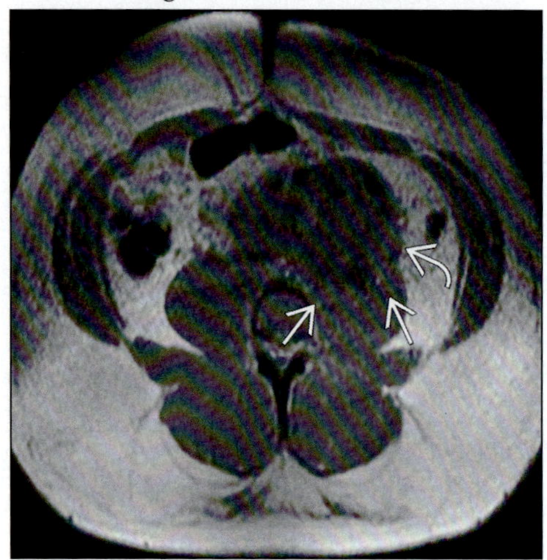

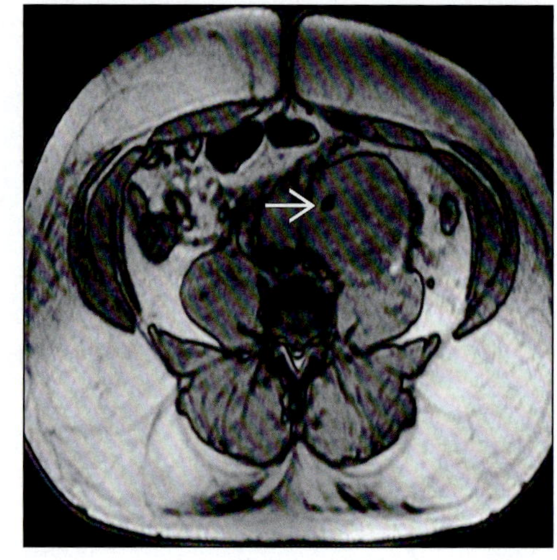

(Left) Axial T1WI in phase MR in the same patient shows heterogeneous retroperitoneal mass ➡. Left psoas muscle was invaded ➡. (Right) Axial T1WI opposed-phase MR in the same patient shows a heterogeneous retroperitoneal mass. Signal drop on the opposed-phase image ➡ in comparison to the in-phase MR sequence corresponds with fat elements in the mass.

Stage IIIC (T1 N3 M1b)

Stage IIIC (T1 N3 M1b)

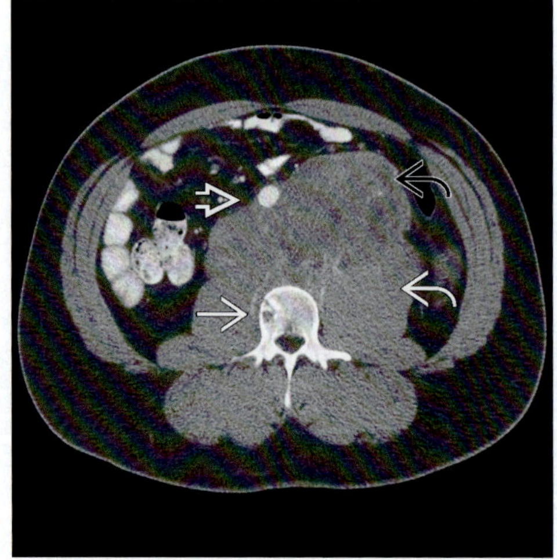

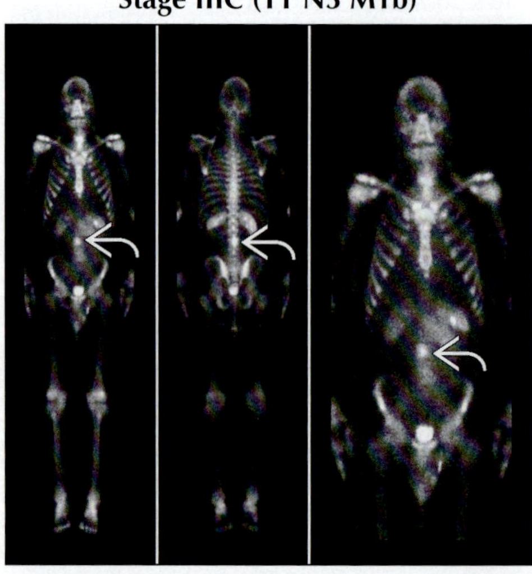

(Left) Axial CECT in the same patient demonstrates a large heterogeneous retroperitoneal mass ➡ displacing aorta ➡ and invading left psoas muscle ➡. Lytic lesion is seen in L3 vertebral body ➡. (Right) Coronal bone scan in the same patient demonstrates uptake in L3 vertebral lytic lesion ➡, consistent with metastatic disease.

Stage IIIC (T1 N3 M1b)

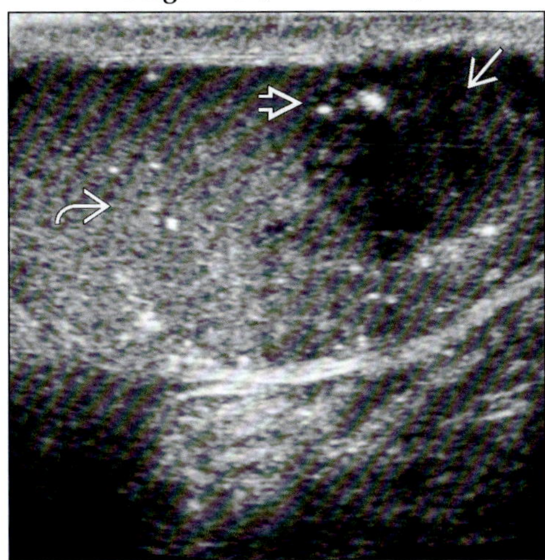

Stage IIIC (T1 N3 M1b)

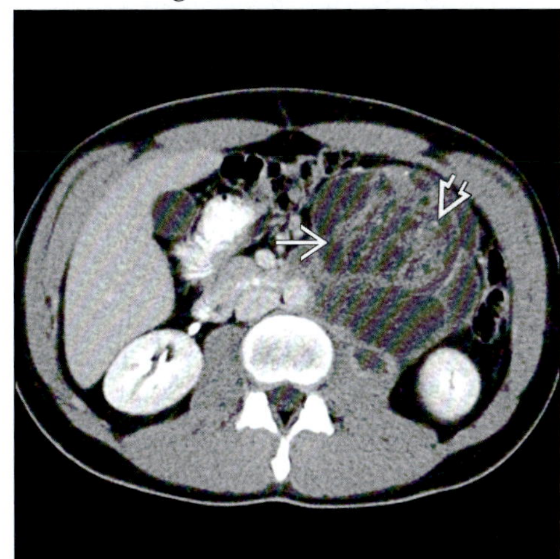

(Left) Longitudinal grayscale ultrasound demonstrates heterogeneous intratesticular mass ➡ with foci of calcification ➡ in the setting of microlithiasis ➡. Pathology revealed teratoma isolated to the testicle, without tunica or spermatic cord invasion. *(Right)* Axial CECT in the same patient shows a large heterogeneous cystic and solid retroperitoneal mass ➡ with calcified foci ➡.

Stage IIIC (T1 N3 M1b)

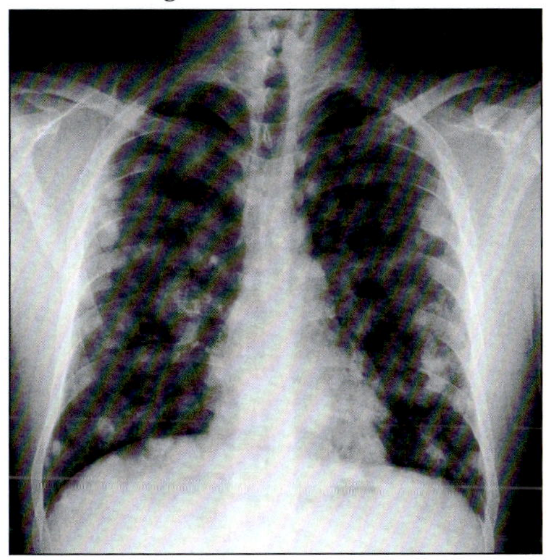

Stage IIIC (T1 N3 M1b)

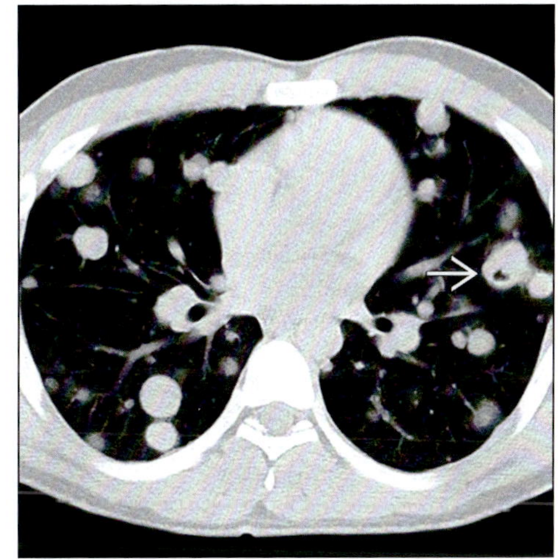

(Left) Chest x-ray in the same patient shows multiple pulmonary metastatic lesions. *(Right)* Axial NECT in the same patient further characterizes multiple pulmonary metastatic lesions, some of which show central cavitation ➡.

Stage IIIC (T1 N3 M1b)

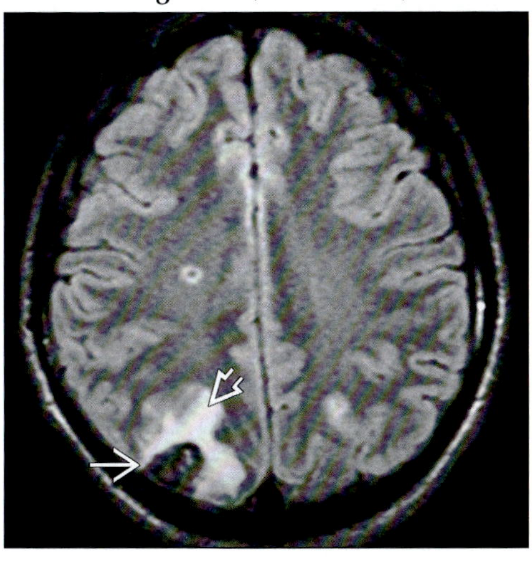

Stage IIIC (T1 N3 M1b)

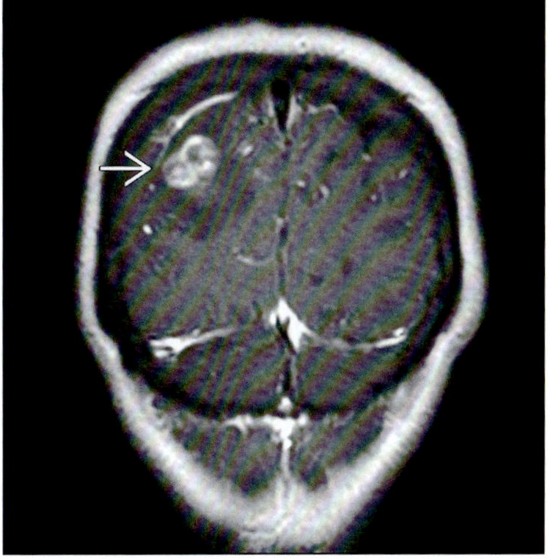

(Left) Axial MR FLAIR in the same patient shows intraaxial metastatic lesion in the right posterior parietal lobe ➡ with surrounding vasogenic edema ➡. *(Right)* Coronal T1WI C+ MR in the same patient shows intraaxial metastatic lesion in the right parietal lobe with peripheral enhancement ➡.

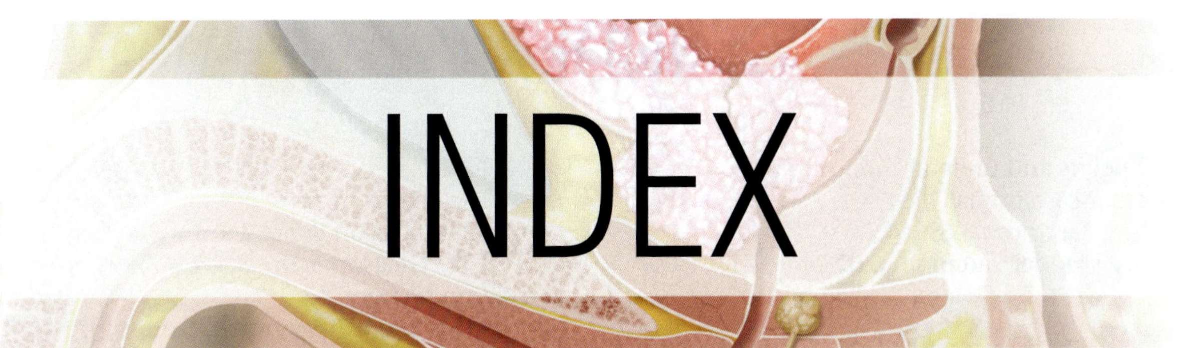

INDEX

INDEX

INDEX

S

T

U

INDEX